4th Edition

Fertility, Cycles & Nutrition

Self-care for improved
cycles and fertility...
naturally!

4ᵗʰ Edition

Fertility, Cycles & Nutrition

Self-care for improved
cycles and fertility...
naturally!

by Marilyn M. Shannon

The Couple to Couple League
International, Inc.
P.O. Box 111184
Cincinnati, OH 45211-1184

Published by:

The Couple to Couple League International, Inc.
P.O. Box 111184
Cincinnati, Ohio 45211
U.S.A.
800-745-8252
www.ccli.org
ccli@ccli.org

Cataloging data:
> L.C.: 2009924234
> ISBN: 978-0-926412-34-7

Shannon, Marilyn M.
Fertility, Cycles & Nutrition: Self-care for improved cycles and fertility...naturally!

Nutrition
Health, reproductive
Menstrual cycles
Natural family planning
Infertility
Pregnancy

Printed in the United States

10 9 8 7 6 5 4 3

Acknowledgments

As with the first edition of this book, thanks go first to John F. Kippley, a founder of The Couple to Couple League for Natural Family Planning. Having the privilege of teaching natural family planning through this organization since 1982 originally sparked my interest in the relationship between nutrition and reproductive health, and it was he who suggested that I undertake the original edition.

Special thanks go to my husband and best friend, Ron, who not only suggested the very popular "80-20" rule for better nutrition (Rule 12, Chapter 1), but who has also been involved with this project from every angle. He has buoyed me up with the inherent moral support that comes from an equal interest in nutrition, as well as with the practical support with our family activities during this busy time.

Our daughter, Rosemary Shannon Imrick, has been the most knowledgeable, quick, and efficient research assistant I could ever ask for! Starting with an extensive search of the literature which yielded over 900 new papers, she quickly enabled me to limit those to about 300 relevant ones. She also assisted with the review and reading of the chapters, for which I am very grateful. She accomplished everything with good humor and high energy while in the last trimester of an amazingly healthy pregnancy. Her second child and first daughter arrived in April, 2008, adding much joy and fun to the time of writing. Health that gives us energy to enjoy our families — this is what this book is all about! Rosemary and her wonderful husband, Michael, are living it.

I gratefully acknowledge the assistance and dedication of our Couple to Couple League editor, Ann Gundlach, who has patiently, professionally, and cheerfully worked with me, beginning with the first edition in 1990, and continuing with this greatly expanded fourth edition. Likewise, I thank CCL's Scott Hofmann, whose layout and design work provided much behind-the-scenes expertise, including the many new tables. Scott and Ann gave us the beautiful cover, which truly says without words exactly what CCL intends for this book to accomplish.

I am gratified and humbled by the enthusiastic Foreword of this edition written by Marie A. Anderson, M.D. of Fairfax, Virginia. I am indebted to John Bruchalski, M.D., of Arlington, Virginia, and to Kaayla Daniel, Ph.D., C.C.N., of Santa Fe, New Mexico, for their careful reviews of the fourth edition. Likewise I thank Mrs. Gerri Laird, of Arlington, Virginia, and Mrs. Giselle Alderson, of Burlington, Kentucky, for their reviews and encouragement.

Mrs. Kathleen Smith of Rockford, Illinois, graciously shared her expertise regarding yeast overgrowth, providing me with the wonderful analogy of the "grass versus weeds" in Chapter 9. Thanks are due also to Mrs. Jane Dawkins of Fort Wayne, Indiana, who prepared the original Tables 1 and 13. I thank Kris Severyn, R.Ph., Ph.D., for the use of her article, "Uterine Fibroids: How I Kept My Uterus," in Appendix C, as well as Laura Brestovansky for her careful proofreading of this edition.

Thank you to the many Couple to Couple League teachers and members who offered such warmth and encouragement during the biennial national CCL Convention held during the summer of 2008. I am truly humbled by your passion for "fertility, cycles and nutrition," your interest in learning more about these relationships, and in sharing what you have learned. Finally, I wish to express my gratitude to those men and women who permitted me to relate their experiences with nutrition and reproductive health. Their anecdotes are contained within these pages.

Grateful acknowledgment is also given for the quoted materials on pages 92 and 93, which are excerpts from *Vitamin B6: The Doctor's Report,* © 1973 by John M. Ellis and James Presley. Reprinted by permission of Harper and Row, Publishers, Inc.

All Bible verses at the start of each chapter are from The New American Bible, 1972-1973 edition, except where noted.

Table of Contents

Foreword

I firmly believe that a patient is their own best health care advocate. As such, I look at myself not only as a doctor, but also as an educator. One of my favorite resources is Marilyn Shannon's *Fertility, Cycles & Nutrition* because it is so pertinent to women's health from a medical perspective. I particularly like the fact that Marilyn first emphasizes good nutrition, before she targets particular problems such as painful cycles, PMS, polycystic ovary syndrome, infertility, thyroid or any of a number of other issues. It is amazing for me to see the number of problems that simply resolve with good nutrition and a healthy lifestyle. What a blessing it is for my patients to learn that they do not have to rely on powerful drugs or hormones to effectively manage their health.

I work with many couples who use Natural Family Planning. The quality of a woman's cycle is foundational. Clear and consistent fertility observations provide the basis for achieving pregnancy if that is desired, or a reasonable amount of abstinence if it is not. For women with healthy fertility-menstrual cycles, the practice of NFP is relatively easy. However, among young women today it is more common to see less than ideal cycles due to a combination of poor diet and lifestyle factors, the effects of contraceptive hormone use, and even environmental influences. I see charts that indicate various problems which can make NFP more difficult for a couple, as well as interfere with the conception of a much-desired child. As a couple begins to chart, NFP observations frequently raise suspicions for underlying illness which may have been longstanding. I find this information essential to my medical practice.

For these reasons, Marilyn Shannon's *Fertility, Cycles & Nutrition* is now a valued "partner" in my Ob/Gyn practice. The book covers such a wide range of issues related to female — and even male infertility — that I find myself recommending it often. Marilyn has thoroughly examined the research and cites reliable, up-to-date references which demonstrate the positive impact of improved nutrition and lifestyle on health, both reproductive and general. I heartily recommend it to my patients for advice targeted to the issues they experience, or for anyone who simply wants to live more healthfully.

Marie A. Anderson, M.D.
Ob/Gyn, Tepeyac Family Center
Fairfax, Virginia

Introduction

UPDATE FOR THE FOURTH EDITION

What amazing changes are occurring in the field of human nutrition! Daily we learn about new links between nutrition and health, whether it is the role of vitamin D in reducing inflammation or preventing cancer, the effect of the omega-3 fatty acids on brain function, or the antioxidant properties of the hundreds of newly-discovered nutrients in brightly-colored plant foods. When it comes to "fertility, cycles, and nutrition," there has been an equal explosion of interest and new research. In response, the 4th edition of this book has been completely rewritten from beginning to end. While many of the chapter subjects and sequences are the same, virtually every topic has been expanded as well as updated, and some new ones have been added.

It has been most heartening to see that without exception, the new research confirms, extends, and strengthens older studies that formed the basis of the first three editions of *Fertility, Cycles & Nutrition*. This means that the new is consistent with the old, but now there are many more options as you attempt to overcome specific reproductive problems. For example, new research on the effect of light on the hormone melatonin, and on melatonin's effect on reproductive hormones (including progesterone), is truly "shedding light" on a fascinating, useful, but poorly understood topic. New specifics of how excessive exercise affects the menstrual cycle is another example of valuable new research confirming and extending the old.

Through the validation that such research provides, what in the recent past was perhaps somewhat "alternative" is rapidly becoming mainstream. For example, the suggestion to use flax oil for various reproductive problems, first suggested in the *Fertility, Cycles & Nutrition* update of 1996, is now a common recommendation. Meanwhile, flax oil's "first cousin" — fish oil — is being investigated vigorously for its effect on pregnancy, prenatal development, postpartum health, and postnatal brain function.

You will notice that the new *Fertility, Cycles & Nutrition* has more physiological explanations than the slimmer volumes of the past. I have included basic explanations of a number of normal and abnormal processes, so that you can see the rationale for the solution to the various problems that we are attempting to solve. One example of this is the explanation of the critical cell division of the ovum (meiosis), which, amazingly, occurs only a few hours before ovulation. This discussion enables the reader to gain a far clearer understanding of age-related infertility, early miscarriage, and even Down syndrome.

The new *Fertility, Cycles & Nutrition*, like the old one, has an inherently Catholic outlook, since the publisher, The Couple to Couple League, is a Catholic organization that teaches Natural Family Planning. But whether or not you are Catholic or Christian, you will still find it a gentle, encouraging, and practical book, whether you are using it to overcome irregular cycles or to increase your chances of having a baby.

Among the nicest and most common compliments I receive about *Fertility, Cycles & Nutrition* are comments like these: "I loaned it to my friend. She never gave it back!" Or, "I've had to buy three or four copies because I keep giving it to my sisters and my friends!" When women lend their books to their sisters and friends, it is because they believe that the book will make a positive difference in their lives. With all my heart, I hope that this edition of *Fertility, Cycles & Nutrition* will make an even bigger difference in your life and health, and in that of your friends and family. I am excited and optimistic that it will do so.

*   *   *

ORIGINAL INTRODUCTION

Couples who are already practicing a healthy lifestyle, including emphasis on holistic nutrition, are often drawn to the practice of natural family planning (NFP). Conversely, those who choose NFP primarily for other reasons often seem to broaden their interests to include more natural approaches to other areas of life and health. For example, interest in alternative childbirth options is high among NFP users, and the rate of breastfeeding is simply phenomenal. Success in the practice of natural birth regulation, without recourse to chemicals, devices or surgery, undoubtedly encourages such couples to work in harmony with nature in other areas such as nutrition.

There are some striking similarities between natural family planning for birth control and holistic nutrition for health or healing. Both may be termed "appropriate technology" in that they rely on the intelligent use of ordinary things (food, vitamins, information) that may be obtained without undue effort or expense. As such, they are all too often overlooked in an environment in which the high technologies of synthetic pharmaceutical agents or surgery are frequently the first choices for birth control or health care. For their success, both NFP and nutrition require a certain amount of personal commitment, bodily self-awareness and discipline of the appetites, either sexual or for food. Yet both offer large rewards for these small sacrifices — and a major one is improved physical health over the long term.

Despite the close kinship between NFP and nutrition, a real gap has existed in relating the two for practical applications. While natural family planning may be practiced successfully despite a wide range of reproductive disorders, experience shows that couples are happier with it when the times of abstinence are not prolonged by various cycle irregularities and when the use of the infertile time is not disrupted by premenstrual syndrome (PMS), prolonged menses, vaginal infections, or the like. For couples using NFP to overcome infertility, excellent nutrition is as essential as the charting of fertility signs and the timing of intercourse.

This book closes the "information gap" between natural family planning and nutrition for reproductive health. The first part, "Good Nutrition for Good Health," reflects my belief that good nutrition is the best health protector, whether we are referring to reproductive health, cardiovascular health, or any other aspect of health. A diet based on a wide variety of whole foods seems simply to be the diet on which human beings thrive with the least problems for the longest time.

The second part tackles specific reproductive problems, starting with PMS. Since PMS shares a common cause with several other disorders, it is recommended reading even for those who are free from it.

The "Further Reading" and "Resources" pages again emphasize the role of individual responsibility; there is no substitute for your own informed awareness of the often controversial new ideas that are currently transforming the world of nutrition.

Part I

Good Nutrition for Good Health

Most likely you have picked up this book to help solve a problem involving your cycles or your fertility. Perhaps you would like to overcome PMS, or have lighter periods or more regular cycles. Perhaps you are having difficulty achieving a pregnancy. In any case, it is tempting to go right to the specifics of Part II to do so, but first, please take some time to review the basics of good nutrition and to consider the benefits of vitamin and mineral supplements. You will gain much more from the recommendations of Part II if you are well on your way to a more natural, holistic diet and balanced supplementation.

Part I of this book encourages you to improve your overall nutrition on a day-to-day basis. You will see that drastic alterations in the foods you eat are not necessary, and that the much-maligned American diet can be used as the foundation for excellent nutrition. Good nutrition is far more a matter of careful selection and emphasis than wholesale change from, say, meat and potatoes to chick peas on rye! Part I also emphasizes that good food does not require hours of time to find or to prepare. Once you know where to shop and what to shop for, it doesn't take any more time than you are now accustomed to. Once you have the food, there are some wonderful appliances that can even reduce your food preparation in some cases to one-tenth the effort it would take otherwise.

The first chapter consists of some practical rules of thumb that will help you to substantially increase the value of your family's meals while continuing to "cook American." The rationale behind each guideline is briefly explained, because I believe that you will be more motivated to make improvements when you understand the value of doing so. Chapter 2 focuses on ways to acquire and prepare great-tasting food conveniently and quickly. Chapter 3 looks at vitamin and mineral supplements and their value to overall health. Chapter 4 answers some common questions about practical matters involving nutrition.

My sincere hope is that you will implement the general dietary improvements of Part I before you attempt to apply the more specific recommendations of Part II. Best wishes on your journey toward a healthier you, a healthier family, and a healthier future!

1

Twelve Rules for Better Nutrition

One who is cheerful and gay while at table benefits from his food. — Sirach 30:25

1: EAT PLENTY OF WHOLE PLANT FOODS: GRAINS, BEANS, NUTS, VEGETABLES, SEEDS, AND FRUITS.

Whole plant foods provide so much good nutrition and such good taste that they are a great place to start when you begin improving your nutrition. Of the three major food classes — carbohydrates, proteins, and natural fats — plant foods are best known as members of the carbohydrate class. However, grains, beans, nuts, and seeds are also good sources of protein, and the nuts and seeds especially contribute healthy natural fats to the diet. All whole plant foods provide an abundance of vitamins, minerals, and other healthful nutrients. When the carbohydrate content is considered, plant foods can be informally subdivided into three groups: starchy carbohydrates, non-starchy "garden" vegetables, and fruits.

STARCHY CARBOHYDRATES. Whole grains, beans, and a few vegetables are traditionally called "starchy" foods. Some examples of these basic foods are whole-grain bread, whole-wheat pasta, oatmeal, brown rice, granola, peas, navy beans, kidney beans, and potatoes. During digestion, they gradually release the sugar glucose, providing a major source of energy for the body. *Gradual* release of glucose is key, though. When these foods are refined, many of their vitamins and minerals are removed, as well as their valuable fiber. Refined carbohydrates are digested too rapidly, disrupting the blood glucose levels without furnishing the vitamins and minerals that nature intended. That's why your emphasis should be on whole, unrefined starchy foods, rather than on white bread, white pasta, or white rice.

NON-STARCHY "GARDEN" VEGETABLES. Most of the plant foods that we call "garden" vegetables are non-starchy, and are not high energy-producing foods. Instead, they contain a tremendous wealth of vitamins, minerals, fiber, and other nutrients. Spinach, lettuce, green beans, cucumbers, zucchini, Brussels sprouts, asparagus, peppers, cabbage, celery, and onions are common examples of the garden vegetables. It is hard to find an unhealthy example!

FRUITS. Delicious, nutritious fruits, such as apples, oranges, strawberries, cherries, peaches, and cantaloupes are sweet because they contain natural sugars. Fresh, ripe, and raw, they contain an abundance of fiber, vitamins, minerals, and other nutrients. But sweet fruits eaten on an empty stomach may release their natural sugars too rapidly, causing blood sugar swings, just like refined starchy foods. Eating them in moderation, or eating them along with protein or fatty foods, is the best way to prevent such blood sugar swings.

PHYTONUTRIENTS. Exciting new research is revealing that the plant foods, especially the brightly-colored fruits and garden vegetables such as tomatoes, carrots, pineapple, broccoli, blueberries, beets, and grapes, are full of hundreds of wonderful natural chemicals called "phytonutrients." Some phytonutrients act as powerful antioxidants, preventing the kind of damage to cells that ultimately results in degenerative diseases, including cardiovascular disease and cancer. Others provide materials for the body's cells that improve the immune system, the eyes' delicate structures, brain function, and even reproductive function.

FIBER. The presence of fiber is another huge benefit of eating whole plant foods. Fiber is the indigestible material that makes foods such as almonds, celery, cabbage, and granola so crunchy. It slows down the release of glucose from the intestines into the blood, contributing to steady blood sugar levels. This is good for your energy level, moods, mental concentration, and long-term health. Fiber makes you feel full, which is helpful to appetite control. It stimulates the contractions of the large intestine, so that waste products and toxins are moved out of the body quickly. "Soluble fiber," such as the sticky stuff that makes oatmeal pans so hard to clean, attracts and holds cholesterol. The cholesterol is then excreted in the feces, an effect that has been shown to lower blood cholesterol levels.

HOW MUCH OF THE WHOLE PLANT FOODS SHOULD YOU EAT? There is no single answer that suits every individual. But most everyone can — and should — eat the non-starchy garden vegetables plentifully. Because they are so low in calories and so high in fiber, vitamins, minerals, and phytonutrients, adding them to every meal and snack is a good goal to aim for. Eaten raw, their crispness gives you something to munch on instead of packaged chips or pretzels. Nuts and seeds, with their proteins and natural fats, are a satisfying substitute for chips and dips as well.

Most people can eat whole, raw fresh fruits daily. In moderation, their tangy sweetness and fiber will really help you if you are trying to overcome a craving for sugary junk foods and drinks. Sweet fruits are best eaten with proteins and fats, though, because on an empty stomach, many of them release their sugars too fast for stable blood glucose levels. Those who are trying to overcome yeast infections and other problems caused by yeast (discussed in Chapter 9) may need to be cautious with the sweet fruits until their health improves.

When it comes to the grains, beans, and starchy root vegetables such as potatoes, many people can enjoy these foods as long as they are truly whole and natural, and are eaten with other protein and fatty foods. However, if you are fighting weight gain, polycystic ovary symptoms (discussed in Chapter 8), water retention, or blood sugar swings caused by a diet of refined sugary and starchy foods, you may need to limit the starchy plant foods such as potatoes, bread, corn, and pasta. If that is the case, don't forget about the seeds, nuts, and the many delicious non-starchy garden vegetables!

2: GET ENOUGH PROTEIN TO MEET YOUR NEEDS.

Protein that you eat enables you to make protein that you need. Muscle tissue contains protein, of course. Connective tissue is formed from thread-like proteins called collagen. Skin cells are waterproofed by a special protein. Even your bones are one-third protein. Cells make a huge variety of different proteins for use as enzymes, hormones, antibodies, clotting elements, and many other functions.

The body's proteins are long but intricately folded chains whose "links" are hundreds of amino acids. Human proteins are made of specific combinations of twenty different amino acids. Nine of the twenty amino acids are "essential," which means they must be available in the diet.[1] The other "nonessential" amino acids can be made by the body from the essential ones.

How does this relate to what you eat? All of the essential amino acids must be present in your food in order for your body first to produce the nonessential amino acids, and then to make the various proteins that it needs. "Complete proteins" are foods that contain all of the essential amino acids. Animal products — milk, cheese, yogurt, other dairy products, eggs, fish, poultry, and red meat — are all complete protein foods.

Those who practice a strict vegetarian diet know that beans and grains together provide all the essential amino acids. While it is not necessary to eat grains and beans at the same meal, there are many traditional dishes that do combine them, perhaps because they taste so good together! For example, beans on a cornmeal taco provide complete protein. A side of rice and beans forms complete protein, as in Mexican cuisine. So does succotash, which is a Native American dish of corn and lima beans. Even the humble peanut butter sandwich is a complete protein food, since the peanut is actually a bean, and wheat is a grain.

A small amount of animal protein eaten with a grain food or beans also provides high quality protein dishes. Pasta dishes made with cheese, chili beans with meat sauce, beef and noodles, chicken chop suey over rice, pork and beans, and cereal with milk are all examples of the practical application of this principle, which has been used around the world by thrifty homemakers since antiquity.

Protein is relatively hard to digest, so its amino acids are slowly released from the digestive tract into the blood. Eaten with whole carbohydrate foods, it greatly slows down the release of glucose into the blood, contributing to steady blood sugar levels over several hours. That's why, if you have a tendency to low blood glucose, called hypoglycemia, you may find that extra protein, especially for breakfast, helps to stabilize your blood sugar levels. This is also why more protein and fewer starchy carbohydrates may be a helpful approach if you are attempting to lose weight. For the same reason, more protein may help you out if you are trying to overcome a craving for sugary or starchy junk foods. The slow digestion of protein makes you feel satisfied longer.

How much protein do you need? There is a wide range of protein intake that is healthy. Many Americans eat more than is necessary for good health, but as the examples above suggest, extra protein is beneficial to some people. If you are pregnant, you need to be careful to get enough protein in the earlier months to combat morning sickness, and during the later months to support your own increasing needs as well as your baby's brain development. You need more protein when you are breastfeeding than when you are not. Growing children need proportionally more protein than adults.

Table 1, "Suggested Daily Food Goals" (pages 8–9), provides a means of checking up on your daily servings of all major food groups, including the proteins. If you are pregnant or breastfeeding, **Table 13, "Suggested Daily Food Goals for Pregnant and Nursing Women"** (pages 146–147), provides a checklist to make sure you are getting enough servings of protein each day.

3: CHOOSE HEALTHFUL FATS AND OILS; AVOID THE TRANS FATS.

You are probably aware that the artificially produced "trans fats" are harmful to your health. Many people, though, are unaware that natural vegetable oils contain essential nutrients which the human body *must* have.

Essential fatty acids. The "essential fatty acids" are only two in number: linoleic acid and alpha-linolenic acid. Linoleic acid is needed in a greater amount and is easy to obtain. It is abundant in most vegetable oils, including corn oil, soy oil, safflower oil, walnut oil, and sunflower oil.

The wonderfully health-promoting alpha-linolenic acid, often termed the "omega-3" essential fatty acid, is needed in lesser amounts, but is considerably harder to get. Small but significant amounts are present in canola oil, soy oil, and walnut oil. Commonly used food oils such as corn oil, olive oil, and peanut oil contain virtually none. Flax oil, which can be taken in capsules, is by far the richest source, as it is more than 50 percent alpha-linolenic acid.

Practically speaking, canola oil is a good choice for your kitchen, because it contains both of the essential fatty acids and is also rich in "monounsaturated" fatty acids which have many health benefits. It is mild-tasting and can be used for cooking at moderate temperatures. Olive oil is another source of the healthful monounsaturated fatty acids, but while it offers a zippy taste and many phytonutrients, it lacks the hard-to-get alpha-linolenic acid.

Because light, oxygen, and heat progressively damage both of the essential fatty acids, it is a good practice to use only "expeller-pressed" oils, which are processed at low temperatures and which are available at health food shops. These oils should be capped tightly and stored in the refrigerator, as much for the darkness as for the cold.

About a tablespoon or two of the healthy food oils daily is all that is needed to obtain sufficient linoleic acid. Avoid low- or no-fat salad dressings, which do not provide the essential fatty acids. And consider taking supplements of flax oil in order to obtain enough of the valuable omega-3 alpha-linolenic acid, a health practice that is particularly beneficial to many aspects of reproductive function. (Supplementing flax oil is addressed in Chapter 3.)

TRANS FATS. When the unsaturated vegetable oils are converted to margarine or shortening to make them solid at room temperature, the essential fatty acids are destroyed. What is worse, they are converted to unhealthy trans fats which interfere with the function of the essential fatty acids. The same occurs when natural peanut butter is partially hydrogenated. As much as possible, avoid these major sources of trans fats: margarine, shortening, peanut butter not labeled "natural," prepackaged pastries, and deep-fried fast foods such as french fries and breaded chicken or fish. Examine labels and avoid packaged foods containing any of the following: "trans fats" or "hydrogenated" or "partially hydrogenated" oils. Be aware that some foods labeled "0 trans fats" actually do contain trans fats.[2]

Making small changes that you will hardly taste, especially avoiding trans fats and using the healthy natural oils and fats, will make a great difference to your long term health. It may even improve your cycles or fertility, as recent research has shown that intake of trans fats contributes to infertility.[3] Use butter instead of margarine. Eliminate shortening from your kitchen. In many cases, vegetable oil such as canola oil can be used in place of shortening. When you fry, use a little canola or olive oil at medium temperatures. If you absolutely can't do without shortening, use a small amount of lard instead. Surprised? Lard, which contains both monounsaturated and saturated animal fat and is a source of cholesterol, is stable when heated. I must mention, though, that I have never had either shortening or lard in my kitchen, and I have not missed either!

SATURATED FATS AND CHOLESTEROL. Saturated fats and cholesterol are found in animal products such as poultry, red meat, milk, butter, cheese, and eggs. These natural fats have important health benefits. They are part of all cell membranes. As such, they are involved in the maintenance of the fatty "myelin sheaths" that insulate neurons, and in the maintenance of a healthy gut lining. They assist with the absorption of the fat-soluble vitamins A, D, E, and K.

Cholesterol is the precursor of the sex hormones estrogen, progesterone, and testosterone, as well as of the other steroid hormones. It also is the precursor of vitamin D, which the body can make if the skin is exposed to sufficient sunshine. Both fats and oils powerfully affect the digestive hormones, slowing down the emptying of the stomach and the absorption of glucose into the blood, thereby stabilizing blood sugar levels. When digestive processes occur gradually, the meal "sticks to your ribs," an old expression that means it digests slowly, releasing nutrients and satisfying hunger over a long period of time.

TABLE 1
SUGGESTED DAILY FOOD GOALS

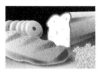 ## Whole Grains

3 servings daily
(1 serving = 1 slice bread or ½ cup cooked cereal)

....

Whole grain bread	Whole grain pasta	Millet
Oatmeal	Whole grain pancakes	Tortillas
Whole grain breakfast cereal	Brown rice	Bagels

 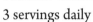 ## Dairy/Eggs

3 servings daily
(1 serving = 6 oz. milk, 2 oz. cheese, 1 egg)

....

Whole milk	Yogurt	Cheese	Kefir	Ice cream	Eggs

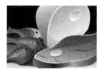 ## Complete Protein

1 serving daily
(1 serving = 3-4 oz. meat)

....

Poultry	Grain + Legume (Peas, beans, peanut
Fish (preferably twice weekly)	butter, nuts, lentils)
Beef, including liver and heart	Dairy + Grain
Pork	Dairy + Legume
Lamb	

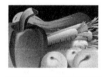 ## Yellow Fruits and Vegetables

1 serving daily
(1 serving = ½ cup cooked or 1 cup raw)

....

Carrots	Sweet potatoes	Mangos	Peaches
Squash	Pumpkin	Apricots	Cantaloupe

This table may be photocopied, covered with adhesive backed clear plastic and taped to

TABLE 1 — CONTINUED.
SUGGESTED DAILY FOOD GOALS

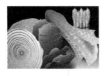 **Leafy Green Vegetables**

3 servings daily
(1 serving = ½ cup cooked or 1 cup raw)

Lettuce	Beet greens	Asparagus
(leaf, Romaine,	Alfalfa sprouts	Chard
Bibb, iceberg)	Cole crops	Kale
Spinach	(cabbage, broccoli,	
Escarole	Brussels sprouts,	
Endive	cauliflower, kohlrabi)	

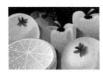 **Vitamin C Source**

1 serving daily
(1 serving = 1 medium fruit or ½ cup berries)

Citrus fruits	Tomatoes	Peppers
(oranges, grapefruits,	Melons	Potatoes
tangerines)	Berries	

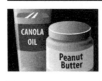 **Unsaturated Oils**

1 serving daily
(1 serving = 1–2 tablespoons)

Monounsaturated	**Polyunsaturated**	**Both**
Olive oil	Soy oil *	Canola oil *
Peanut oil	Walnut oil *	Sesame oil
Unprocessed peanut butter	Safflower oil	
Avocado oil	Sunflower oil	
	Corn oil	

* Source of the essential omega-3 alpha-linolenic acid.

your refrigerator. Check off the boxes daily with a dry erase marker.

If you have a hard time believing that saturated fats or cholesterol can be healthy, here is an interesting finding: In the recent, very large Nurses' Health Study, using one or two servings of whole milk products daily correlated with significantly higher fertility in women compared to using skim (low fat) milk products.[4] While most likely there are several different explanations for this finding, it should at least reassure those who are nervous about consuming naturally saturated fats and cholesterol, even in moderation.

FISH OILS. What about the healthy fatty acids abundant in fish oils, abbreviated EPA and DHA? Your body can actually make EPA (eicosapentaenoic acid) and DHA (docosahexaenoic acid) if you have the hard-to-get omega-3 alpha-linolenic acid discussed above, along with several vitamins and minerals. EPA and DHA are best known for their heart-healthy effects, but they also stimulate the immune system, promote proper brain function, decrease inflammation, and perform other vital functions in virtually every cell. Eating fatty fish is one way to obtain these wonderful nutrients, but now that contaminant-free fish oils are available in capsules or as lemon-flavored liquids, they are recommended as supplements in Chapter 3.

4: SUBSTITUTE MORE NUTRITIOUS INGREDIENTS FOR LESS NUTRITIOUS INGREDIENTS IN YOUR FAVORITE RECIPES AND DISHES.

More nutritious foods are simply fresher and closer to their natural state than are other less healthful foods. Whole, unprocessed foods, whether from animal or plant sources, are rich in vitamins and minerals. Since they do not contain additives, they minimize the problem of harmful chemicals. Their natural fats supply the body with essential fatty acids, or fuel, and satisfy the appetite as well. Their starches and sugars, snugly wrapped in the natural packaging called fiber, are slowly digested and released to the blood. **Table 2, "Foods to Emphasize"** lists such foods, and **Table 3, "Food Substitutions,"** gives examples of many nutritious foods that can easily be used in place of nutritionally inferior foods in your familiar recipes, salads, and other dishes.

TABLE 2, FOODS TO EMPHASIZE		
Whole grain cereals, breads and pasta	Natural peanut butter	Eggs
Brown rice	Millet	Milk
Kidney beans, navy beans, pinto beans, lima beans, peas, and lentils	Fresh vegetables	Yogurt
	Fresh fruits	Natural cheese
	Red meats	Butter
	Poultry	Expeller pressed oils
Nuts and edible seeds	Ocean fish	Herbal teas

TABLE 3, FOOD SUBSTITUTIONS	
Prefer	**Instead of**
100% whole grain bread, sour dough bread, or bread made with rye, oats, barley, or small amounts of other flours	White bread or "wheat" bread
Brown rice or millet	White rice or instant rice
"Old-fashioned" rolled oats	Quick-cooking or instant oatmeal
Granola	Boxed breakfast cereals
Bran muffins	Sweet rolls
Whole grain pasta (wheat, rice, or vegetable)	White pasta
Sweet potatoes, acorn squash, butternut squash, turnips	White potatoes
White potatoes	Frozen or boxed potato foods
Dark green leafy vegetables	Light green vegetables
Romaine lettuce, leaf lettuce, Bibb lettuce, endive, spinach, or escarole	Iceberg lettuce
Fresh vegetables	Frozen vegetables
Frozen vegetables	Canned vegetables
Deep yellow, orange, red, or purple vegetables	Pale-colored vegetables
Freshly made salads	Packaged salads
Homemade coleslaw	Packaged coleslaw
Brussels sprouts, broccoli, lima beans, beets, or peas	Green beans
Whole, ripe, raw fruits	Canned fruits, fruit juices
Poultry, beef, lamb, ocean fish, organic liver or heart	Processed meats
Natural cheese	Processed "cheese food"
Natural peanut butter	Processed peanut butter
Olive oil, canola oil	Shortening
Butter	Margarine
Fruits	Sugary desserts
Air-popped popcorn, trail mix	Packaged chips
Herbs and spices	Salt or monosodium glutamate (MSG)

Nutritionally inferior ingredients are those that contain trans fats, added sugar, white flour, excess salt, or artificial colors, sweeteners, flavorings, and preservatives. These ingredients are all too common in prepackaged or processed foods. Vitamins, minerals, essential fatty acids, and fiber have been lost from such foods during processing. Food additives may disrupt blood sugar levels, essential fatty acid metabolism, or vitamin and mineral balance. **Table 4, "Foods to Limit,"** lists such foods.

TABLE 4, FOODS TO LIMIT		
Sugar	Margarine	Soy foods and soy milk
Artificial sweeteners	Shortening	
Soft drinks	Processed peanut butter	Prepackaged foods
Fruit juices	Processed cheese	Aluminum-containing baking powder
White flour	Bacon, wieners, ham, lunch meat, sausage	
Refined vegetable oils		

5: EAT MORE RAW FOODS, AND COOK OTHER FOODS GENTLY.

Cooking food has value beyond making it taste good. Heating food kills bacteria and parasites, makes the food easier to digest, and makes certain nutrients more available. Unfortunately, it also destroys some vitamins. For example, several B vitamins, vitamins C and E, and the essential fatty acids are all harmed by cooking.

Fruits, vegetables, seeds, and nuts are foods that can be eaten raw, and they are ideal to satisfy your sweet tooth or your need to munch on something crunchy. In general, eat your fruits raw, not cooked or bottled as a juice. This is one of the simplest and tastiest pieces of nutritional advice around! For example, a raw apple is a delicious food which provides fiber that slows down the release of its natural sugars. Prefer that juicy, crispy apple to apple sauce or bottled apple juice, both of which are likely to contain added sugar. Similarly, a real orange contains many more nutrients than pasteurized orange juice. A number of vegetables are good eaten raw, either alone or in big salads. **Table 5, "Foods to Eat Raw,"** lists foods that are delicious as well as healthy when eaten raw. Notice also how many raw foods are brightly colored. Naturally colorful fruits and vegetables contain a wealth of wonderful phytonutrients!

Vegetables that do need cooking can be steamed or heated in a little boiling water. Leave vegetables such as green beans, cauliflower, and asparagus a little crisp when you cook them. You will add a gourmet touch as well as better nutrition by doing so.

When it comes to fish, poultry, and red meat, thorough cooking is necessary for tenderness, good taste, and safety. When meats are cooked it is healthier to use longer cooking times with lower temperatures rather than higher temperatures. Longer, slower cooking is also the secret to juicy, tender roasts.

TABLE 5, FOODS TO EAT RAW

Vegetables	Fruits	Seeds and Nuts
Carrots	Apples	Pumpkin seeds
Celery	Oranges	Sunflower seeds
Cucumbers	Grapefruits	Almonds
Green peppers	Tangerines	Walnuts
Tomatoes	Nectarines	Brazil nuts
Snap peas	Blueberries	Hazelnuts
Green onions	Blackberries	Pecans
Radishes	Raspberries	
Spinach	Pears	
Romaine lettuce	Plums	
Leaf lettuce	Grapes	
Endive	Cherries	
Mung bean sprouts	Peaches	
Broccoli	Apricots	
Cauliflower	Watermelon	
Green or red cabbage (coleslaw)	Honeydew melon	
Mushrooms	Cantaloupe	

6: EAT A GREATER VARIETY OF FOODS.

The best, freshest, most toxin-free natural food cannot build health alone. Other than mother's milk for a young baby, no complete food exists. The dozen or so basic foods that Americans eat — beef, chicken, milk, potatoes, bread, pasta, and so forth — do not supply all of the dietary factors that produce optimal health. Ongoing research identifying hundreds of beneficial molecules in whole plant and animal foods indicates that there are many more nutrients which have not yet been discovered. The greater the variety of nutritious foods you eat, the greater the chance you have of acquiring such beneficial dietary factors, even those as yet undiscovered. Use Tables 2, 3, and 5, as well as the information on shopping for food in Chapter 2, for ideas for new foods that you may wish to try.

7: SHARPLY LIMIT YOUR SUGAR INTAKE.

Table sugar and brown sugar are calorie-rich, vitamin-poor, and rapidly absorbed. When you snack on a candy bar or soft drink, especially on an empty stomach, your blood sugar is suddenly jolted upward. Your pancreas reacts immediately to this stress by secreting the hormone insulin. Insulin quickly lowers blood sugar levels by allowing glucose entry into the body cells (including the fat cells, where any excess is stored as saturated fat). When this blood sugar jolt is repeated again and again, the pancreas overreacts. It becomes overly efficient, and the stress of high blood glucose brought on by the rapid absorption of sugar results in insulin overproduction and low blood glucose in a short time. This is "reactive hypoglycemia." Its symptoms include fatigue, irritability, depression, headaches, and the inevitable craving for more sugar. As you will see in Part II, hypoglycemia contributes to PMS (Chapter 5), and high insulin levels adversely affect the ovaries, interfering with cycle regularity and promoting polycystic ovary syndrome (Chapter 8).

Sugar depletes the body of hard-to-get B vitamins as well as the minerals chromium, zinc, manganese, and magnesium, all of which are necessary to metabolize it. It lacks the important fiber found in whole, unrefined carbohydrate foods. It feeds yeast organisms, promoting vaginal yeast infections and "yeast overgrowth" problems (Chapter 9).

Even though fruits do provide vitamins, minerals, fiber, and phytonutrients, very sweet fruits such as ripe bananas, ripe peaches, or grapes may trigger reactive hypoglycemia, especially if you eat them on an empty stomach. Sweet fruit juices and canned fruits are even more likely to do so. Honey is sweeter than table sugar and contains some vitamins and minerals, but it also can interfere with blood sugar levels.

Used in small amounts, however, sugar, honey, and molasses do serve a useful role, because they encourage you to eat healthy foods that you otherwise might not enjoy. For example, health-building foods such as yogurt or cooked oatmeal are rather grim without a little sweetener. The goal should be to link sugar to nutritious foods — to bran in bran muffins, to beans in baked beans, to fresh greens in salad dressings, to cranberries in cranberry relish, and so forth.

Sugar is less harmful on a full stomach since other foods, especially protein and fats, slow down its absorption out of the intestines and into the blood. Because of this, a useful guideline that allows you to "cheat" a bit is to serve your treats and sweet fruits as desserts after a meal, not as snacks by themselves. You can also choose small servings of desserts that have plenty of protein and natural fat in them, such as ice cream, custard pudding, pumpkin pie, or dark chocolate-covered nuts.

It is better to prepare your meals starting with basic foods such as vegetables, pasta, meat, fish, grains, or dairy products, but when you do buy packaged items, be careful to read the labels. Processed and prepackaged foods contain more sugar than you would ever pour into your home-cooked dishes! The amount of sugar in prepared foods is often disguised by adding several different types of sugar; for example, "high fructose corn syrup," "corn syrup," and "fructose."

Watch out also for artificial sweeteners, which may be added to otherwise healthy foods such as yogurt. Artificial sweeteners may actually increase your craving for sugar, and may even cause your pancreas to secrete extra insulin.[5] For a complete understanding of the problems with sugar, corn syrup, and the various types of artificial sweeteners in packaged and processed foods, read *Get the Sugar Out!* by nutritionist Ann Louise Gittleman (see "Further Reading").

8: DRINK PLENTY OF PURE WATER INSTEAD OF SOFT DRINKS AND CAFFEINATED BEVERAGES.

What's in your water? Or in the water where you work? It is hard to generalize, but depending on where your water comes from, agricultural runoffs, industrial wastes, or bacterial contamination could affect your drinking water. Despite these problems, it has become much easier to acquire purified drinking water conveniently and economically. The popular habit of carrying drinking water is an excellent and encouraging trend. Carrying ice-cold water is also the best way to overcome the bad habit of relying on soft drinks to quench your thirst.

Water treated by reverse osmosis is probably the purest. Such water can be obtained in many communities through home delivery or pick-up. Once you invest in some one-, three-, or five-gallon water containers, it is very economical to buy water purified by reverse osmosis at vending machines located within supermarkets. Home distillers or reverse osmosis units are more expensive, but are effective answers to unsatisfactory tap water. Or consider obtaining a high-quality filter for your kitchen tap. Get yourself your own refillable stainless steel water bottle and drink to your health!

Before you dismiss the idea of paying for healthful drinking water, consider the price of soft drinks: $2.20 to $8.00 per gallon! But you pay much more for soft drinks with your health. Sugar dissolved in water is absorbed extremely rapidly, especially on an empty stomach. That triggers a rapid insulin spike, followed by reactive low blood glucose. No wonder that daily drinking of sugary sodas has been linked to infertility in women.[6] Even artificially sweetened drinks have been implicated in weight gain, and increased blood glucose and insulin.[7] Elevated insulin is well known to interfere with the function of the ovaries, as explained in Chapter 8. Drink water instead of sugary sodas or diet sodas.

CAFFEINE. Caffeine is a good slave but a bad master. When you use it only occasionally or in moderation, it provides a lift that many people enjoy. However, it affects the nervous system, and can cause anxiety and irritability. It can deprive you of a good night's sleep, sometimes just in small amounts, because it powerfully reduces the "sleep hormone," melatonin. Used to excess, caffeine depletes the body of B vitamins and raises blood glucose by over-stimulating the adrenal glands. The latter effect triggers the insulin response, ultimately causing hypoglycemia, fatigue, and the craving for more caffeine.

Caffeinated beverages are a factor in premenstrual syndrome (PMS), at least for some women.[8] In amounts exceeding 300 mg per day (about two to three cups of coffee), using caffeine relates to a delay in achieving pregnancy.[9] A higher incidence of miscarriage once pregnancy occurs has been found related to consumption of more than 200 mg of caffeine per day (about 2 cups of coffee).[10] Higher intakes increase these risks.

Coffee is the most familiar source of caffeine, but soda pop, non-herbal teas, and chocolate also contain caffeine or related compounds which have similar effects. **Table 6, "Caffeine Content of Selected Beverages,"** contains a chart of the caffeine levels found in coffee, tea, and other beverages.

Caffeine affects blood vessel constriction, so if you are trying to cut back on a heavy-duty caffeine habit, it is better to reduce your caffeine consumption gradually — over a period of two or three weeks — to avoid withdrawal headaches. If you don't want to give up sipping on a hot drink, you can still enjoy flavor, aroma, warmth, and low calories by selecting phytonutrient-rich green teas, white teas, or other herbal teas. Some of these may contain small amounts of caffeine, but small amounts are not problematic, according to the studies referenced above.

TABLE 6, CAFFEINE CONTENT OF SELECTED BEVERAGES	
Beverages, 8 oz.	Caffeine content in milligrams (mg)
Coffee, drip	115-175
Coffee, brewed	80-135
Coffee, instant	65-100
Tea, iced	47
Tea, brewed (ave.)	60
Tea, instant	30
Tea, green	15
Hot cocoa	14
Beverages, 12 oz.	
Mountain Dew	54
Diet Coke	45.6
Pepsi-Cola	37.5
Diet Pepsi	36
Coca-Cola Classic	34

(Source: *www.wilstar.com/caffeine.htm*; from National Soft Drink Association, U.S. Food and Drug Administration, Pepsi.)

9: MAKE YOUR MEALS TASTY AND SIMPLE.

Nutritious, tasty, simple to prepare — these describe the ideal meal. So far the focus has been on better nutrition. However, if you emphasize the principle of improving the ingredients of your familiar, favorite dishes, you will already have one important element of good taste: familiarity. You naturally tend to like what you are used to, and the freshness, naturalness, and gentle cooking of nutritious foods will automatically add gourmet taste. Good food tastes good!

Once you get rid of prepackaged foods with their sugary additives, you'll discover that natural foods are often quite sweet. Constant consumption of soft drinks, baked goods, desserts, and artificial sweeteners stimulates rather than satisfies your sweet tooth. Conversely, when you cut down on sweet junk food, your sensitivity to sweet taste will noticeably improve. The sweetness of carrots, cabbage, whole wheat bread, meat, and even grapefruit will pleasantly surprise you. Eliminating added sugar also enables you to enjoy the actual taste of the food itself. Strawberries, apples, watermelons, and other sweet fruits will taste like the treats they really are!

Simplicity is a major consideration since so many homemakers are so very busy. The rule of thumb of using a greater variety of foods is of real value here. Many of the convoluted, time-consuming recipes in cookbooks are only an attempt to create variety where it really doesn't exist. For example, it is easy to scrub and microwave a white potato. So why peel it, boil it, mash it, fry it or au gratin it? Instead of depending on so many inconvenient ways to disguise the same old foods, offer real variety in your meats, grains, beans, fruits, and vegetables, and prepare them simply. Instead of that potato, why not rice, baked squash, sweet potato, corn on the cob, or baked beans? Refer again to Tables 2 and 3 for some ideas for increasing variety.

BREAKFAST. Hot cereals are traditional breakfast foods. However, if you use cold cereal, make it a point to use whole-grain cereals, rather than the over-advertised junk foods that have replaced real grain foods. Rolled oats, granola, bran muffins, multi-grain pancakes and homemade waffles are all excellent foods. Whole wheat cereals are nutritious, but wheat is so commonly used as bread that it is an excellent idea to avoid it in breakfast grains to increase your variety of food. Our family particularly likes an organic breakfast granola called "Honey Gone Nuts," distributed by Breadshop's Natural Foods. It is a substantial, chewy, wheat-free granola, complete with oats, seeds, walnuts, and almonds.

Whole fruits contain natural sugars, but they also offer freshness and fiber. Freshness and fiber are much reduced in bottled fruit juices. Why not improve your nutrition by eating a delicious orange or tangerine instead of drinking orange juice? Or purple grapes instead of grape juice? Grapefruit instead of grapefruit juice? As a habit, prefer the whole fruit to the fruit juice, and you will add real zip to your breakfast!

A good source of protein and some fat, along with the fruits just mentioned, will enable your breakfast to give you a long, steady release of glucose, keeping you energetic and alert until lunchtime. Eggs are a protein and fatty food that really do "stick to your ribs." Milk is another good protein food. Cottage cheese, hard cheese, and yogurt are also excellent sources of protein. Putting butter, peanut butter, or cashew butter on whole wheat toast slows the release of glucose from the toast. If you prefer meat for breakfast, try some of last night's leftovers, but avoid commercially processed meats such as bacon and sausage.

LUNCH. Lunch is great for sandwiches of whole grain bread packed with tuna salad, chicken salad, toasted cheese, natural peanut butter, leaf lettuce, tomatoes, sloppy joes, and so forth. Expand your lunch menu with soups, tacos, wraps, corn bread, yogurt, fruit, last night's leftovers, or perhaps another breakfast food such as multi-grain pancakes. You can also microwave a sweet potato and eat it with butter as part of your lunch.

DINNER. If you serve a traditional American-style dinner, you probably prepare the evening meal around meat, potatoes, a vegetable, and a salad. This pattern gives you something to work with! Broaden your protein menu with ocean fish, tuna, chicken, turkey, or other poultry. Use the "potato position" for brown rice, sweet potatoes, corn, peas, baked squash, beans, or whole grain pasta. Then cook up a couple of hefty servings of dark green or yellow vegetables — whatever is in season or on sale. Make your salad last but serve it first, and make it big!

Casseroles, stews, soups, chili, chicken and rice, lasagna, and baked beans are nutritious and economical ways to improve your nutrition. In reality, such foods combine two or three of the four basic dishes above. Your favorites can be improved by substituting better ingredients for poor ones (Table 3) and adding the vegetables at the last minute.

I do not serve dessert with dinner except on special occasions. This not only eliminates extra sugar, but it also simplifies dinner preparation considerably. On the other hand, if your family is accustomed to dessert, why not try a seasonal fruit? A slice of cantaloupe or watermelon, apples sprinkled with cinnamon, sections of seedless oranges, or a dish of fresh pineapple, blueberries, cherries, or strawberries after a meal is a good way to satisfy your sweet tooth without disrupting your blood sugar or spending valuable time on preparation. *Get the Sugar Out!* by Ann Louise Gittleman contains many other ideas for low-sugar desserts (see "Further Reading").

SNACKS. Children, pregnant and nursing mothers, and anyone who tends toward hypoglycemia (often characterized by fatigue or irritability which improves after eating, or migraine headaches in the morning or late afternoon) may find snacks just about a necessity. A combination of carbohydrates, protein, and fats makes the best snacks. The carbohydrates get the blood sugar up in a short time, while the protein and fat slow the release of sugars into the blood, so that the blood glucose remains neither too high nor too low over a long period of time.

Yogurt, peanut butter on bread, seed-nut-raisin trail mixes, granola cereal with milk, cheese and whole-grain crackers, toasted cheese sandwiches, or hard-boiled eggs on a salad make good snacks. Sugary foods, including sweet fruits, are the worst snack foods, because they cause wide swings in the blood glucose when they are eaten without other food. Mothers of toddlers who wake up frequently at night or who resist bedtime may find that a hearty protein-rich snack before bed solves the problem. A protein-rich bedtime snack may also help prevent morning headaches in some individuals.

10: MAKE GOOD CHOICES WHEN YOU EAT AWAY FROM HOME.

Breaking all the rules occasionally at a fast food restaurant can be fun, but if you must eat lunch or another meal away from home regularly, eating out can make improved nutrition harder to achieve. The truth is, you can get excellent, delicious, highly nutritious meals at fine restaurants, but you will pay real money for their fresh, whole, gently-handled ingredients! Here are some suggestions for those who are away from home during the day.

1) EAT BREAKFAST AT HOME EVERY DAY, AND MAKE IT SUBSTANTIAL. Have French toast, homemade bread with peanut butter, whole grain granola with milk, or eggs and fruit. Or eat a breakfast that seems like lunch — sandwiches, soup, cottage cheese, or leftovers from last night. Avoid the coffee-and-donut breakfast, which is a recipe for blood sugar swings that drain your energy, disrupt your concentration, and rattle your nerves. Before you leave home, fill up your stainless steel water bottle with some ice cold water, unless you are lucky enough to have purified drinking water at your workplace or school.

2) PACK UP SOME GOOD FOOD AND TAKE IT ALONG FOR LUNCH. If you have access to a microwave oven, plan on last night's casserole, chili, lasagna, stew, or spaghetti. Or pack whole-grain sandwiches or cold chicken to go. Fruits, salads, yogurt, hard-boiled eggs, or tuna salad are other possibilities.

3) RELY LESS ON VENDING MACHINES FOR SNACKS. Take a trip to the grocery store and find some snack items. Trail mixes of raisins, seeds, and nuts, or yogurt, whole-grain granola bars, natural cheese, whole grain crackers, baby carrots, celery, or fruits are all possibilities. Use vending machines for milk, yogurt, trail mixes, and other nutritious foods only.

4) MAKE GOOD CHOICES AT FAST FOOD RESTAURANTS AND CAFETERIAS. Even fast food restaurants usually have salads available. Make digging into a vegetable salad a habit if you must eat out often at a fast food place or cafeteria. Choose meats that are not processed; for example, broiled fish, hamburger, chicken, or steak, rather than ham, hot dogs, bacon, or lunch meats. Can you get a baked potato? A bean burrito? Chili? A chef salad? Fresh fruits? Avoid the soft drinks, french fries, breaded chicken nuggets, breaded fish, processed cheese, and sweet desserts.

5) **MAKE IT A PRIORITY TO EAT THE EVENING MEAL AT HOME.** There's no place like home for lots of things, including good nutrition. Eat dinner together as a family.

11: ENLIST YOUR FAMILY'S COOPERATION.

Make no mistake about it — if your spouse or children rebel at your efforts to improve the family's nutrition, it is an uphill battle. I have no specific advice for the recalcitrant spouse other than to appeal to his maturity, reason, and especially to his taste buds. As the mother of nine children, I can offer some suggestions to encourage children to good nutritional habits and attitudes. First, keep junk food out of the house. Children can then be permitted to choose their own breakfasts, lunches, and snacks. A corollary to this is to limit the small screen. There are better reasons than nutrition for doing so, but restricting the TV and computer will also prevent your children from being tantalized by the shameless advertising of worthless foods. As a significant side benefit, they will also get more exercise.

Next, let the children participate in every phase of food preparation, from gardening to actual cooking. Then brag about it at dinner: "Vahn picked the asparagus. Monica floured the fish." The child who helps prepare the food is already prejudiced in its favor. I frequently set the table or act as "gofer" while my helpers make salads, scrub vegetables, or cook pancakes. My husband and I also take the children shopping and have them select the fresh vegetables, seafood, and other items.

Actively teaching children about nutrition is an immense aid. Kids are impressed to find out that protein helps them grow big, or that vitamins keep them healthy. Of course, your own example is your best teaching aid; picky parents have pickier children! And to the extent that you as a parent avoid junk food, you will be pleased at how naturally your children follow your lead.

I believe that just as you teach your children about the dangers of smoking at an early age, you should also teach them not to drink sugary (or diet) beverages at all. Yes, your children may be slightly ahead of the crowd if they avoid soft drinks and boxed juices, but many schools are now getting the message that these are prime culprits in the epidemic of childhood obesity, poor food choices, brain fog, and poor academic performance. What a help it is that bottled water is now "cool" to carry!

BABIES. If you have not had children yet, you can plan beforehand to get future babies off to an excellent start in nutrition, and save many problems later on. Sheila Kippley's wonderful *Breastfeeding and Natural Child Spacing* covers early solid feeding as well as the best nutrition, breastfeeding. I believe that my children's enthusiasm for salads, cole slaw, vegetables, rice, fish, and yogurt is an outgrowth of their early feeding, which I learned from the first edition of Sheila Kippley's book. I never used baby food; in fact, I never even mashed my babies' foods, and I've never spoonfed them anything (other than yogurt, which is just too messy to qualify as a finger food). Another good resource for introducing solids to breastfed babies is *The Art of Breastfeeding* by Linda Kracht and Jackie Hilgert. Chapter 6, "Breastfeeding the Older Baby and Baby-led Weaning," has specific advice for introducing solids. (See "Further Reading".)

Around the time my children were six months old and could sit up in the high chair with the family, I gradually introduced them to finger foods such as soft cooked carrots, broccoli, asparagus, green beans, raw bananas, and tiny pieces of meat. Why spoon-feed a baby who loves to use his hands to put everything into his mouth? I've concluded that pureed baby foods spoil a child's taste for textured food such as salads and vegetables for years. The recognizable green beans and peas that inevitably appear in the diaper are probably nature's way of preventing the young child from obtaining too much nutrition from adult food at the expense of his mother's milk.

It is obvious that having babies sit at the table, watching Mom and Dad eat, whets their appetite for adult food. Togetherness at the table has a role in good nutrition! I have also noticed that babies who are permitted to feed themselves finger foods at the table are not nearly as prone to put small objects into their mouths. Instead, they seem to graduate quickly from their fingers to a fork — not a spoon — just like they see Mommy and Daddy using.

THE FAMILY. Finally, strive for harmony at the dinner table. Such harmony has a value even beyond its role in family bonding. It is a real factor in good nutrition. Tension at the table, the American habit of eating in a rush, or other unpleasantness stimulates the "fight-or-flight" response. The fight-or-flight response interferes with digestive secretions and diverts the blood supply away from the digestive organs. Both digestion and absorption of a meal are decreased when the fight-or-flight response is activated. On a practical level, we have taught our children not to criticize food at the table, which spoils the meal for others and offends the cook! Instead, they may quietly pass up the occasional foods that they dislike, a practice that we have found goes a long way toward avoiding conflict at the dinner table.

A gracious mealtime, followed by a bit of relaxation, quiets the fight-or-flight nerves and encourages the "rest-repose" division of the nervous system, stimulating all aspects of the digestive and absorptive processes. Body and spirit are truly inseparable! The parents who set the tone of the dinner by inviting the Lord's presence, and then complimenting their children on their salad making, table setting, or pleasant manners, are helping to nourish both body and spirit.

12: USE THE "80-20" RULE.
This final guideline means that as you try for better nutrition, work toward a goal of 80 percent improvement. Having done that, don't worry about the imperfect 20 percent! It is simply not realistic to commit the time and effort to locating and preparing organically grown foods of prime freshness all the time. As you will see in Chapter 3, taking vitamin and mineral supplements helps to compensate for the inevitable inadequacies of the modern diet.

Completely avoiding all junk food all the time would restrict you from many memorable celebrations: cookouts with friends, birthday parties, weddings, Christmas. Your children are far more likely to accept your leadership in matters of nutrition if they understand that you are reasonable; that treats are not forbidden — but that they are *treats*.

Summary – Chapter 1

TWELVE RULES FOR BETTER NUTRITION

1) Eat plenty of whole plant foods: grains, beans, nuts, vegetables, seeds, and fruits.

2) Get enough protein to meet your needs.

3) Choose healthful fats and oils; avoid the trans fats.

4) Substitute more nutritious ingredients for less nutritious ingredients in your favorite recipes and dishes.

5) Eat more raw foods, and cook other foods gently.

6) Eat a greater variety of foods.

7) Sharply limit your sugar intake.

8) Drink plenty of pure water instead of soft drinks and caffeinated beverages.

9) Make your meals tasty and simple.

10) Make good choices when you eat away from home.

11) Enlist your family's cooperation.

12) Use the "80-20" rule.

2

Obtaining & Preparing Nutritious Food

Like merchant ships, she secures her provisions from afar. She rises while it is still night, and distributes food to her household. —Proverbs 31:14-15

When nutritious ingredients have replaced refined foods in your home, it is easy to use them in the same recipes you have always used. And when your home contains no junk food, you can snack healthfully on whatever you choose from the kitchen. The hurdle that many homemakers face, though, is to find out where to get the best foods conveniently and economically.

This chapter addresses the issue of where to get healthy food, and then how to prepare it. It assumes you are as busy as you really are! It also includes reviews of two very useful cookbooks, either one of which will give you practical help in the matter of preparing good meals quickly and well.

—— OBTAINING NUTRITIOUS FOOD ——————

If you are presently eating the worst of the American diet — processed meats, packaged mixes, frozen main dishes, and sweet grocery store baked goods — you can improve your nutrition immensely while still shopping at the same supermarket. But there are other sources of healthful foods which may offer better nutrition and sometimes lower prices. The following are thumbnail sketches of the nutritional possibilities of the supermarket as well as alternative food sources.

SUPERMARKETS

It is obvious that the explosion of interest in holistic nutrition has paid off well for the consumer at the grocery store. Many whole, natural foods are now stocked in entire sections of the larger stores. Brown rice, whole-grain macaroni, beans, whole-wheat flour, granola, and natural peanut butter are readily available. The huge produce sections, with many organically-grown fruits and vegetables, make it easy to increase the assortment of fresh fruits and vegetables that you use. The variety of hormone-free poultry, quick-frozen ocean fish, eggs from free-range chickens, and nutritious ethnic foods offered at most supermarkets is large and growing.

Even if a grocery store does not contain expanded sections of natural foods or produce, it can still remain the basic place to shop. Experienced nutrition-conscious homemakers "shop the walls." That is, they favor the basics — produce, frozen vegetables, dairy items, meat, and fish — along the walls and bypass most of the processed foods on the shelves in the center of the store.

PRODUCE. In the produce department, it is easy to be overwhelmed by so many new and unfamiliar fruits and vegetables, so plan to browse a little some day soon. Challenge yourself to try just one new item each time you shop. Go ahead and bring home a kiwi or two. Or treat the family to a fresh pineapple. What about a bunch of fresh beets? Or some bright green Romaine lettuce or other leafy salad greens? Could you jazz up your chili sauce with some red or yellow peppers? Those bright colors and spicy tastes are sure signs of foods rich in phytonutrients. What is on sale lately? Asparagus? Strawberries? Cherries? Artichokes? Acorn squash? Watermelon? Cranberries? It is both nutritionally and economically sound to increase the variety of your fresh produce purchases by selecting whatever is in season or on sale.

FROZEN FOODS. Look around the frozen foods section for the frozen vegetables: green beans, corn, peas, lima beans, and mixed vegetables. Prefer fresh vegetables to frozen, but frozen to canned. Avoid the frozen, prepackaged dinners or side dishes. With the right cookbook, as you will see, you will be soon making your own main dishes that are tastier, cheaper, and healthier in every way!

DAIRY. In the dairy department, select natural yogurt and natural cheeses such as cottage cheese, cheddar cheese, or mozzarella cheese. Avoid processed "cheese foods." Choose butter instead of margarine. If you are attempting to overcome infertility or cycle irregularity, favor full-fat dairy products over no-fat ones. In some groceries, you many be able to get organically produced cows' milk, or goats' milk if you are allergic to cows' milk. Some grocery stores now offer "DHA-containing" chicken eggs. DHA is the fatty acid that supports brain function and development, so reach for those!

MEATS. In addition to beef and chicken, what other meats might you wish to try? Turkey? Lamb? Pork? Notice the labels — it is now possible to get meats that are labeled "hormone-free" and "antibiotic-free." Try to buy raw poultry that does not have flavored "juice" added to it. If you use meat on sandwiches, avoid the processed luncheon meats and make sandwiches from cold turkey, chicken or beef. Skip ham, bacon, hot dogs, and sausage also.

FISH. Basic, unbreaded fish fillets are healthier than the breaded, frozen kind. Besides, it is extremely fast and easy to cook raw fish. You can just dip it in a little flour and seasoning, and pan fry it in a little canola oil for a couple of minutes on each side. If you live inland, as I do, you may have trouble finding frozen fish that is not breaded or precooked, or the "fresh" fish is not very fresh at all! If this is the case, try stocking up on frozen fish fillets during Lent, when even stores that usually do not carry frozen perch, whiting, or whitefish fillets will have good buys on quick-frozen, unprocessed ocean fish.

Look for "wild-caught" ocean fish instead of farm-raised fish. Fish do not make their own healthful fatty acids (abbreviated EPA and DHA); instead, they eat algae that contain the EPA and DHA. Farmed salmon, for example, are fed grains that alter their fatty acid content, detracting from the value of farmed salmon compared to wild-caught salmon[1] If you are concerned about contaminants in fish, you can check out the Natural Resources Defense Council's website: *www.nrdc.org/health/effects/mercury/guide.asp*. As of this writing, perch, whiting, whitefish, and pollock are on the "least mercury" list. So are many other fish, including freshwater trout.

ON THE SHELVES. In the center of the store, be sure to examine the ethnic foods section. Here you can find taco shells, dry beans, peas, and lentils for soup. How will you use them? Take a look at the wrapper; almost always you can find a recipe on it. I buy canned kidney beans and pinto beans for chili, and canned tomato sauce, which I use to make my own spaghetti, chili, or lasagna sauce. I use canned chunk light tuna occasionally for tuna noodle casserole or tuna patties. I also pick up commercially prepared condiments — ketchup, mayonnaise, tartar sauce, and mustard — from the shelves.

HEALTH FOOD SHOPS

Good health food shops are actually miniature grocery stores that specialize in food supplements as well as organic and natural foods. It is helpful to understand these two terms before you purchase foods labeled as such. "Certified organic" refers to foods that are grown on mulched or manure-enriched fields without the use of chemical fertilizers, herbicides, or pesticides. With reference to animal products, it means that the animal was fed from such plant foods, and that no hormones or antibiotics were used. Certified organic foods do not include genetically modified foods or irradiated foods.[2] "Natural" means unprocessed. "Natural" rice has not been refined after harvesting, but it has been grown using conventional farming methods and chemicals. Organic foods are the best, and their higher prices reflect the difference. They will contain more vitamins and minerals and less pesticide or herbicide residues than other foods.

Health food shops are usually more expensive than grocery stores, so they may appeal more to smaller families than to larger ones. But they are good places to get to know, because they carry several desirable items not found in most supermarkets. If you bake your own bread, in addition to organic flour, you can easily pick up baking yeast, iodized sea salt, gluten, and nutritional yeast. You can find expeller-pressed canola oil, walnut oil, and extra-virgin olive oil, aluminum-free baking powder, and lecithin. You can get organic rye or buckwheat flour and whole-grain pasta. You will also find tasty breakfast cereals based on whole, organic grains.

Some health food shops stock raw seeds and nuts. Some carry fresh-baked breads made with organic ingredients. Many feature locally-grown organic produce and DHA-rich eggs. Some may have organic milk. If you are hoping to buy top-quality bottled salad dressings, the health food shop most likely will have them. If you need gluten-free foods, or if you have allergies that restrict what you can eat, you will find health food shops a real blessing. They most likely will have foods labeled just for you. Take a little time to look around, and ask the shopkeeper how to use unfamiliar items that interest you.

Health food shops are probably best known for their large selection of vitamins and minerals. In addition, they will have flax oil in capsules or bottles, as well as purified, good-tasting fish oil to take as a supplement. Bottles of "probiotics," which are friendly bacteria in capsules, can be purchased at health food shops. Other healthy oils, herbs, and teas are worth considering also.

If the nearest health food shop is inconveniently far away or too expensive for your budget, at least use it to purchase expeller-pressed vegetable oils, aluminum-free baking powder, iodized sea salt, whole grain flours, and pasta. I prefer the privately-owned health food shops to the typical shopping mall chains, since the former usually emphasize whole foods to a greater degree than the latter. Both, however, are generally better sources of food supplements (vitamins and minerals) than are pharmacies.

FOOD CO-OPS
Food co-ops are member-owned groceries that are found in many communities. They typically sell a wider variety of natural and organic foods than the health food shops, and they can offer reduced prices to members as a result of direct bulk purchasing and no-frills shop keeping. These are excellent places to buy your grains, beans, flours, oil, honey, bran, nuts, peanut butter, breakfast cereals, and pasta. Co-ops are wonderful for those who wish to eat nutritiously on a shoestring budget, because if you are willing to work a few hours per month, you will get additional price reductions on your purchases. Chances are you will be able to bring your little ones to the shop as you work, as there is probably a corner space filled with toys to keep small hands occupied.

I get much of the nonperishable food for my large family from our local food co-op. My monthly list includes the following, almost all of which is organically produced: bread flour, wheat gluten, baking yeast, nutritional yeast, and lecithin (these last two for increased nutrition in our daily bread), expeller-pressed salad oils, natural peanut butter, brown rice, granola cereal, other multi-grain cereals, oatmeal, bran, cornmeal, and whole wheat, whole rice, and vegetable pasta.

BUYING CLUBS
A "buying club" is another convenient way for cost-conscious homemakers to acquire natural or organic foods. It is especially practical if your family is large or if you have space to store nonperishable items, because most of the items are sold in fairly large quantities. A buying club is generally a small food co-op handled by a single family from their home. The member families order from the managing family a few days ahead of the monthly pick-up date, and on pick-up day they drive to the managing family's home to pick up and pay for their groceries. Pick-up day, in fact, is often a time to visit for a few minutes

with friends who also belong to the buying club. To find the buying club nearest your home, try this website: ***www.unitedbuyingclubs.com***.

FARMERS' MARKETS

Are you aware that many cities and towns feature wonderful farmers' markets where you can buy fresh produce brought in by nearby farmers? These markets are the next best thing to your own garden. The huge farmers' market in Milwaukee where I used to shop was filled with a great variety of incredible bargains. We lived there as budget-conscious newlyweds, and my temptation was always to buy more than the two of us could possibly eat. We would visit the farmers' market on a Saturday morning, going home with brown bags filled with too much of everything.

These popular markets are usually open for a limited number of hours and days during the growing season only. Even if you don't garden, you will get a sense of the natural order of the seasons as the type of produce changes through spring, summer, and fall: asparagus, spinach, green onions, and leaf lettuce early in the spring; soon peas, broccoli, radishes, turnips, strawberries, zucchini, and cucumbers; then the big explosion of beans, corn, tomatoes, peppers, eggplants, apples, pears, peaches, cantaloupe, watermelons, and everything else. Inevitably, autumn slows down to potatoes, onions, cabbage, and pumpkins.

Spend some time at your local farmers' market some Saturday morning. Shop carefully, and you will certainly find gratifying freshness and even organically grown items. Make it a point to try something new every time. Ask the friendly vendors how they prepare, say, a rutabaga or a bunch of fresh kohlrabi. The best thing about farmers' markets is that they are such fun to visit, especially if you would like to experience the old-time "down-home" way of getting to know the hard-working folks who grow your food. Not only are your purchases good for you, but they also support local family farmers and return money to the community.

COMMUNITY SUPPORTED AGRICULTURE

Is the term "Community Supported Agriculture" or the abbreviation CSA new to you? CSA is a new but rapidly-growing option that is a classic "win-win" situation for all involved. CSAs vary, but they can be summarized as groups of consumers who partner with a farmer to distribute the cost of production as well as the fruits of the soil among the members.

CSAs are good for the farm families, because they make a market and take financial pressure off the family farmers. They are good for the consumers, who have fresh, often organic, reasonably-priced produce, eggs, poultry, and red meat available in the natural timing of the seasons. They are good for the land, because organic farming practices enrich the soil. They are even good for production animals, which are permitted to graze to provide the recommended "pastured" meat that you may have heard about but have not been able to obtain. They are good for the community, because they create bonds between city and farm folks, and they recycle money within the community. They are good for the environment, because they cut the waste of trucking food from far away.

CSAs are eminently logical — why should Americans, who live in one of the most agriculturally blessed nations on earth, need to truck in food from across this huge nation? Isn't it more sensible to obtain it from across town?

Please look into the website ***www.localharvest.org*** to find out where there are local organic farms near you, and how to become a "shareholder" or "subscriber" in this type of cooperative venture.

GARDENING

Your own garden is good for the soul as well as the body, and it can be a wonderful family project, providing true quality time for dads, moms, and kids all at once. Give yourself a couple of summers to get good at it, and please don't invest in a tiller or herbicides or even a spade until you read *Gardening Without Work* (see "Further Reading") by the late Ruth Stout. This book explains in a highly readable way the art of mulch gardening — using spoiled hay, straw, fall leaves, or grass clippings to prevent weeds, retain moisture, and fertilize the soil. It is the easy way to garden! Using a modified version of this method, we till our large garden only once every two or three years. We do use small amounts of conventional fertilizer and the low-toxicity plant product rotenone as a pesticide. You can learn more about mulch gardening by searching for "Ruth Stout Gardening" on the internet.

My suggestion for beginners is to plant whatever grows the best with the least care. Asparagus is on the top of my list. This hardy vegetable will produce for you the fourth year after planting, and will feed your family scrumptiously and effortlessly for years early each spring while you are just putting in the spinach seeds! High fencing for tall pole beans and edible pod peas (Sugar Snap, an incredible raw treat) will maximize your yields and minimize your bending. Nothing is easier to grow than sweet corn, and nothing compares with ripe corn picked as the water boils, or corn roasted on an outdoor grill. Beets, turnips, lettuce, onions, broccoli, Brussels sprouts, cabbage, cucumbers, and of course tomatoes are other easy-to-grow plants with high nutrient returns. If you have room for some berry bushes, fruit trees, or grape vines, put some in. For example, one of the easiest fruits to grow is the Concord grape, which needs no spraying and thrives for years.

PRIVATE FARMERS

There are growing numbers of families who own small amounts of land and are attempting to raise chemical-free vegetables, fruits, meat, eggs, honey, and dairy products for their own family as well as to sell for extra cash. If you have the land to do this, why not give it a try? If you are a young couple still not settled in your own home, I strongly encourage you to consider a few acres zoned for agriculture.

If such an undertaking is out of the question, I can assure you that there are homesteaders around who would enjoy the extra cash of raising a free-ranging, antibiotic- and hormone-free lamb, goat, or steer for you. No, you do not end up with a four-footed potential steak in your suburban garage! They take the animal to a custom butcher, and you literally pick up the pieces, all cut and wrapped according to your specifications. Rabbit, chicken, and other poultry are available in this way also. Our own family keeps a flock of chickens for organic eggs and meat, and our children sell our extra eggs. We also keep a small herd of dairy goats for milk and meat, and usually raise a few ducks and geese and several lambs each summer for a bit of variety. There are many other small farmers like us who may have produce, organic eggs, honey, or meat animals to sell. You can contact them through your local 4-H office, local advertising tabloids, or at your farmers' market.

—— PREPARING NUTRITIOUS FOOD ——

THE RIGHT COOKBOOK

The right cookbook could be the most important "ingredient" of all for preparing healthful meals. The ideal cookbook should use all natural ingredients; it should provide lots of options so that recipes can be adapted to your taste or pantry supplies; it should cover a wide variety of nutritious foods; it should contain mostly quick and easy recipes; and every single recipe must be delicious! Here are my recommendations; either or both of these will fill the bill:

Saving Dinner: The Menus, Recipes, and Shopping Lists to Bring Your Family Back to the Table, by Leanne Ely, is a cookbook that will jump-start you on your way to real, natural, tasty homemade dinners, and a great variety of them (see "Further Reading"). This book not only offers very quick-to-cook dishes, but also gives you weekly menus and even shopping lists. The book is set up by season, focusing your emphasis on fresh, natural, and thrifty ingredients. There are many nice touches — for example, the summer menus do not use the oven at all! The sidebars offer helpful tips on soaking beans, cutting squash, and marinating meat. It contains no dessert menus, but with all the tasty foods to start with and the spices for added flavor, you will not miss dessert. Some homemakers may wish to follow the menu plans closely, but for most others, just the recipes are more than enough to help you to bring the family back to the table. For a preview, go to *www.savingdinner.com.*

Whole Foods for the Whole Family, published by La Leche League International (see "Further Reading"), was written by and for busy mothers who wish to eat holistically while still "cooking American." It is somewhat more comprehensive than *Saving Dinner* and offers more instruction for those who have never had much experience in home cooking. It has many, many basic recipes, but it also has sections on making your own whole-wheat bread, peanut butter, sprouts, yogurt, and even baby food. It explains how to cook brown rice, millet, dried peas, and beans. It features many meatless main dishes and many ethnic dishes. There are also desserts that require very little added sugar and are loaded with nutrients. The book includes an appendix that lists recipes that are easy to make, easy to freeze, especially quick to prepare, and so forth. Browsing through it is a delight; you learn about basic nutrition, and it teaches you elementary kitchen skills that you despaired of ever learning. I love this book!

KITCHEN APPLIANCES

Once you have acquired nutritious whole food, whether from grocery or garden, you will be storing it, preparing it, and serving it. Many of the tools that are already in your kitchen are well-adapted to these tasks. Others that you may not use are also worth considering.

The refrigerator is basic, of course, and the bigger the better. Many natural, unprocessed foods must be refrigerated — for example, salad oils and peanut butter. You will need space for all your fresh produce. A deep freezer is especially useful for those who garden or raise their own meat. A microwave oven makes it easy to cook white potatoes, sweet potatoes, and other vegetables. It is great to reheat a plate of food quickly, but it is no substitute for the ordinary stove and oven.

FOOD PROCESSOR

Nothing will help you increase your consumption of good food like a Cuisinart® food processor. It turns out huge amounts of green salads and cole slaw in seconds. It slices fresh beets, tomatoes, and stew vegetables such as carrots and celery. It chops onions, cold chicken for salad, tuna for tuna patties, and potatoes for potato pancakes. It can be used to make peanut butter, mayonnaise, salad dressings, and natural pumpkin pie. It can chop mozzarella cheese or cheddar cheese into a fine topping. It grinds meat for those who butcher their own animals. I have also noticed that the smaller pieces that it produces seem to help my young children really enjoy their salads.

A good food processor such as the Cuisinart® will repay you for years in big, fresh salads with minimal clean-up or maintenance. I use my medium-sized Cuisinart® just about every day, and have done so for as long as I have had one. I can recommend this brand heartily; my first one lasted for 17 years of almost daily use.

BREADMAKER

A breadmaker is the most incredible little robot ever introduced into a kitchen. You drop in the ingredients, set the timer, and in three hours you take out a fresh, fragrant loaf of bread. There is virtually no clean-up, because the pan releases the bread with hardly a crumb left behind. You can set the breadmaker to have the bread ready any time: the next morning, before supper, or as you go out the door to take dinner to a friend. Most important, the breadmaker can make 100% whole-wheat bread with all natural ingredients and no artificial preservatives or trans fats. For better nutrition, you can even fortify your bread with nutritional yeast and lecithin from your health food shop or co-op.

Bread that can be perfectly sliced (just like store-bought bread) is essential if your family is going to use homemade bread daily. If it is crumbly or if it squashes as you try to slice it, it will not be good for sandwiches. That is why you will need to add gluten to 100 percent whole wheat bread, as is noted in the recipe below. I have not invested in one of the slicing templates that promise to enable you to slice the bread uniformly, because I have not had any difficulty with this. I do have a good serrated bread knife, though.

If you do not have a recipe that suits your taste and nutritional goals, you will need to modify a recipe. A problem with breadmakers is that your friend's favorite recipe will not necessarily work well in your brand of breadmaker. You might try the basic whole-wheat recipe for your own machine, and then adjust it for better nutrition. Or try mine (below) and alter it as needed. In general, bread that is too high and sinks in the middle needs less water, less honey, less gluten, less yeast, or more salt. Bread that is too heavy may need more water, honey, gluten, yeast (or another brand of yeast), or less salt. My recipe is based on an original one for whole-wheat bread that came with my first breadmaker, but it has been modified beyond recognition. Do not give up on your ideal bread too soon — it may take half a dozen or more bad loaves before you create the perfect recipe.

Once you have the ideal recipe, do not change it. In my home, all of the family members who make the bread have the recipe below memorized, so that

Marilyn Shannon's Bread Recipe

This is my one and only bread recipe, made for my Breadman breadmaker. I hope it will work well for your willing little kitchen servant.

- 1 1/2 cups warm water
- 3 3/4 cups hard organic whole wheat flour
- 2 tablespoons gluten
- 1 tablespoon nutritional yeast
- 1-2 tablespoons granular lecithin
- 2 teaspoons salt
- 2 tablespoons butter
- 3-4 tablespoons honey
- 2 teaspoons granular baking yeast

Instructions: Drop ingredients in, set timer, and savor the fragrance of baking bread in your kitchen in a couple of hours. When the buzzer sounds, remove the steaming loaf. Invite your husband to the kitchen table with you to enjoy a warm slice, covered with melted butter. "Give us this day our daily bread." Makes one 2-pound loaf.

it is simple to start a delicious loaf of bread right before we go to bed. I also store the right-sized measuring cup or measuring spoon in each container of ingredients, so that it is hard to make a mistake.

YOGURT MAKER

Using a yogurt maker will save many dollars spent on yogurt and will produce better yogurt than you can buy. Several different brands of electric yogurt makers are available inexpensively through department stores. Some make one large batch of yogurt; others make it in individual one-cup servings. Many health food shops carry powdered yogurt starter, which ensures good tasting yogurt every time.

If you have never made yogurt, here is the process. First, you scald the right amount of milk in a saucepan to kill off bacteria. Then the milk is allowed to cool down to a temperature compatible for the friendly bacteria that will convert the milk to yogurt. If you are in a hurry, you can set the pan in a sink of cold water. Once the temperature has dropped enough (according to your yogurt thermometer), you stir in the yogurt starter. You place the mixture in the yogurt maker, plug it in, and in a few hours or overnight you remove the warm yogurt. Once it cools in the refrigerator, it is ready to eat with some jam, honey, or fruit as a sweetener. Homemade yogurt is generally thinner than the grocery store type. Do not be disappointed if that is how it turns out. Your yogurt maker will come with recipes to help you use more of this wonderfully nutritious food.

POPCORN POPPER

Our popcorn popper is used so frequently that it stays out on the counter, along with the toaster, breadmaker, and food processor. The air-popped popcorn avoids overheated oil, though it is not quite as crispy as the oil-popped variety. Popcorn topped with melted butter really does make a quick, easy, delicious, nutritious snack.

WATER PURIFICATION SYSTEM

Are you remodeling your kitchen? If so, why not install a reverse osmosis water purification system? It will provide convenience and an improvement in your health, especially if you have city water or a shallow well. And what a great way to motivate yourself to kick the bad habit of drinking soft drinks!

If a reverse osmosis system will not fit into your budget, what about a filter for your kitchen tap? Look for a high-quality one that removes both organic and inorganic contaminants, and change it as often as specified by the manufacturer. Then, purchase good quality stainless steel water bottles for family members who work or go to school outside the home. That way, all of you can carry your "homemade" water with you, instead of buying plastic bottles of very expensive and not necessarily contaminant-free water.[3]

POTS, PANS, AND BAKEWARE

Stainless steel pots with tight-fitting lids are ideal for basic cooking tasks such as steaming vegetables. Your stainless steel teakettle is another staple item; let it remind you of all the tasty and healthful teas that you can enjoy with family or friends, or just for an afternoon pick-me-up. A really big stainless steel soup pot is useful if there are to be leftovers. My new one holds four gallons, and I love using it to make stew or chicken and rice or spaghetti sauce for my large family. A big, covered stainless steel roasting pan is another essential item. Each Sunday before church, we put a roast in the oven — usually our own lamb, goat meat, duck, goose, or chicken, surrounded with potatoes, carrots, and onions. The roasting pan does the rest until we come home and make the gravy. Stainless steel cookie sheets, muffin pans, and cake pans are nice to have for your homemade desserts and muffins, which are more nutritious and better-tasting than store-bought treats — plus you get the fun and family time of making them yourselves!

A high-quality non-stick frying pan may encourage you to cook more frequently at home, since it is so easy to use and so quick to clean. I now own a new Starfrit® brand frying pan with a powdered ceramic surface. My son-in-law, an excellent and health-conscious cook, though, insists that his properly seasoned cast iron frying pan is as easy to clean as any non-stick type. I do not recommend department-store coated cookware, because high temperatures cause breakdown of the coating, releasing potentially harmful products.[4] However, the recently available powdered ceramic-coated cookware is much safer, and concerns about coated cookware may soon be a thing of the past.[5]

A pressure cooker is a great aid to bean cookery and for preparing stew meats. A slow cooker (crock pot) is not only good for stews and soups that you start in the morning, but it is also wonderful to take to potluck dinners, full of whatever you'd like to serve hot.

CANISTERS, CONTAINERS, AND OTHER KITCHEN ODDS-N-ENDS
Extra canisters are important for your flours, brown rice, millet, beans, whole-grain pasta, herbal teas, and popcorn. Glass dishes with tight-fitting plastic lids are just what you need to keep your leftovers in top shape. A good bread knife and cutting board are essential equipment for breadmaking. A hand-held pepper mill filled with peppercorns will enable you to season your food like a gourmet cook. If you take lunch with you, invest in insulated containers to keep hot things hot and cold things cold.

DINNERWARE
Finally, may I suggest something not directly related to food preparation? You need a beautiful set of dinnerware. (Yes, even if you, like us, have young children.) A beautifully set table with a lovely tablecloth and centerpiece adds such graciousness to your meals. Better yet, it encourages you to prepare your best meals for your family as well as for your guests.

Summary — Chapter 2

Good food sources

SUPERMARKETS: Still a great place to shop, and getting better.

HEALTH FOOD SHOPS: Get acquainted with one near you.

FOOD CO-OPS: Economical, especially if you work in it a few hours per month.

BUYING CLUBS: Good for large, cost-conscious families.

FARMERS' MARKETS: Fresh and fun.

CSAS: A win-win for all involved.

GARDENING: Good for the soul, as well as for the body.

PRIVATE FARMERS: Find one nearby for organic meat and eggs.

Recommended supplies

COOKBOOK: Not an appliance, but you need Leanne Ely's *Saving Dinner* or La Leche League's *Whole Foods for the Whole Family*.

REFRIGERATOR: Make it big and store your flour and oils in it also.

DEEP FREEZER: For frozen vegetables and meats.

FOOD PROCESSOR: Cuisinart® for salads and many other tasks.

BREADMAKER: If you have one, use it!

YOGURT MAKER: Provides the best quality and cheapest yogurt.

POPCORN POPPER: Fun and nutritious snacks.

WATER PURIFICATION SYSTEM: A wonderful addition to a kitchen.

POTS WITH TIGHT-FITTING LIDS: For steamed vegetables. Stainless steel soup pot, roasting pan, cookie sheets, muffin and cake pans, ceramic non-stick or cast iron frying pan.

PRESSURE COOKER: For bean cookery and stews.

CANISTERS: For all those grains, beans, rice, and flours.

STORAGE DISHES WITH TIGHT-FITTING LIDS: Keep your leftovers fresh.

DINNERWARE: For a beautifully set table, every day.

3

Basic Supplements to Consider

God also said: "See, I give you every seed-bearing plant all over the earth and every tree that has seed-bearing fruit on it to be your food." — Genesis 1:29

Do you get discouraged by much of what you read or hear about modern food? Have you concluded that it is simply not possible to get top-quality nutrition out of the food you buy and prepare? Are you in a situation where it is difficult for you to make your own food at home? Are you concerned about sprays on plants used for food and the diet of animals used for food? Would you like to be in the best health possible before you get pregnant? There is a way of compensating for the inadequacies of our modern diet and even for the toxins in the environment: taking vitamin, mineral, and essential fatty acid supplements.

I rank the prudent use of vitamin, mineral, and essential fatty acid supplements as a health practice second only to wholesome food in the benefits it provides. The purpose of this chapter is to provide a brief overview of vitamins, minerals, and essential fatty acids; to explain the rationale for taking them as supplements; and to recommend a plan of supplementation which is within the limits of safety, comprehensive enough to be beneficial, and flexible enough to be tailored to your individual needs. The chapter ends with several practical suggestions to help you get the most benefit from taking supplements.

DEFINING VITAMINS, MINERALS, AND ESSENTIAL FATTY ACIDS

Vitamins and minerals are sometimes called "micronutrients" because they are needed only in tiny amounts compared to the "macronutrients": carbohydrates, proteins, and fats. In terms of how much you need, the two essential fatty acids fall somewhere in between the micronutrients and macronutrients. Nevertheless, in this book "micronutrients" refers to vitamins, minerals, and essential fatty acids, because these three classes of essential nutrients can be added to the diet in pill form; that is, as supplements.

VITAMINS are complex, carbon-based molecules synthesized by other living creatures but necessary to human life and health. As such, they must be obtained in the diet. Vitamins are divided into fat-soluble and water-soluble types: vitamins A, D, E, and K are fat-soluble; the various B vitamins and vitamin C are water soluble. Vitamins are absorbed from the intestines and ultimately enter the blood.

Cells receive vitamins from the blood and use them for a variety of essential functions. Some are used to liberate energy from food molecules, some assist in cell division, some prevent oxygen damage to cellular parts, some enable various cell structures to be synthesized, and some help to rid the body of toxins. Many perform these tasks by serving as "co-enzymes"; that is, they enable the cells' enzymes to do their job of sparking the multitude of chemical reactions taking place within cells. If you envision an enzyme as a razor, the thin strip of metal which does the actual cutting is analogous to a vitamin which serves as a co-enzyme. The enzyme cannot work without it.

MINERALS are simpler than vitamins. They occur in the non-biological world, though most dietary minerals come from plant and animal foods. Calcium, phosphorus, and magnesium are minerals used in relatively large amounts in our bodies, because they are major components of bone. Potassium, chloride, and sodium are also abundant in the body. The others that our bodies require are "trace minerals," needed only in minute amounts. Iron, zinc, copper, chromium, selenium, and iodine are examples of trace minerals. Minerals are absorbed from the intestines into the blood, but many are more difficult to absorb than are vitamins.

Some minerals, such as magnesium, zinc, and selenium, perform a large number of functions in many different cell types. Iron is a mineral well known for its role in red blood cells, where it carries oxygen, but it is also used by almost all other cells to liberate energy. Like the vitamins, many minerals serve as cofactors for various enzymes within cells. Without the mineral as co-factor, the related enzyme cannot perform its vital function of enabling cellular activity to proceed at its normal, rapid pace.

ESSENTIAL FATTY ACIDS are relatively long, thin, carbon-based molecules which are termed unsaturated because they do not contain as much hydrogen as is chemically possible. There are only two essential fatty acids, linoleic acid and alpha-linolenic acid. Alpha-linolenic acid, also called the "omega-3" essential fatty acid, is the precursor molecule of docosahexaenoic acid (DHA) and eicosapentaenoic acid (EPA), which are longer, more complex, and more fragile fatty acids used abundantly in brain tissue and in the reproductive glands.

Essential fatty acids are most abundant within the seeds of certain plants. Linoleic acid is found in most natural plant food oils, such as corn oil, soy oil, sunflower oil, sesame oil, and safflower oil. Because it is unsaturated, it is chemically reactive and is subject to damage from light, oxygen, and heat. Linoleic acid is easy to obtain through the diet, so it is not necessary to supplement it.

Alpha-linolenic acid is harder to get, and is less stable than its more plentiful relative. Small amounts are found in canola oil, soy oil, walnut oil, and pumpkin seed oil, but flax oil is by far the most plentiful source of it. People who eat expeller-pressed, unheated flax oil regularly on their salads can get alpha-linolenic acid in a natural food form. Or, high-quality flax oil can be obtained from a health food shop and taken by the teaspoon. It should be kept in the refrigerator and used within two or three weeks of opening, so do not purchase it in large bottles. As many people do not like the taste of flax oil, supplementing it in capsules is a simple way of obtaining alpha-linolenic acid, and I recommend this practice highly. In my counseling as a Couple to Couple League volunteer, I have found supplementing flax oil very helpful to virtually all of the reproductive problems discussed in Part II.

You can purchase fish oils, generally cod liver oil, as a source of EPA and DHA. It is possible to get fish oils that are certified free of toxic heavy metal, including mercury, cadmium, lead, and other contaminants. These oils can even be purchased with lemon flavor, making the stereotype of terrible-tasting cod liver oil of the past obsolete. The fish liver oils are also sources of modest amounts of vitamins A and D.

The EPA and DHA in fish oils are not essential, however. Human beings can make EPA and DHA from the omega-3 alpha-linolenic acid, such as is plentiful in flax oil, if vitamins B3, B6, C, and the minerals magnesium and zinc are available in the diet.[1] Should you supplement fish oil in addition to flax oil? If you are supplementing flax oil as well as the vitamins and minerals, or if you eat fatty fish weekly, you may consider fish oil optional. However, a recent review of many research articles confirms that supplementing the diet with fish oil is beneficial to a long list of reproductive problems, including menstrual pain, infertility, pregnancy problems such as gestational diabetes and pre-eclampsia, postpartum depression, menopausal problems, and osteoporosis. Fish oil supplements also have a very positive effect on the brain development of children born to mothers who took such supplements.[2]

WHY SUPPLEMENT?
Why should you take supplements? There are a number of reasons to do so.

SUPPLEMENT TO MEET INDIVIDUAL NUTRIENT NEEDS. Based simply on the wide genetic variation of humans and the definition of average, almost everyone is likely to have higher than average needs for one or more of the 50 or so essential nutrients. You may not absorb particular nutrients well from the digestive tract, a problem that increases with age — even while your need for calories is decreasing. Entire groups of individuals are known to have higher requirements for particular nutrients than even a *balanced* diet may provide: pregnant and nursing women, dieters, smokers, drinkers, the elderly, oral contraceptive users, those who exercise vigorously, and those with acute or chronic illnesses. Some therapeutic drugs deplete micronutrients; for example, over-the-counter pain medications lower levels of vitamin C, folic acid, and iron. Eating refined sugar depletes the body of B vitamins and several minerals.[3] Supplements help ensure that you are getting enough of all the nutrients that you, as a unique individual, need for your particular circumstances.

SUPPLEMENT TO HELP YOUR BODY GET RID OF TOXINS. Vitamins and minerals help the body to detoxify harmful substances formed within the cells through normal metabolism, as well as those taken into the body because of their presence in the environment. For example, folic acid, vitamin B_6, and vitamin B_{12} enable the body to reduce the levels of homocysteine, a harmful byproduct of the metabolism of certain amino acids. Vitamins A, C, and E, and beta-carotene are well known as antioxidants, which neutralize dangerous free radicals that are formed in cells. Vitamin A helps the body to detoxify contaminants such as dioxin and polychlorinated biphenols (PCBs). Selenium helps protect against toxic heavy metals such as lead. Many vitamins and minerals are needed as part of enzyme systems that the liver uses to change various metabolic wastes, hormones, prescription drugs, and environmental toxins into forms that make them less potent and easier to excrete.[4]

SUPPLEMENT TO MAKE UP FOR NUTRIENT DEFICIENCIES IN MODERN FOODS. When you consider typical American food, a balanced diet providing sufficient vitamins and minerals becomes more illusion than reality. When people eat only a few different kinds of food, the chance for adequate intake of each vitamin, mineral, and fatty acid diminishes. Even if you are eating abundant fruits, vegetables, and whole grains, many nutrients are lost when foods are harvested in an under- or over-ripe state or when they are stored, preserved, heated, peeled, juiced, or exposed to air. Vitamin E, for instance, is damaged by exposure to oxygen, heat, and light. Even raw fruits and vegetables are not as nutrient-rich as they might be, since most are grown on depleted soils replenished with only a few minerals, and cultivated year after year. The domestic crops themselves are hardly "natural" — many have been extensively bred for traits such as high yield, drought resistance, uniform size, or firm texture, but not for vitamin and mineral content. Supplements are a practical way of compensating for nutrient loss that occurs as a result of modern methods of producing, preserving, and preparing food.

SUPPLEMENT TO COMPENSATE FOR AN INADEQUATE DIET. How many people are actually eating a "balanced diet" *on a daily basis*? Even though there is considerable controversy regarding what a "balanced diet" really is, most nutritionists agree that large numbers of men, women, and children are not eating healthy foods daily. The huge numbers of fast food restaurants which line American roadways tell a dismal tale. The problem of recycling millions of aluminum beverage cans reflects a bigger problem with human nutrition. My own experience as a college instructor has driven this point home to me: many, many young adults simply do not eat anything close to the diet they know they should. Supplementing the micronutrients helps overcome the deficiencies of a "hit-and-miss" diet.

SUPPLEMENT TO IMPROVE HEALTH PROBLEMS. A prime reason to consider careful supplementation of vitamins, minerals, and essential fatty acids is to overcome specific health problems. Scientific literature contains numerous studies demonstrating the benefits of specific micronutrients on a variety of human illnesses. These studies are published in respected, peer-reviewed journals by medical doctors and other credentialed investigators; double-blind studies are well represented along with promising open studies. Some of the books recommended in the "Further Reading" section contain extensive citations of current research involving nutritional healing for many human diseases. Part II of this book cites such studies involving reproductive disorders.

SUPPLEMENT FOR OPTIMAL HEALTH. Sensible supplementation can help you toward the goal of optimal health. Optimal health refers to more than just the absence of disease. It refers to a state characterized by abundant energy, emotional stability, and the ability to participate vigorously in life's work and recreation. While optimum health is a subjective condition, improved energy level and sense of well-being are common reports among supplement users and undoubtedly contribute to their widespread and continuing popularity. Chances are great that you have already been taking supplements yourself, even before reading this book.

We are currently seeing immense growth in interest in the role of micro-nutrients in health and healing. This trend has been given quite a boost as the "baby boom" generation enters its mature years, demanding alternative information on how best to preserve vigorous good health and to prevent degenerative diseases. The real question is no longer *whether* to supplement, but how to do so effectively and safely.

BASIC SUPPLEMENTS TO CONSIDER

Table 7, "Basic Supplements to Consider" (pages 44–45), is a general plan for supplementing the micronutrients effectively, comprehensively, and safely. In many cases the suggested amounts of the vitamins and minerals in this plan are substantially higher than the well-known "Daily Values" (DVs) that are part of food labels. DVs are formulated to cover the minimal nutrient needs of the majority of healthy individuals, and to prevent classic deficiency diseases such as scurvy, beriberi, pellagra, and rickets. They are not formulated for overcoming specific health problems, nor are they intended to represent optimal intake. For example, published studies of vitamins and minerals used to overcome physical disorders, such as PMS or male or female infertility, often involve nutrient levels considerably higher than the DVs.

Among nutritionally-oriented medical doctors who are actively involved in healing through nutritional alternatives, a consensus seems to have developed regarding the amounts of the various vitamins and minerals that are commonly supplemented. The amounts of supplements listed in Table 7 are in the general range suggested by clinically experienced, nutritionally-oriented physicians, including Guy Abraham, M.D., who used double-blind studies to establish the link between PMS and nutrition;[5] the late William G. Crook, M.D., who pioneered medical and nutritional treatment of yeast overgrowth;[6] Phyllis Balch, C.N.C., author of *Prescription for Nutritional Healing*;[7] Julian Whitaker, M.D., author and founder of the Whitaker Wellness Institute in Newport Beach, California;[8] the late John Lee, M.D., who is so well known for his research on natural progesterone for women that it is easy to overlook his constant emphasis on better nutrition;[9] Dean Raffelock, D.C., and Robert Rountree, M.D., whose clinical experience with pregnant and postpartum women has led them to strongly recommend nutritional supplementation;[10] and Susan Lark, M.D., women's doctor and author.[11]

Far more critical than comparing supplement dosages to the rock-bottom DVs is relating them to their toxic levels. Footnotes have been added to Table 7 where research has indicated a potential for toxicity. The *Nutrition Almanac* (see "Further Reading") also contains information on vitamin and mineral toxicity.

If you are contemplating pregnancy, you should discuss your vitamin and mineral supplements with a nutritionally-aware health care practitioner. However, I have made every effort to recommend only supplement amounts that are safe before and during pregnancy and breastfeeding.

GUIDELINES FOR SUPPLEMENT USE
The following guidelines are offered to enable you to reap the considerable benefits of nutritional supplements and to minimize the possible risks.

1) PROPER DIET IS A HIGHER HEALTH PRIORITY THAN SUPPLEMENTATION. Supplements cannot compensate for a sugar-laden diet, a diet full of trans fats, a low-fiber diet, or a low-protein diet. Whole plant foods are full of an astonishing array of health-promoting molecules called phytonutrients, which are not part of vitamin and mineral supplements.

2) SEEK REALISTIC NUTRITIONAL COUNSELING WHEN YOU SUPPLEMENT. If you are in ordinary good health, that may just mean approval from your family doctor or gynecologist. If you suffer from a serious disorder such as diabetes, celiac disease, or liver, kidney, or cardiovascular disease, make every effort to find a physician who is aware of the specific risks as well as the specific benefits that supplements may hold for you. A nutritionally-oriented doctor can address any possible potential for overdose, but moreover, he or she may be able to recommend supplements to improve your particular health problem. See the question and answer related to this in Chapter 16 for more information about locating a nutritionally-aware physician.

3) STRIVE FOR BALANCE WHEN YOU SUPPLEMENT. High doses of some nutrients can cause increased requirements for others. The B vitamins deserve special attention in this regard. While "balanced" B complex supplements in the suggested amounts are readily available, tablets of the B vitamin folic acid of 1,000 micrograms (mcg; equal to 1.0 mg) or more are still obtainable by prescription only. (Folic acid may mask vitamin B12 deficiency in strict vegetarians and those with gastrointestinal abnormalities, but it is one of the safest and most valuable vitamins to supplement.) In the higher potency B-complex vitamin supplements, such as the 50 or 100 mg/mcg amounts, folic acid is too low for balance, and should be taken separately in 400 or 800 mcg tablets, which are widely available without prescription (see Table 7).

Other nutrients which must be properly balanced include calcium and magnesium; to take the former without the latter is to invite magnesium deficiency. Copper and zinc must also be balanced with one another. Magnesium and vitamin B6 are both involved in similar cellular work. Vitamins B6, B12, and folic acid work together in the body to reduce the buildup of a toxic metabolite called homocysteine. Vitamin A increases the need for vitamin E, and vitamin E's activity is enhanced by selenium. Calcium cannot be absorbed and used in the bone without adequate amounts of vitamin D, magnesium, manganese, zinc, and folic acid. The hard-to-get essential fatty acid alpha-linolenic acid, found abundantly in flax oil, cannot be converted to its active forms without vitamins B3, B6, C, and the minerals magnesium and zinc. Vitamin E is required to prevent the oxidation of the essential fatty acids.

Because of the interaction of nutrients and the need for balance, I strongly recommend that any program of supplementation include all of the essential nutrients listed in Table 7. Even if research indicates that only one micronutrient has reversed a physical problem that you are attempting to overcome, this principle of balanced supplementation still holds true.

4) ALWAYS TAKE SUPPLEMENTS ON A FULL STOMACH, PREFERABLY IN DIVIDED DOSES WITH BREAKFAST AND LUNCH. Taking micronutrient pills between meals can unnecessarily irritate your stomach or intestines, and may decrease the absorption of some nutrients, especially the fat-soluble ones. Some people find that taking supplements with their evening meal causes them to have too much energy to fall asleep at night. Take your vitamins with breakfast and lunch, when you will appreciate the energy boost later in the day.

5) BEGIN TAKING SUPPLEMENTS GRADUALLY. The most common side effect of taking vitamin and mineral supplements is an upset stomach. If you begin gradually and you do discover that they upset your stomach, you can back off and increase them even more slowly. It may take a couple of weeks to work up to what you want to take.

6) PREFER NATURAL VITAMINS TO SYNTHETIC VITAMINS. Vitamin E is a complex molecule that occurs in either a "right-handed" form or in a mirror image ("left-handed" form). Human cells prefer the "right-handed" molecule. Synthetic vitamin E is a mixture of both. Natural vitamin E, manufactured by living organisms, is the "right-handed" form, and is more usable to the body as such. On a vitamin bottle, natural vitamin E is listed as "d-alpha tocopherol," while synthetic vitamin E is labeled "dl-alpha tocopherol." (The "d" actually stands for the Latin word for "right," and the "l" in "dl" for the Latin word for "left.") Other vitamins are chemically the same whether derived from natural sources or synthetic. However, "natural" vitamins often include other molecules that occur together with the known vitamin and may enhance the cells' ability to use the actual vitamin efficiently. For example, vitamin C is often found together with complex molecules called "bioflavinoids." "Natural" vitamins are also less likely to have food colorings or preservatives in them.

7) USE TIMED-RELEASE VITAMINS TO HELP PREVENT LOSS OF THE SUPPLEMENT INTO THE URINE. Taking vitamins often results in bright yellow urine, revealing that the vitamins indeed have been absorbed out of the intestines and into the blood, and providing evidence that the kidneys are extremely efficient at

removing excess from the blood. Timed-released vitamins slow the absorption of the nutrients into the blood, and prevent some of the inevitable urinary loss, though it is usual to have bright yellow urine if you supplement. Timed-release vitamins may also decrease digestive upset.

Instead of timed-release formulation, you may prefer a supplement labeled to take several of the capsules or pills daily. Taking them throughout the morning and afternoon with meals or snacks is another strategy to reduce urinary losses.

8) LOOK FOR "AMINO ACID CHELATES" TO ABSORB MINERALS MORE EFFECTIVELY. Minerals are more difficult to absorb than are vitamins. The "chelated" forms of minerals are more absorbable than other forms, because chelation means that the mineral has been bound to another molecule, often an amino acid, and "hitches a ride" across the intestinal wall along with the amino acid or other molecule. Not all minerals listed in a good multimineral supplement will be chelated, but at least the iron should be, as in this form it is less likely to destroy other nutrients. Health food shop brands of supplements are usually formulated with these considerations.

To give another particularly useful example, plain magnesium oxide can be quite laxative if it is not well absorbed. While some magnesium oxide is usually well tolerated, look for magnesium as a "chelate": magnesium aspartate, magnesium gluconate, or magnesium citrate. These forms are better absorbed and far less laxative than magnesium oxide alone. When it comes to calcium, calcium citrate is a highly absorbable form, as are calcium lactate, calcium gluconate, and calcium malate. Calcium carbonate, which is not a chelated form, is the least expensive form of calcium. However, it is not as absorbable as other forms of calcium.[12]

9) READ SUPPLEMENT LABELS CAREFULLY. Examine the list of vitamins and minerals, and then the actual amount of each. Ask for complete labels on prescription vitamins, especially typical prenatal vitamins, which are surprisingly low in potency. Pharmaceutical house multivitamins are closely tied to DVs and are generally less potent than the health food shop brands, so I suggest that you obtain as complete a multivitamin/multimineral supplement as possible from a health food shop. Even so, you will probably have to round out these supplements with additional folic acid, vitamins C and E, and magnesium, according to your particular health goals.

10) BECOME AWARE! Refer to the books listed in the "Further Reading" section to gain knowledge and confidence in the value and safety of supplements.

A NOTE ON VITAMIN BRANDS
For the convenience of the reader, this book recommends several brands of multivitamin/multiminerals: Optivite PMT and Androvite for Men, by Optimox Corp.; Professional Prenatal Formula, by LifeTime; and ProCycle PMS, by Women's Health America. Since the publication of the second edition of *Fertility, Cycles & Nutrition* in 1992, the Couple to Couple League has

recommended these because of their relative completeness, modest cost, and availability, and in particular the solid research behind Optivite and the similar ProCycle. In this edition we also recommend the proprietary herb/vitamin/mineral mix Fertility Blend, which contains the herb *Vitex agnus castus*. I have no financial interest at all in any of these, nor have I ever. Other brands with similar natural vitamins, chelated minerals, and potencies (amounts) may be equally helpful. In all cases, obtain the approval of your health care provider.

TABLE 7, BASIC SUPPLEMENTS TO CONSIDER

Vitamins	Daily amount	Comments
A (Retinyl palmitate)	5,000-20,000 IU	Use 8,000 IU maximum if pregnant or seeking pregnancy.[a]
B1	25-100 mg	
B2	25-100 mg	
B3 (Niacin)	25-100 mg	
B6 (Pyridoxine)	25-300 mg	Over 500 mg/day has been associated with neuropathy. Taking with other B vitamins and magnesium reduces potential for toxicity. Tested for safety during pregnancy. Seek nutritional counseling for amounts over 300 mg.[b]
Pantothenic acid	25-100 mg	
Choline	25-100 mg	
Inositol	25-100 mg	
Para-amino benzoic acid (PABA)	25-100 mg	
B12	25-2,000 mcg	Safe and recommended for pregnancy.[c]
Folic acid	400-4,000 mcg	Rarely, masks vitamin B12 deficiency; take B12 also. Safe and beneficial for pregnancy.[d]

a Rothman, K., and Moore, L. "Teratogenicity of high vitamin A intake" (*NEJM* 1995, 333:1369-1373). Beta-carotene, which is not pre-formed vitamin A, can be taken in amounts far higher than the guideline given here.

b Shrim, A., Boskovic, R., Maltepe, C., et al. "Pregnancy outcome following use of large doses of vitamin B6 in the first trimester" (*J. Obstet. Gynecol.* 2006, 26: 749-751); Guy Abraham, M.D., also reports this upper level safe and beneficial during pregnancy when used as part of a multivitamin/multi-mineral containing other B vitamins and magnesium: Beck, S., Abraham, G. "Optivite PMT and Gynovite Plus Total Dietary Programs for Premenstrual Syndrome and Menopause" (Optimox Corp., 1992, p. 27)

c Raffelock, D., Rountree, R., and Hopkins, V. *A Natural Guide to Pregnancy and Postpartum Health* (New York: Avery, 2002, p. 131). These authors recommend up to 5,000 mcg vitamin B12 per day.

Vitamins	Daily amount	Comments
C	1,000-3,000 mg	Chewing it may increase tooth decay.
D3 (Cholecalciferol)	400-1,000 IU	
E	400-800 IU	Prefer natural to synthetic.

Minerals	Daily amount	
Calcium	500-1,000 mg	Raises the need for magnesium.
Magnesium	500-1,000 mg	
Iron	0-30 mg	
Iodine	150 mcg	
Copper	2-3 mg	
Zinc	25-50 mg	
Manganese	10 mg	
Chromium	100-200 mcg	
Selenium	100-200 mcg	
Potassium	from diet	

Essential Fatty Acids	Daily amount	
Flax oil	5-10 1-g capsules (1-2 teaspoons)	Requires vitamin E.
Fish liver oil	5 1-g capsules (1 teaspoon)	Should be certified contaminant free. Optional if flax oil is supplemented. Requires vitamin E.

d Wilson, R. "Pre-conceptual vitamin/folic acid supplementation 2007: The use of folic acid in combination with a multivitamin supplement for the prevention of neural tube defects and other congenital anomalies" (Joint SOGC-Motherisk Clinical Practice Guideline, *JOGC*, Dec., 2007, 1003–1013); Goh, Y., and Koren, G. "Folic acid in pregnancy and fetal outcomes" (*J. Obstet. & Gynaecol.* 2008, 28:3–13) Folic acid supplementation in amounts up to 5,000 mcg is recommended to prevent neural tube defects. This amount does not mask vitamin B12 deficiency.

Summary — Chapter 3

➤ Vitamin, mineral, and essential fatty acid supplements help overcome nutrient deficiencies that may result from an individual's higher than average requirements. Some help to detoxify metabolic and environmental toxins. They also compensate for foods that are raised on depleted soils, bred for qualities other than high nutrition, cooked or otherwise processed. They help to overcome the effects of the widespread habits of poor nutrition, such as eating at fast food restaurants and drinking canned beverages. Studies show that vitamins and minerals can prevent or improve some diseases. Supplements can help you to achieve optimal health.

➤ Table 7 provides a plan for supplementing vitamins, minerals, and essential fatty acids. In order to supplement safely and effectively, the following guidelines should be used:

1) Proper diet is a higher health priority than supplementation.

2) Seek realistic nutritional counseling when you supplement.

3) Strive for balance when you supplement.

4) Always take supplements on a full stomach, preferably in divided doses with breakfast and lunch.

5) Begin taking supplements gradually.

6) Prefer natural vitamins to synthetic vitamins.

7) Use timed-release vitamins to help prevent loss of the supplement into the urine.

8) Look for "amino acid chelates" to absorb minerals more effectively.

9) Read supplement labels carefully.

10) Become aware! Refer to the books listed in the "Further Reading" section to gain knowledge and confidence in the value of supplements.

➤ This book recommends several brands of multivitamin/multimineral supplements: Optivite PMT, ProCycle PMS, Professional Prenatal Formula, Androvite for Men, and Fertility Blend.

4

Questions & Answers Part I:
Good Nutrition for Good Health

She was able to eat for a year, and he and her son as well; the jar of flour did not go empty, nor the jug of oil run dry. — 1 Kings 17:16

FOR ONE WEEK I TRIED INCREASING MY FAMILY'S WHOLE GRAINS BY SWITCHING TO OATMEAL FOR BREAKFAST INSTEAD OF OUR USUAL BOXED CEREALS. IT GAVE MY HUSBAND AND ME SUCH BAD GAS THAT I DO NOT THINK WE WILL EVER TRY IT AGAIN!

This situation can happen to anyone who tries to make a major dietary change. Your digestive tract is accustomed to one type of food, and suddenly, it has to deal with something far different. A gradual change is the right answer as you move from refined foods to whole foods. It may also help to add good-quality yogurt to your diet, since yogurt contains healthy bacteria which can replace the gas-producing bacteria now thriving in your intestines. Better yet, get a probiotic supplement from a health food shop. Such supplements contain millions of "friendly" bacteria to crowd out the bad ones in your intestines. Just follow the directions on the bottle. Pharmacies also carry natural remedies for gas, such as "Beano," a source of enzymes which are helpful in preventing gas from any plant food, not just beans. Many people eat oatmeal without gas problems, and chances are you can, too.

MILK AND MILK PRODUCTS JUST DO NOT AGREE WITH ME. WHAT SHOULD I DO FOR CALCIUM SINCE I AVOID MILK PRODUCTS?

It is not just the calcium; equally as important is the protein and natural fat in dairy products, especially if you are pregnant or breastfeeding. You can easily get calcium from supplement pills, but you must get your protein from your food. Each cup of milk or yogurt contains about 8 grams of protein, and an ounce of cheese contains about 7 grams. A three-ounce serving of lean meat or fish contains about 15 to 18 grams of protein. An egg contains about 6 grams of protein. A peanut butter sandwich made with two pieces of whole wheat bread and two tablespoons of peanut butter contains about 10 grams of protein. Therefore, a serving of meat or fish can replace the protein of two servings of dairy, or a large egg and a peanut butter sandwich can replace the protein of two servings of dairy food.

But back to calcium: The cole crops — cabbage, broccoli, cauliflower, brussels sprouts, and kohlrabi — and dark leafy greens are good sources of calcium, but it is still prudent to supplement calcium. Calcium supplements should also contain magnesium, preferably in an amount equal to or nearly equal to the calcium. Vitamin D, along with magnesium and dietary fat, is necessary to assist with the absorption and use of calcium. (See Table 7 for amounts.)

It is worth mentioning that there are two basic reasons for the statement that "milk just does not agree with me." You may be lactose intolerant, which means that you do not produce enough of the digestive enzyme that breaks down lactose (also called milk sugar). If that is the case, you can purchase tablets of lactase, the enzyme that you are lacking. Products such as "Lactaid" will do the job.

Milk allergies are the other likely possibility. A reaction to the protein in milk is not the same as lactose intolerance, and is best dealt with by avoiding milk to the extent that you need to. Or, if you are allergic to cows' milk but are not lactose intolerant, you may be able to use goats' milk instead. Some individuals who cannot tolerate pasteurized milk can enjoy raw milk, if they can obtain it.

I WOULD LIKE TO EAT MORE BEANS, SINCE THEY ARE A HEALTHY FOOD, BUT DO YOU HAVE ANY IDEAS HOW?

I bet you are eating more beans than you realize. Peanuts are actually a bean, so natural peanut butter qualifies. So do peas. Then there are chili beans, and beans in Mexican cuisine, baked beans, and lima beans. Though not beans, tree nuts are another important source of vegetable protein, so that snacking on all kinds of nuts is another way to emphasize vegetable protein. And one final point: if you are trying to eat more vegetable protein and less animal protein, if you are a typical American, you are likely eating animal protein far in excess of what you really need. Between milk, cheese, eggs, and meat, it is possible that just using moderation in the animal proteins will help get a healthy balance established between animal and plant proteins.

DO YOU RECOMMEND SOY FOODS FOR BETTER FERTILITY?

No, I do not. In the past I was never a fan of tofu, soy nuts, or soy milk, mainly because I am a proponent of a diet containing both plant and animal foods. I considered foods with soy protein to be primarily of interest to people who practice a vegetarian or vegan diet.

However, in the past several years, two changes have taken place. First, soy has grown immensely in popularity, its "isoflavones" touted as a source of weak estrogens for menopausal women looking for alternatives to artificial hormone replacement therapy. But second and more important, a number of studies now show that soy products such as soy milk and tofu have adverse physical effects. Soy foods are difficult to digest, and even contain enzymes that interfere with protein digestion. Unfermented soy foods contain an anti-thyroid factor that can interfere with healthy thyroid function, as discussed in Chapter 7, under the section "Low Thyroid Function." Poor thyroid function, which is not always recognized clinically, is a well-established and common cause of cycle irregularity and infertility. There are other concerns with soy foods, including their possible involvement with some types of breast cancer. If you are interested in a brief summary of these concerns, see nutritionist Ann Louise Gittleman's book, *Before the Change*, in which she explains why she no longer recommends unfermented soy foods. She does consider two servings per week of the fermented soy foods tempeh and miso to be acceptable.[1] Fertility researchers Jorge Chavarro, M.D. and Walter Willett, M.D., despite being generally favorable to plant-based protein sources, echo these concerns. They recommend that women limit soy foods to two to four servings per week.[2]

When it comes to men, a recent study of infertile men showed that soy foods lowered men's sperm concentrations, and the higher the intake of soy foods, the lower the sperm concentrations.[3] The isoflavones are the apparent culprits in this effect. Because of these concerns, I have placed soy foods and soy milk in Table 4, "Foods to Limit." "Limit" does not mean "avoid 100%"; for example, occasional eating of soy foods hidden in granola bars is not likely to affect you, unless you have an allergy to soy.

DOES THAT MEAN THAT I SHOULD AVOID THE SOY OIL IN MY SALAD DRESSINGS?

No, the cautions above involve whole soy products. Moreover, for many people soy oil in salad dressings is unfortunately the only source of the omega-3 essential fatty acids, particularly for those who do not supplement either flax oil or fish oil, as recommended in Chapter 3.

WHAT IS THE BEST WAY TO GET MORE OF THE BENEFICIAL OILS IN MY DIET?

Heating food oils damages their valuable fatty acids, so frying foods in oil is not the best way to increase your consumption of beneficial oils. When you do sauté fish or eggs, just use a little olive oil or canola oil and medium heat.

To use healthy oils without heating them, which is what you are probably asking about, here are some ideas: Mix olive oil into pasta after cooking to prevent it from sticking. Use a little olive oil over cooked vegetables. Add olive or unheated canola oil to commercial salad dressing — shake it up and pour it over your salad. Or make your own salad dressings, using the cookbooks recommended in Chapter 2. By the way, be sure to store your salad oils tightly capped in the refrigerator. They are damaged by light, heat, and oxygen. (The only exception to this is olive oil. In the refrigerator, it becomes too thick to pour, though it liquefies again at room temperature.)

Because the omega-3 essential fatty acid alpha-linolenic acid is not abundant in the above-mentioned oils, taking supplements of flax oil and/or fish oil in capsules is a health practice that I recommend strongly. Keep in mind also that vitamin E is an antioxidant that helps protect the fat-soluble nutrients in the body's cells. It should be part of your daily vitamin supplement.

I AM OVERWHELMED WHEN I THINK OF GIVING UP FOODS WITH CAFFEINE AND SUGAR. I DON'T REALLY KNOW WHERE TO START.

Do not plan on giving them up; instead, plan on cutting down on them. A really good idea is to promise yourself that you will have them only after a full meal, or only after a nutritious, protein-rich snack followed by a big glass of cold water. This will almost automatically reduce the amount of these that you eat or drink, and it will also limit the swings in blood sugar that create the craving for more. And do not underestimate the value of a salad with salad dressing, a handful of nuts, or a hard-boiled egg in satisfying your appetite and reducing sugar cravings. In fact, the late Dr. Robert Atkins, in addressing this very issue, wrote that while many people can binge on sugary foods, such as eating thirty cookies, who has ever binged on ten hard-boiled eggs? His point was that proteins and fats (such as are in hard-boiled eggs) are just too filling.[4]

Keeping sweets out of sight or even out of the house or workplace is a great help, and limiting what you do eat to small portions is another strategy. Let's face it — most of us have a compulsion to finish the piece of food we start eating, so picking up one bite-sized piece of candy is better than trying to eat only one bite of a full-size candy bar.

Another way of dealing with sugar cravings is to use raw fruit to satisfy it. Along with the fruit sugar, you will get fiber and many other nutrients. Just be careful that you do not overdo it, such as eating a large bunch of very sweet grapes on an empty stomach. But you can eat quite a few strawberries or blueberries or a large apple without defeating your purpose, as these do not contain as much sugar.

For variety, try dark chocolate-covered almonds, peanuts, or cashews. They are crunchy, and also contain protein and natural fat, and so are very filling. The slight bitterness of dark chocolate is reminiscent of coffee — and there is a little caffeine lift in it, too.

If it is "sugar water" you crave, meaning soda pop, why not go cold turkey, substituting unsweetened iced tea or ice water? Yes, it is breaking one habit and replacing it with a new one, but the fruit or dark chocolate-covered nuts just mentioned can really help out. Dissolved sugar, as is in pop and sweetened juices, is the worst offender when it comes to blood sugar swings.

I certainly consider eating a good diet a higher nutritional goal than taking supplements, but in this case I think starting general supplements a week or two before you begin to break your sugar and caffeine habit will make it easier to change. This is true because certain micronutrients, notably the B vitamins and minerals, tend to regulate blood glucose levels. "Hypoglycemia" in Chapter 5 mentions specific nutrients which may help to reduce these cravings by improving blood glucose control. See also "Yeast Overgrowth" in Chapter 9, since intense sugar cravings may relate to yeast problems.

IS NUTRASWEET A SAFE SUBSTITUTE FOR SUGAR?

NutraSweet (aspartame) has caused a variety of adverse reactions in some individuals. Headaches, seizures, visual disturbances, dizziness, fatigue, depression, confusion, and memory loss are among the most common complaints. Dry mouth and intense thirst, creating a craving for more, is another common report. Women have reported heavy or scant menses and worsened PMS while using aspartame-containing products. These reproductive disturbances may occur because phenylalanine, which comprises about 50 percent of the aspartame molecule, stimulates the secretion of prolactin from the pituitary gland. Excess prolactin secretion is well known to affect the fertility-menstrual cycle.[5]

H.J. Roberts, M.D., a distinguished physician from Florida, published an extensively referenced book documenting these and many other less common reactions. *Aspartame (NutraSweet): Is It Safe?* explodes the general belief that NutraSweet has been thoroughly tested and found safe. He points out that one of aspartame's breakdown products is the poisonous methyl alcohol. He urges pregnant and breastfeeding women to completely avoid it, and urges parents to prohibit their children from using it — no small challenge, as this strange chemical is available in thousands of products. Skeptics would do well to read and heed Dr. Roberts' book. (See "Further Reading.")

WHAT ABOUT OTHER SWEETENERS?

If you are planning to frequently use the new substitutes for sugar, my advice is short — don't. Small amounts may be acceptable, but how much can you get away with and still have optimum health? If you are only going to use a little, such as an occasional sweet drink, sweeten it with sugar or honey. Nutritionist Ann Louise Gittleman's *Get the Sugar Out!* explains the problems with the various artificial sweeteners, including aspartame (NutraSweet, Equal, Canderol) and the very similar sucralose (Splenda). She does recommend stevia, which is a sweet herb that can be used to sweeten drinks or foods.[6]

I AM CONCERNED ABOUT THE MERCURY AND OTHER CONTAMINANTS IN FISH, AS I AM HOPING TO BECOME PREGNANT.

The benefits of fish far outweigh the possible mercury issues. For example, a large study showed that pregnant women who consumed very little fish had a higher risk of their children having developmental problems compared to the children of women who ate more than the amount recommended by the government while they were pregnant. In effect, the study showed that the risk from the loss of the nutrients in fish (among them protein and DHA), was greater than the risk of harm from exposure to traces of contaminants.[7]

However, I recommend that you have it both ways — eat fish with the least contamination. The guidelines change, so check the website of the Natural Resources Defense Council: *nrdc.org/health/effects/mercury/guide.asp*. Fish that my family enjoys include whitefish, whiting, and perch, which as of this writing are on the "least mercury" list. Canned chunk tuna, which we use once a month or so, is on the "moderate" list, to be eaten fewer than six times per month.

I'M SO FRUSTRATED BY EVERYTHING I READ: IF IT'S MILK, IT'S GOT HORMONES. IF IT'S FISH, IT'S FULL OF MERCURY. IF IT'S EGGS, IT'S CHOLESTEROL. IF IT'S FRUIT, IT'S TOO SUGARY. OR IF IT'S NOT TOO SUGARY, IT'S BEEN SPRAYED. I EVEN READ THAT POTATOES PRODUCE MORE "SUGAR SHOCK" THAN CANDY.

Whoa! Don't let this kind of perfectionism discourage you from getting started with better nutrition. It is better to improve your diet to the extent you can than to skip the nutritious whole foods you mentioned because of these kinds of concerns. You may wish to reread Chapter 2, "Obtaining & Preparing Nutritious Food," which addresses at least some of your concerns. Taking vitamins, as recommended in Chapter 3, helps the body to compensate for the various inadequacies of the food we eat.

Rule 6 from Chapter 1, "Eat a greater variety of foods," is particularly helpful if you are concerned about unwanted additives or toxins that may be in foods that you buy. Not only will you get more vitamins and minerals, but you will also limit your exposure to what you are trying to avoid. How much variety? The late, great nutritionist, Adelle Davis, who wrote in the 1950s, suggested in her book *Let's Cook It Right*, that a homemaker should have thirty different menus for dinner.[8] You can see how following that old guideline would keep your consumption of tuna fish, for example, well within the recommended limits of safety discussed above.

Actually, eggs are back on the healthy list, after several years of caution because of the high cholesterol content of their yolks. And while it is true that a plain cooked potato, by itself, really does increase blood glucose levels rapidly, who eats one all by itself? You have it as a side dish with meat, usually with butter, gravy, sour cream, or a cheese sauce. Protein and fatty foods significantly slow down the release of glucose from a food like a potato or a sweet fruit. Potatoes are also a good source of potassium, vitamin C, and iron. Fruits are much more likely to be eaten alone on an empty stomach, which is why it is worth reminding you that it is better to eat them with other foods, preferably protein or fatty foods.

WHAT IS MILLET? HOW DO I USE IT?

Millet is an exceptionally nutritious, fiber-rich grain that is an excellent source of B vitamins and magnesium. It is a staple in many parts of the world. You may recognize it as bird seed — those round, little yellow seeds that many bird feeds feature. It cooks exactly like rice, only faster (one cup of grain to two cups of water or so, bring to a boil, cover, simmer for about twenty minutes), and can be used in any recipe that calls for rice. Its flavor is mildly reminiscent of lima beans, but like rice, you eat it with a sauce. It is good with Chinese dishes or as chicken and "rice."

MY FOOD BUDGET IS STRETCHED TO THE LIMIT. ANY SUGGESTIONS ON WAYS TO CHANGE TO ALL THE GOOD FOOD YOU RECOMMEND WITHOUT INCREASING WHAT I AM ALREADY SPENDING?

Using food dollars prudently is a growing issue for everyone, not just those on the tightest budgets. I think everyone agrees that fast food is more expensive than basic home-cooked meals, especially if you factor in the soft drinks. In the supermarket, substituting basic whole food that you prepare at home instead of prepackaged items will definitely save you a few dollars. It is the fresh produce that increases your food bill the most as you try to eat more fresh fruits and vegetables.

Here are some ideas to help you make those dollars cover everything they should. First, the cheapest sources of protein are beans, eggs, milk, and chicken. Whole milk is a better buy than skim milk. In my hometown independent grocery store, even hormone- and antibiotic-free chicken is sold, usually on Mondays, at a reduced price, along with "reduced for quick sale" red meat. Might there be a store like that near you? Do you have room in your freezer if you find some really good buys?

Whole grain pasta is not much more expensive than the white variety, and tomato sauce to make your own meat sauce is another inexpensive, nutritious item. Brown rice is wonderfully nutritious. Look for a breadmaker on sale after Christmas, and then make your own bread.

Potatoes, onions, and cabbage are very good buys in the produce department, and usually other seasonal items are on sale. Meanwhile, your own garden can help out in a big way, especially if you freeze your beans, peas, broccoli, and sweet corn. Your local farmers' market is another place to find bargains, particularly at the very end of the day or of the week.

Unhealthy junk food is a major waste of food dollars. Instead, indulge in the family fun of making treats in your own kitchen. Peanut butter or oatmeal cookies, no-bake cookies, tapioca pudding made with plenty of eggs, homemade ice cream, or buttered popcorn are examples that give families entertainment as well as a treat!

Make a conscious effort to cut down on food waste to save dollars. Do not let that lettuce or celery in your vegetable crisper go bad. Put leftovers right up on the top refrigerator shelf where you will see them immediately, and use them for breakfast or lunch the next day. Make French toast with day-old homemade bread, or make smaller loaves if you consistently have leftover bread. If it is something that is not the best as leftovers, such as fish fillets, ask your family members how many they would like before you start defrosting.

A freezer will save you many food dollars, so be sure to have a signal light or some other means of being alerted in case it ever loses power.

Finally, here is a website that is made for nutritionally-oriented homemakers who are on a tight budget: *www.savingdinner.com* (click on "Frugal").

I DON'T THINK I CAN AFFORD SUPPLEMENTS. ANY THOUGHTS ABOUT THEIR EXPENSE?

Comprehensive multivitamin/multimineral supplements are more costly than one-a-day-type vitamins. I personally feel that "time is money"; that is, the extra productive time I have because of the added energy they give me is well worth the monetary investment. But I took this question to a friend of mine, a divorced mother of three young children who works only part-time for their sake. She is on the tightest budget of anyone I know, but she always serves holistic food to her family. She replied:

"I buy health food store vitamins before I buy anything else. It is my highest priority for off-budget items. I can't afford to be sick, or miss work, or miss school. My kids and I hardly ever get sick any more. I would be sick four or so times a year with the flu before I took vitamins."

As the admen say, good nutrition doesn't cost, it pays. For many people, insurance and paid sick leave mask the true financial cost of poor nutrition.

WOULD YOU PLEASE EXPLAIN THE DIFFERENCE BETWEEN FLAX OIL AND FISH OIL? SHOULD I CHOOSE ONE OR THE OTHER, OR CAN I TAKE BOTH?

The analogy I use to explain how they are alike and how they differ is this: Imagine that cake is essential to your body. There are two ways that you can get cake, because you cannot "make it from scratch." First, you can get a whole cake at a bakery. Or, you can get a cake mix and add water and butter and eggs. Then you can make the cake yourself. Fish oil, which contains the fatty acids EPA and DHA, is the whole cake; that is, it contains the finished products. EPA and DHA are long, highly unsaturated fatty acids that our cells use for a number of vital processes. Flax oil is the cake mix. It contains an abundant amount of the hard-to-get alpha-linolenic acid, the "omega-3" essential fatty acid. If B vitamins and minerals (the water, butter, and eggs of the analogy) are available, the cells are able to convert alpha-linolenic acid into DHA and EPA.

Besides the pre-made DHA and EPA, cod liver oil (but not all fish oils) contains modest amounts of vitamins A and D. It is available purified of contaminants, and in lemon or other flavors. It is very valuable! In addition to the hard-to-get alpha-linolenic acid, convertible to EPA and DHA, flax oil contains phytonutrients called lignans, which are weak estrogens that, at least in males, act as anti-estrogens. In women they may block the function of stronger estrogens, a beneficial function.

My experience in counseling the use of flax oil has been very positive in virtually every aspect of female reproductive health, whether it is in overcoming infertility of unknown cause, lightening heavy menstrual periods, or reducing hot flashes or vaginal dryness. On the other hand, fish oil is still better studied, and I particularly recommend it to pregnant and nursing mothers.

Which one should you choose? Because of my counseling experience, I have a preference for flax oil over fish oil, but taking both is also an excellent practice. A teaspoon or two of flax oil (5-10 grams or five to ten 1 g capsules) and one teaspoon of fish oil (5 grams) are just fine if you want to get the overlapping benefits of both. Just be sure to take vitamin E also, about 400 IU daily, as these unsaturated nutrients are vulnerable to oxidation, and vitamin E is a major antioxidant.

I STARTED TAKING FLAX OIL, AND I THINK IT HELPED ME GET PREGNANT AFTER IRREGULAR CYCLES AND INFERTILITY. BUT IT GAVE ME A RASH AROUND THE CORNERS OF MY MOUTH. I WOULD LIKE TO KEEP TAKING IT, BUT IS THERE ANY SUBSTITUTE FOR IT THAT I MIGHT NOT BE ALLERGIC TO?

Yes, you can get pumpkin seed oil at health food shops. It has alpha-linolenic acid, though not in the same high amount as in flax oil. You will need more capsules to get the same amount of the alpha-linolenic acid. Ask the shopkeeper for a comparison of their brand of pumpkin seed oil with flax oil. Another possibility is fish oil capsules or oil. Just make sure it is certified contaminant free, and use about 1 teaspoon (5 capsules) daily.

VITAMINS UPSET MY STOMACH. DO YOU HAVE ANY SUGGESTIONS?

This is one of the most common reasons why people do not take vitamins. First, always take vitamins with a meal, and start very gradually with the lowest dose. Some people find that freezing their vitamins makes them go down more easily with less stomach upset. This may just help you to swallow the pills, or it may delay the dissolving of the vitamin long enough to make a difference.

But let's also consider why you have a sensitive stomach. Some people get upset stomachs because they have excess stomach acid, but others actually get upset stomachs because they do not produce enough acid to begin digesting their food. A little self-help trial to see which might explain your digestive upsets is to try the following: squeeze a fresh lemon into a glass of water, and have a few sips of it with food that causes your stomach to be upset. If it makes your stomach feel worse, you may be producing too much acid. There are many over-the-counter remedies for acid stomach. If, to your surprise, it makes you feel better, or does not bother you, it may be that you do not produce enough acid to activate digestive enzymes in your stomach. The acidic lemon juice may be helping out, so try having lemon juice in water with your meals. Some people with sensitive stomachs are also helped by digestive enzymes which can be purchased at health food shops.

EVER SINCE I STARTED TAKING VITAMINS, MINERALS, AND FISH OIL, I HAVE BEEN DREAMING VIVIDLY PRACTICALLY EVERY NIGHT. IS THIS A COINCIDENCE?

It is a sign of good mental function to remember dreams, and vitamin B6 and fish oil are probably the two nutrients that promote dreaming the most, though other B vitamins might be involved. If you do not care to "spend the night at the movies," as my husband puts it, take those supplements first thing in the morning. Cut down on the amount that you take if that does not work.

WHAT KIND OF VITAMINS SHOULD YOUNG CHILDREN TAKE?

My opinion is that nursing babies and toddlers are fine with the vitamins they get through their mother's milk, assuming she uses supplements, including fish oil and/or flax oil. (The quality of the mother's milk is improved by such supplements.) For older children, health food shops have chewable vitamins, and vitamin C is especially helpful for their immune systems. However, make sure that your children brush their teeth immediately after taking chewable vitamin C, since it can promote tooth decay if left on the teeth. Avoid vitamins with food colorings in them.

I have my youngest children take a half-teaspoon or a bit more of lemon-flavored cod liver oil daily to give them the EPA and DHA that are so important to their immune systems and brain function. They do not have a problem with the taste, as it really is very mild tasting, and we started it at around two years of age. It is now easy to purchase contaminant-free fish oil at health food shops, so look for this on the label. Our youngest child, who is adopted and was never breastfed, received a little fish oil daily in one of her bottles. It also helped with the problem of constipation, which is common in bottle-fed babies.

Dr. Julian Whitaker, founder of the Whitaker Wellness Institute in Newport Beach, California, recommends chewable vitamin pills for children beginning around age four. He suggests that the supplements include 125-250 mg of vitamin C, 25-50 IU of vitamin E, 2,000-4,000 IU of A and beta-carotene, 10-20 mcg selenium, 50-100 mg calcium, 200-400 IU vitamin D, 200-400 mcg folic acid, 5-10 mg B6, and 50-100 mg B12. He additionally recommends supplemental DHA from fish oil.[9]

Once girls and boys are over 100 pounds, you can consider giving them an adult dose of a multivitamin/multimineral, or at least nearly an adult dose.

I HAVE FOUR SMALL CHILDREN, AND EVEN THOUGH THEY ARE GOOD KIDS, I FEEL CONSTANTLY "STRESSED OUT" BY THE SHEER AMOUNT OF WORK AROUND THE HOUSE. CAN NUTRITION MAKE A DIFFERENCE?

The well-nourished person can perform a tremendous amount of work, day in and day out, without reaching "wit's end." Cutting down on caffeine is the first step because it contributes to that anxious feeling. The mineral magnesium is probably the most noticeably nerve-calming nutrient, followed by the

B vitamins, especially B6, vitamin C, zinc, and flax oil. Calcium supplemented without magnesium may cause nervousness and anxiety in some people, so be sure to supplement calcium with equal or almost equal amounts of magnesium. The nutritional strategies for keeping blood sugar up help to give you the energy to tackle the day's activities — see Rule 7 in Chapter 1 and the discussion of hypoglycemia in Chapter 5. Vitamin E may also boost your energy.

I know that many people would suggest that you hire household help for this common problem, but the price of one morning's help can buy you a month's supply of vitamins. I would choose the latter without hesitation, though I do not intend to diminish the role of diet, exercise, and adequate rest. The physical stress of multiple pregnancies, nursing, being on your feet constantly, and being "on-call" 24 hours a day — it is incomprehensible to me that anyone would advise women like you (or me) that they can function well without serious attention to the best nutritional support they can get.

ARE YOU IMPLYING THAT EVERYONE OUGHT TO TAKE VITAMINS IN THE AMOUNTS YOU SUGGEST IN TABLE 7?

No. If you are completely satisfied with your health, your energy level, and your mental outlook, and you eat as healthfully as you reasonably can, you very likely do not need more than a one-a-day vitamin/mineral supplement. My observation is that young adult men form the largest group in this category. This may explain why some women tell me that their husbands fail to understand the relationship between fatigue, moodiness, and nutrition — they simply have never experienced it.

Whether or not to take vitamins should not be an all-or-none decision. For example, those who are reasonably satisfied with their health, energy level, and moods may want to take a middle road by supplementing vitamins, minerals, and essential fatty acids at a low level as an "insurance policy." Others who have improved their health through diet and supplements may be able to maintain their good health through excellent diet and perhaps a low level of supplementation. In other words, taking food supplements (or not taking them) should relate to your perceived need, which changes with age, illness, pregnancy, stress level, and diet.

There are many good multivitamins available through health food shops and other outlets, and in the following sections of this book I mention four by name: Optivite, Androvite, ProCycle, and Professional Prenatal Formula. One of the reasons I recommend these is that the full dose for each is four to six tablets per day. This gives the users a great deal of flexibility in finding their own middle ground between high levels of supplements and none at all.

I AM TRYING TO IMPROVE MY OVERALL HEALTH, NOT JUST MY CYCLES. ANY OTHER SUGGESTIONS BESIDES BETTER NUTRITION, WHICH I AM ALREADY TRYING? I ALREADY GET SOME EXERCISE EVERY DAY.

Yes — get enough sleep! This is so very important, but I think it is neglected because it does not take a whole book or a medical expert to explain it. It is all too easy to cheat yourself out of an hour or two of sleep at night because you are too busy and caffeine seems to make up the sleep deficit. However, it makes a terrific difference to how you feel, to your sense of well-being, to your energy, and to your stress level. Yes, you may be able to "get by" on six hours of sleep a night, but you should aim for what makes you feel energetic and rested all day long. For many women, that is eight or possibly even nine hours, especially if you are wakened at night by child care, a full bladder, or other disturbances to your sleep. If you are pregnant or breastfeeding, a nap in addition to eight or nine hours at night may be just what you need to feel great. If you need more motivation than feeling energetic and rested to make yourself get enough sleep, consider this: inadequate sleep is associated with weight gain in women, and on average, the less women sleep, the more weight they gain.[10]

I am convinced that many women do not recognize their own symptoms of chronic sleep deprivation because it is so much a part of their lives. I think many just consider themselves as having low energy, or being stressed or irritable by temperament, when lack of sleep is actually the underlying cause of these symptoms.

Here are some ideas to help you get the sleep you need: First, acknowledge that you need enough sleep, probably eight hours a night, and perhaps more. Next, consider how you can get it. Can you wake up later in the morning? Take a morning, afternoon, or early evening nap? Go to bed earlier? What can you cut out or delegate to make more time for sleep?

You will feel better, think better, look better, and enjoy life more if you go through it in a rested state. You will be more cheerful. You will manage stress better. Your immune system will work better. And you will be more productive if you spend the time you need sleeping, because it will increase your energy and mental focus during your waking time.

What if you have trouble falling asleep? Caffeine, vitamin pills, and sweets before bedtime can be stimulating. Do not take them any later than early afternoon if you have difficulty sleeping. Skip anxiety-producing news or scary movies before you go to bed. Try to go to bed and get up at more or less regular times. Make sure your bed is firm enough or soft enough. Making sure that your room is warm enough or cool enough is another consideration. Working on improving factors like these can improve your sleep quality, but there is simply no substitute for the quantity that you need to protect your health and feel your best.

Keep your room very dark — even pitch black if necessary — if you have trouble falling asleep or sleeping well. Why? When the lights go out, the hormone melatonin is released from the pineal gland, which is buried deep in the brain. Conversely, when the lights go on, the pineal gland receives the message from your eyes, and your melatonin output drops. This interesting hormone is a natural sleep aid, but even dim light can reduce its production, more in women than in men. You make less melatonin as you age, and it drops quite a bit during premenopause. This means a very dark room may become more important to your sleep quality as you grow older. Consider room-darkening blinds and clocks without lighted displays. This topic is developed further in Chapter 9 under the heading "Sensitivity to Night Lighting."

Julian Whitaker, M.D., recommends 500 mcg (0.5 mg) to 3 mg of melatonin about 30 to 60 minutes before bedtime for those who need a natural sleep aid.[11] If you decide to try this, start with the lower amount, and work up if you need more. Too much may make you feel sluggish. Melatonin, which is available over the counter at health food shops, is a potent antioxidant and may even have a protective role against cancer. Nevertheless, if you may become pregnant, obtain your doctor's approval before trying it. Do not use it if you are breastfeeding.[12]

The most practical advice that I have seen for getting enough sleep is a whole chapter devoted to this topic in *The Schwarzbein Principle II*, by Diana Schwarzbein, M.D., an endocrinologist who has written a nutritionally-oriented book which focuses on overcoming the effects of stress and poor diet. (See "Further Reading.")

Women's health advocate and author Virginia Hopkins, though, says it best: "Take your vitamin ZZZ's!"[13]

Part II:

Overcoming Reproductive Problems & Challenges

INTRODUCTION TO PART II

As the title implies, the main purpose of this book is to offer suggestions on how to assist the natural fertility processes to function normally through better nutrition. Therefore, Part II truly forms the core of this book. However, please keep three things in mind as you review the nutritional information that follows in the next twelve chapters.

First, a nutritious diet as described in Part I is always a higher priority than taking supplements for good nutrition. Second, when you look up a particular cycle problem, often only a small number of vitamin or mineral supplements are listed as potentially helpful. While these should be stressed, all of the vitamins, minerals, and essential fatty acids listed in Table 7 should be taken together to prevent imbalances as you supplement. Where a range of doses is given in Table 7, you can use the higher levels for micronutrients that are listed as helpful to your situation, but take lower levels of the others.

Finally, I mean it sincerely when I say that the suggestions that follow on these pages are not meant to replace the counsel of your health care provider. Nutrition and professional health care are by no means mutually exclusive, and more and more doctors and other health professionals are deeply interested in the value of a good diet and nutritional supplements. A doctor's ability to diagnose, treat, and advise are great blessings. However, once a diagnosis is made, healing through nutrition should ordinarily be considered the *first* resort. If intervention through drugs or surgery becomes necessary, the value of excellent nutrition is even greater.

FEMALE REPRODUCTIVE BASICS

Whether you are reading this book to have more regular cycles, to overcome infertility, or to reduce your chance of a miscarriage, reviewing the basic events of the menstrual cycle will increase your understanding of how, why, and where nutrition can make a difference. What follows is a simplified summary of those events and their causes. I especially encourage you to read the section entitled "Maturation of the ovum," which contains information that is unfamiliar to many women. The vocabulary in bold here will also be used in the chapters of Part II.

PRE-OVULATION PHASE. During the first part of the menstrual cycle, as the menstrual flow is ending, the pituitary gland at the base of the brain secretes **follicle stimulating hormone (FSH)**. FSH stimulates a **follicle** (a small sac of cells containing an unfertilized ovum) in one of the two ovaries to begin to mature. As the follicle develops, it grows larger and secretes increasing amounts of estrogen. Estrogen causes the inner lining of the uterus, the **endometrium**, to thicken in preparation for a possible pregnancy. Estrogen also causes the cervix of the uterus to secrete a mucus discharge which is necessary for normal fertility and sperm migration. Depending on the quality of the mucus, natural family planning (NFP) providers refer to it as "less fertile" or "more fertile"; if it is absent the term "dry" is used.

OVULATION. When estrogen from the enlarging follicle rises to a critical point, it stimulates the pituitary gland to increase the secretion of a second hormone, **luteinizing hormone (LH)**. LH then stimulates more estrogen, and estrogen stimulates more LH, and therefore both hormones rise steeply for approximately two days. The spike of LH, called the LH surge, triggers ovulation. **Ovulation**, of course, is the release of the ovum from the follicle. That unfertilized ovum will be picked up by tiny "fingers" on the end of the fallopian tube, and microscopic hairs in the wall of the tube will move the ovum slowly toward the uterus. It will live only eight to twenty-four hours if it is not fertilized. After that, it will die, and it is so very tiny that no remains of it will be observed. If conception is to occur, the ovum must be fertilized within those eight to twenty-four hours, an event that happens in the outer one third of the fallopian tube. Sperm must be able to swim "upstream" in order to fertilize the ovum.

POST-OVULATION PHASE. After ovulation, whether or not conception has occurred, the empty follicle gets a new look and a new name. It becomes yellowish and is called the **corpus luteum**, Latin for "yellow body." It secretes estrogen and especially progesterone, which prepares the endometrium for possible implantation of a newly conceived child.

Progesterone additionally causes the early, waking, "basal" temperature to rise slightly, a sign that can be observed and recorded on the NFP chart. The presence of progesterone, combined with decreased estrogen levels, also causes a distinctive change in the cervical mucus discharge. After about two weeks, if pregnancy has not occurred, the corpus luteum stops secreting progesterone, and the drop in this hormone causes the inner lining of the uterus to be shed in the process of menstruation.

Keep the term "corpus luteum" in mind because it is used frequently in scientific discussion of the fertility cycle. The post-ovulatory phase of the cycle is called the **luteal phase**, and inadequacy of the corpus luteum's ability to secrete progesterone is called **luteal phase deficiency**. It is useful to realize that what happens before ovulation, during the pre-ovulatory phase, sets the stage for the post-ovulatory time of the cycle. For example, if the follicle fails to develop properly before ovulation, it will become an inadequate corpus luteum after ovulation, and the result will be luteal phase deficiency.

The understanding of the normal fertility-menstrual cycle is at the heart of NFP. Women who chart their mucus and temperature signs gain an extremely accurate awareness of where they are in their fertility cycles, and the benefits of this extend well beyond family planning. For example, if a woman is troubled by PMS, which is associated with the luteal phase, she will know from her fertility observations exactly when to expect such symptoms. Or, if a woman's thyroid function is low, her basal temperature will be abnormally low, even if blood tests fail to reveal it. If she is not ovulating, she will know, because she will not see the post-ovulatory temperature rise, even if she still has menstrual bleeding. (Such "cycles" without ovulation are called **anovulatory cycles**.) If her luteal phase is abnormally short she will easily see it on her chart, and will recognize it as luteal phase deficiency.

MATURATION OF THE OVUM. While many women find that much of the above information is simply a review, I know from years of NFP consulting that most women are not aware of the critical events that occur within the unfertilized ovum during the *two days* before ovulation. Considering what follows will give you a better understanding of certain types of infertility, certain types of miscarriage, and certain types of birth defects, notably Down syndrome.

At ovulation, the unfertilized ovum contains only half as much genetic information as most other body cells. It is said to be haploid. In the human, that means it contains only 23 single chromosomes, whereas most other body cells contain 46 chromosomes in 23 pairs, and are called diploid cells. This is by design. When a haploid ovum is fertilized by a sperm, which is also haploid, the newly conceived human being has 46 chromosomes, and will begin to develop.

However, the millions of ova (plural of ovum) which develop in the ovaries of a baby girl long before she is born are all diploid cells, with 46 chromosomes! These diploid ova must become haploid cells before fertilization can occur. The time line for a diploid ovum to become a haploid ovum is one of the most remarkable physiological sequences in the human body. The process involves cell division by the diploid ova, and for reasons beyond the scope of this discussion, this cell division occurs in two separate events, called meiosis I and meiosis II. **Meiosis I**, called "reduction division," is the critical cell division that actually reduces the ovum from its diploid state (46 chromosomes) to its haploid state of 23 chromosomes.

Long before a baby girl is born, her ova begin meiosis I, but they are arrested in it. That is, the process is begun but is not completed. Once puberty occurs, usually only one ovum per cycle, within the developing follicle, will complete the all-important meiosis I. Amazingly, it does so during the two days just before ovulation. Truly a last-minute preparation for the big date!

Why is this so vital? If meiosis I occurs normally, normal fertilization is likely. If, however, the cell division is faulty, the unfertilized ovum will not end up with exactly 23 chromosomes. If this occurs, the ovum is genetically imperfect. It may not be able to be fertilized at all, so that pregnancy cannot occur.

In some cases such an ovum can be fertilized, but because of missing or extra chromosomes, development of the newly conceived child cannot proceed normally. The tiny child dies within a few days or weeks in what is sometimes called, unfortunately, a "blighted ovum" or "empty sac" pregnancy. Sometimes it is simply called an "early miscarriage," and is said to be caused by a "random genetic error." Despite the terminology, it is the loss of a child and often a great sorrow to the parents.

Very occasionally, when meiosis I occurs abnormally during those two days before ovulation, the result is an unfertilized ovum with two number 21 chromosomes. Should this ovum be fertilized by a normal sperm, the newly conceived child will have three number 21 chromosomes. This condition is Down syndrome, or trisomy 21, and unlike other similar genetic errors, it is mild enough that the baby, with extra love and care, can usually survive and grow and live to adulthood, despite some mental and physical disabilities.

What does it take for that ovum to complete meiosis I correctly? Answering that question has many implications. If the ovum can complete meiosis I properly during the two days before ovulation, infertility of certain types will decrease. Early miscarriage without development of the child will decrease, and even the incidence of Down syndrome might also decrease.

It is known that the hormones FSH and LH stimulate the ovum to complete meiosis I. It is also known that folic acid, vitamin B12, and zinc are involved in cell division. So are other B vitamins, notably vitamin B6, and the mineral magnesium, and the essential fatty acids. Vitamin C is necessary for folic acid function. As the ova age within a woman's body, infertility, miscarriage, and the incidence of Down syndrome all increase. The ova are older, and may not complete meiosis I as well as younger ones did. Still, providing them with all of the micronutrients that they need to undergo their cell division before ovulation occurs is the most fruitful way to overcome infertility and miscarriage related to the quality of the ova. Table 7 in Chapter 3 provides recommended amounts of these nutrients, and more specific information is provided in Chapter 9, under the heading "Age-Related Infertility."

MALE REPRODUCTIVE BASICS

Unlike the woman's, a man's reproductive cells — the sperm — are produced in abundance beginning at puberty and continuing well into old age. This process occurs in the walls of the seminiferous tubules, which are the microscopic tubes coiled within each testis. There the sperm begin to form after meiosis of the precursor cells.

SPERM PRODUCTION. Meiosis, the special cell division that only ovum and sperm can undergo, makes the sperm haploid (23 chromosomes in the human). Sperm lose cellular material so that their heads contain little more than the nucleus with its genetic material. The tip of the head forms an **acrosome**, which contains enzymes capable of digesting the covering material that surrounds an ovulated ovum. They develop a tail. They are the only self-propelled cells in the human species, and their ability to deliver their genetic material to the ovum depends on the whipping movement of their tails. Between the head and tail, a flexible midpiece contains tiny energy-producing units, the mitochondria.

Sperm production, though occurring at a very rapid pace in terms of numbers — perhaps one hundred million per day — is not particularly fast for each individual sperm. It takes two months for the sperm to develop from start to finish. Part of this time is spent outside the testes, in a coiled tube atop each testis called the **epididymis**. Both the testes and the epididymides (plural) must have a temperature lower than the core temperature of the body, or sperm production will not take place.

From the epididymis, the sperm enter the vas deferens, which is the thin, muscular tube that enables the sperm to enter the pelvis. Immediately prior to ejaculation, the sperm are pushed through the vas deferens. Each vas deferens enters the prostate gland, where it empties into the urethra. Three large glands, the two **seminal vesicles** and the **prostate gland**, secrete fluids into the urethra, forming the majority of the semen.

Both the production of sperm and the production of the hormone testosterone by the testes are stimulated by the hormones FSH and LH, the same hormones found in women. As you would probably guess, they do not have a cyclic pattern of secretion as they do in women.

FERTILIZATION. Released into the female reproductive tract, the vast majority of the sperm cells soon die. Only a small minority are able to swim up into the fallopian tube. If an ovulated ovum is present, many sperm bury their heads into it; it is many times larger than the sperm cells. Together their acrosomes release enough enzymes to digest the covering. One sperm penetrates the ovum, and its nucleus soon fuses with the nucleus of the ovum. Conception, or fertilization, has occurred, and the newly conceived human being has all the genetic information it will ever have.

SPERM NUTRIENT NEEDS. Sperm need many nutrients to function efficiently. They require folic acid, zinc, vitamin B_{12}, and a number of other nutrients in order to provide for the constant, ongoing meiosis. They use B vitamins to generate energy. Selenium is necessary for the function of the midpiece. Vitamin C and E are essential antioxidants. Because of their small amount of cellular material, they are not able to neutralize the byproducts of their energy use efficiently, and so they must rely on other antioxidants. The cell membrane and the acrosome must be relatively fluid, not stiff, so that the sperm can fuse to the ovum during conception. This requires, among other nutrients, the two essential fatty acids. Meeting the nutritional needs of sperm production is the focus of overcoming male infertility.

SUMMARY. The reproductive cells of both sexes require a number of micronutrients to undergo their cell division, and especially in the case of the sperm, to produce energy and neutralize cellular wastes. Providing the body with these nutrients is the most fruitful self-care method of overcoming infertility

5

Premenstrual Syndrome (PMS)

Her ways are pleasant ways, and all her paths are peace. — Proverbs 3:17

Back when I was in my thirties, premenstrual syndrome (PMS) was a topic of great interest among women. Mood changes, fluid retention, craving for sweets — the premenstrual blues were talked about, written about, and researched. In fact, the first talk I ever gave at a Couple to Couple League Convention was on nutritional self-care strategies for PMS, and that presentation led to CCL's request that I write the first edition of this book. Now, however, with few exceptions, it is difficult to find new research or new books to help out with this all-too-common problem.

What has happened to research on PMS? I think the answer is this: The baby boom generation, who are in the midst of the change of life, have a growing interest in menopause. Their concern with PMS, which affects women who have menstrual cycles, has declined. With half of all American women past menopause and many more soon to follow, the researchers have followed the demographics. Perimenopause, the transitional time before menopause, has replaced PMS as the hot topic when it comes to women's health issues.

Despite the current focus on menopause, though, PMS still exists. And as one women's doctor has written, "Perimenopause can be more about PMS than about menopause."[1] That is, the changes of the perimenopause time include PMS, and need to be recognized as such. While it is true that PMS tends to become more severe as women approach menopause, it bothers many younger women as well, even teens. Fortunately, the nutritionally-oriented research from the not-too-distant past is still very helpful for improving PMS. As you will see, no matter what your age, you can be optimistic that you can help yourself to overcome or improve PMS through better diet, specific vitamins and minerals, and some other self-help practices beyond nutrition.

DEFINING PMS

PMS is a actually a broad term, referring to a large group of symptoms which all have one thing in common — they occur mainly during the post-ovulatory (luteal) phase of the cycle, beginning two to three days to a week or so before the menstrual period begins. Severe PMS may start earlier and last into the next cycle, though most often it disappears when the menstrual period begins. PMS does not include menstrual cramps or heavy bleeding, topics which are discussed in Chapter 6. The symptoms of PMS can be classified into four categories, as summarized below in Table 8.

TABLE 8, SYMPTOMS OF PMS, FROM MOST TO LEAST COMMON*	
PMT-A: ANXIETY	Characterized by anxiety, mood swings, irritability, and nervous tension.
PMT-H: HYDRATION	Characterized by water retention, weight gain, swelling of the extremities, breast tenderness, and abdominal bloating.
PMT-C: CRAVINGS	Characterized by cravings for sweets, cravings for carbohydrates, increased appetite; sometimes associated with headaches, fatigue, palpitations, and the "shakes."
PMT-D: DEPRESSION	Characterized by severe depression, forgetfulness, crying, confusion, and insomnia.[2]

* This classification was developed by Guy Abraham, M.D., who prefers the term "premenstrual tension" (PMT).

There are longer and more detailed lists of PMS symptoms, but most relate to the ones classified above. Premenstrual flare-up of acne is the only common symptom that does not easily fit into one of these four categories.[3] Women who are bothered by PMS usually experience more than one symptom, and their symptoms may change from cycle to cycle.

NUTRITION AND PMS

Gynecologist Guy Abraham, M.D., undertook pioneering studies on PMS and nutrition in the 1980s. His research is still truly remarkable for its holistic approach. He compared the daily diet of women who had PMS to the diet of women free from it. He observed the effect on PMS of consuming sugar and refined flour versus eating whole grains and vegetables. He considered the role of the healthy essential fatty acids versus the trans fats. Based on these studies, he developed a practical diet plan to improve the symptoms of PMS. At the same time, he researched the role of vitamins and minerals in PMS. Instead of recommending only one or two supplements, he formulated a complete multivitamin/multimineral for PMS, called Optivite PMT, and then tested it under double-blind conditions.

Dr. Abraham's contributions to women's reproductive self-care can hardly be overstated. Because his supplement recommendations tend to normalize the levels of estrogen and progesterone during the luteal phase, his PMS plan may also benefit women with short luteal phase, menstrual cramps, infertility, recurrent miscarriage, and endometriosis. For PMS as well as for these problems, the nutritional strategy detailed below is the practical self-help that the Couple to Couple League has recommended since 1990, with much positive feedback from women like you.

PROPOSED CAUSES OF PMS

Here are some of the nutritionally-related causes of PMS, as originally proposed by Dr. Abraham. Understanding this research, though it is somewhat technical, is valuable because it helps you to realize how and why nutrition makes a difference, not just in symptoms, but even more important, in the balance of estrogen, progesterone, and other hormones.

ABNORMAL LUTEAL FUNCTION (LUTEAL PHASE DEFICIENCY). Some women, especially those with anxiety and related symptoms (PMT-A), have estrogen levels that are too high and progesterone levels that are too low in the luteal phase of their cycles. This is a common hormonal imbalance, and is often called "estrogen dominance." Nutrition that tends to correct this imbalance by lowering estrogen and raising progesterone is beneficial to PMS, and it may also improve the other reproductive problems mentioned above.

B vitamins and diet play a role in regulating estrogen levels. If B vitamins are lacking, the liver cannot effectively inactivate estrogen, and estrogen rises.[4] Conversely, dietary fiber, which is the indigestible portion of whole plant foods, has the beneficial effect of reducing estrogen levels, apparently by "shielding" estrogens which are excreted in the bile from being reabsorbed back into the blood.[5] Women without PMS were far more likely to take vitamin supplements regularly, especially B vitamins, and were found to eat twice as much dietary fiber compared to women troubled by PMS.[6]

Estrogen dominance can also be improved through nutritional means that raise progesterone. Excess estrogen itself decreases progesterone, so reducing elevated estrogen promotes better progesterone levels. Consumption of excess animal fats is implicated in PMS because these fats contain arachidonic acid, the dietary precursor of a harmful "local hormone," the prostaglandin $PGF_2\alpha$. This prostaglandin depresses the function of the corpus luteum, which produces the progesterone in the luteal phase.[7] Dr. Abraham found that women without PMS consume as much fat as those with PMS, but they use more vegetable fat, while women with PMS consume more animal fat.[8]

Naturally decreasing the hormone prolactin can help PMS. Prolactin, produced by the pituitary gland, is higher in some women with PMS than in women without it. High levels of prolactin decrease progesterone levels, contributing to estrogen dominance and PMT-A.[9] The hypothalamus controls prolactin primarily through inhibition, not stimulation, and prolactin will rise abnormally if it is not properly regulated. Vitamin B6 reduces prolactin levels by stimulating the production of dopamine, which decreases prolactin release.[10] Magnesium is also necessary for the synthesis of dopamine, and so can contribute to normal levels of prolactin. Zinc is another nutrient that suppresses elevated prolactin levels.[11]

Vitamin B6 (pyridoxine) supplements can elevate progesterone levels, which is key to overcoming abnormal luteal function.[12] This vitamin alone has significantly reduced the symptoms of PMS, especially anxiety, in double-blind studies.[13] Vitamin C, in a large, recent study on infertility, has also increased progesterone levels significantly.[14] Dr. Abraham's complete diet and the supplement Optivite PMT, which includes large doses of both vitamin B_6 and vitamin C, as well as magnesium and zinc, has lowered high luteal phase estrogen and raised low luteal phase progesterone to normal levels while reducing the symptoms of PMS.[15]

ABNORMAL FLUID RETENTION. The premenstrual fluid retention (PMT-H) that bothers many women with PMS is responsible for bloating, weight gain, and breast pain or tenderness. These symptoms relate in part to the hormone aldosterone, secreted by the adrenal glands, which sit atop each kidney. Aldosterone causes the kidneys to retain salt and water, and it is elevated during the luteal phase. Excess aldosterone secretion, which occurs in some women with PMS, increases loss of the mineral magnesium.[16] Magnesium works together with vitamin B_6; both B_6 and magnesium are necessary for the synthesis of dopamine, which in addition to lowering prolactin, also helps the kidneys to rid the body of salt and water.[17] That is, magnesium and vitamin B_6 have a diuretic effect.

Intracellular magnesium levels have been found to be lower in women with PMS than in other women.[18] Women with PMS also consume more dairy products than do women without this disorder. High consumption of dairy products, with their unbalanced calcium to magnesium ratio of 10:1, inhibits the absorption of magnesium.[19] Reviews of experiments on the effect of magnesium supplements for PMS conclude that magnesium alone is beneficial for PMS.[20] Moderate use of dairy products combined with plenty of green vegetables and whole grains naturally tends to balance calcium and magnesium.

Even when aldosterone levels are normal or low, high consumption of sugar, which is common in women with PMS, causes fluid retention within a day or two of a sugar binge.[21] Such sugar consumption depletes magnesium. And while excessive salt promotes fluid retention, adequate salt prevents over-secretion of aldosterone.[22]

HYPOGLYCEMIA. Women with PMS consume more sugar and refined carbohydrates than do others.[23] In addition to promoting fluid retention, sugar and refined carbohydrates trigger over-secretion of insulin. Insulin rapidly lowers the blood glucose, resulting in reactive hypoglycemia and symptoms such as craving for sweets, headache, mood swings, and shakiness or faintness. (See Rule 7 in Chapter 1 for an explanation of the relationship between sugar consumption, insulin, and hypoglycemia.)

Insulin secretion is regulated with help from a beneficial local hormone, prostaglandin E_1, so a deficiency of this prostaglandin may contribute to carbohydrate cravings (PMT-C). This prostaglandin is derived from linoleic acid, which is plentiful in many vegetable oils. However, for the dietary linoleic acid to be converted to the helpful prostaglandin E_1, magnesium, vitamins B_3, B_6, and C, and zinc are all necessary. Trans fats, as in margarine, block this vital conversion. These damaging fats also favor the synthesis of the harmful prostaglandin $F_2\alpha$.[24] Conversely, alpha-linolenic acid, found abundantly in flax oil, is the precursor of the healthy "E$_3$" series of prostaglandins, which increase the production of the beneficial prostaglandin E$_1$, while blocking the production of the harmful F$_2$$\alpha$.[25]

Besides limiting sugary foods, both avoiding trans fats as well as taking in the healthy fats and oils, as explained in Rule 3 in Chapter 1, help to keep insulin levels normal. The undesirable insulin over-response to sugar can also be reduced by decreasing the ratio of calcium to magnesium. Dr. Abraham's preferred ratio of supplemental calcium to magnesium is 1:2, opposite the 2:1 ratio of these two minerals which is usually suggested by nutritional advisors.[26]

PMS DIETARY RECOMMENDATIONS

Dr. Abraham's nutritional recommendations integrate the above research into practical advice for women with PMS. He recommends plenty of vegetables, whole grains and beans, fish, and poultry, moderate use of dairy products, and limited red meat. Refined sugar, trans fats, excess salt, as well as alcohol and caffeine, are to be restricted.[27] He suggests olive oil, safflower oil, and flaxseed oil to obtain the healthy monounsaturated fats and the two essential fatty acids.[28]

These recommendations, first published in 1983 and updated in 1990, are similar to the 2008 dietary guidelines of *The Fertility Diet,* based on the Harvard School of Public Health's large Nurses' Health Study on ovulatory infertility in women. Both recommend whole plant foods, which are rich sources of magnesium, vitamins, and other minerals. Both have generous protein allowances, but encourage increased use of plant proteins. Both recommend healthful oils. Both emphatically discourage consumption of sugar, refined carbohydrates, and trans fats.

However, Dr. Abraham counseled limiting dairy products to two low-fat servings daily,[29] while *The Fertility Diet* recommends one to two servings of full-fat dairy products daily. Based on the new research finding that use of full-fat dairy products improves fertility (and therefore hormonal balance), I favor the use of whole-fat dairy products rather than low-fat ones.

That said, as you improve your diet to overcome PMS, use the "Twelve Rules for Better Nutrition" in Chapter 1. They are intentionally flexible, so tailor healthy food choices to your own needs and preferences. For example, you may find that extra protein in the form of meat or eggs, especially for breakfast, helps you to have more stable blood sugar and less sugar craving. On the other hand, your sister may find that high fiber snacks during the day do the same for her.

THE CAFFEINE CONNECTION. Dr. Abraham recommends limiting caffeine-containing beverages "because of their deleterious effects on breast cysts and mastalgia [breast pain]."[30] There are conflicting studies on the effect of caffeine on PMS symptoms, but some studies have found a strong association between PMS and caffeine consumption.[31] Caffeine can make hypoglycemia worse, and many women find that it contributes to nervousness or anxiety.

Dr. Abraham has noted that women with PMS seem to crave chocolate, which contains a caffeine-like substance — as well as high levels of magnesium![32]

ASPARTAME (NUTRASWEET). Aspartame, the artificial sweetener chemical of NutraSweet, contains 50 percent phenylalanine. Phenylalanine stimulates the secretion of prolactin from the pituitary gland.[33] High prolactin levels are involved in luteal phase deficiency, which relates to PMS. Avoid aspartame, as well as other artificial sweeteners.

THE ORIGINAL PMS SUPPLEMENT: OPTIVITE PMT

OPTIVITE PMT, the multivitamin/multimineral supplement which Dr. Abraham formulated and tested, is an integral part of improving PMS. The full dose, which is six tablets, contains 300 mg of vitamin B6 along with substantial amounts of the other B vitamins and a high dose of vitamin C. It contains magnesium but not calcium, and a significant amount of the mineral zinc. It should be taken all month long, not just during the luteal phase of the cycle. (See Appendix A for the complete contents of Optivite PMT.)

In an open study of Optivite, the most improvement was obtained among women with PMS when they took six to twelve tablets of Optivite daily for three or more cycles.[34] Results of three double-blind studies showed that three tablets daily of Optivite were ineffective against PMS, but six tablets per day were more effective than dietary improvement alone. "Once-a-day" type vitamins, used as a placebo, were useless for PMS.[35]

The multi-nutrient approach of Optivite, along with improved diet, is preferable to supplementing with any single nutrient. Even though vitamin B6 alone has been shown to reduce PMS,[36] the B vitamins work as a group, and are more effective if taken together. Vitamin B6 also depends on magnesium for its best function. Significantly, a recent study on infertility has shown that vitamin C (750 mg/day) raises progesterone while improving fertility.[37] Optivite contains 1,500 mg of vitamin C per full dose; undoubtedly this nutrient, which has been in Optivite since its original formulation, has been partially responsible for its effect on PMS and other reproductive problems.

Optivite reduces the levels of estrogen and increases the levels of progesterone in women with PMS who had the high estrogen levels and low progesterone levels that are common with PMS.[38] Mainly because of this effect, I recommend Optivite for PMS, and for self-care of any other problem of estrogen dominance, including luteal phase deficiency, some types of infertility, and early miscarriage.

In over 100,000 women who have used Optivite for several years, no cases of vitamin or mineral toxicity have been reported.[39] While high doses of vitamin B6 alone can be toxic, Dr. Abraham credits this safety record to the balance of the micronutrients within the supplement. The other B vitamins and magnesium enable the body to process the B6 normally, decreasing the possibility of overdose. His advice for women to use the lowest effective dose is another probable reason for this safety record.[40] Nevertheless, you should discuss your vitamin and mineral supplements with your health care provider, and you should not exceed 300 mg of vitamin B6 per day. Instead, if six tablets of Optivite do not help your symptoms, increase magnesium to a total of 1,000 mg per day.[41]

My experience is that women with PMS begin to find relief, often within the first cycle of use, by taking six tablets of Optivite daily (which supplies 300 mg of B6) along with an additional 500 mg of magnesium and three to six capsules of flax oil daily.

Optivite is available from the American Pro Life Enterprise or from the Optimox Corporation. (See "Resources.") The package insert suggests up to six tablets per day plus 500 mg of additional magnesium. Since it is limited in folic acid (200 mcg), if pregnant you should obtain additional folic acid for balance (at least an additional 200 mcg/day, and as much as 4,000 mcg/day if it is suggested for other reproductive problems).

OTHER VITAMIN SUPPLEMENTS FOR PMS

PROCYCLE PMS. Women's Health America (WHA) formulates ProCycle PMS, another excellent vitamin/mineral supplement specifically for PMS. It is much like Optivite, with 300 mg of vitamin B6 and 1,500 mg of vitamin C per full dose. It contains more folic acid (800 mcg) than Optivite and twice as much vitamin D3, vitamin E, selenium, and chromium as Optivite. It contains 300 mg of magnesium compared to Optivite's 200 mg. Unlike Optivite, it contains no iron. This may seem like a disadvantage, but actually, many women are not anemic and do not need supplemental iron, and often it is the iron that causes stomach upset when you take a vitamin/mineral supplement.[42] While Optivite is labeled for six tablets daily, ProCycle PMS is labeled for four tablets to achieve a full dose, making it more convenient to take. ProCycle is available through Women's Health America. (See "Resources"; see Appendix A for contents of ProCycle PMS.)

GENERAL SUPPLEMENTS. Instead of Optivite or ProCycle, you may prefer to modify the general supplement program suggested in Table 7 (Chapter 3) for PMS. For example, Professional Prenatal Formula, which I recommend as a comprehensive supplement for women generally, can serve as your PMS multivitamin/ multimineral, as long as you add 100-200 mg of additional vitamin B6, and 500 mg of additional magnesium. Professional Prenatal Formula is available through the American Pro Life Enterprise. (See "Resources"; see *www.lifetimevitamins. com* for contents.)

In all cases, supplementing 5–10 one-gram capsules of flax oil to gain the valuable alpha-linolenic acid, and/or 1 teaspoon of fish oil, as discussed in Chapter 3, should be part of your PMS nutritional strategy.

OTHER OPTIONS FOR PMS

While improved diet, as outlined in Chapter 1, and Dr. Abraham's supplement recommendations provide the most comprehensive self-help for PMS, there are other approaches to PMS that may interest you. They are listed below, more or less in the order that I recommend them.

CHASTEBERRY EXTRACT. An old remedy for "female complaints" has been rediscovered recently and tested in a large, well-controlled scientific study for its effectiveness against PMS symptoms. It is chasteberry extract, also called "Vitex" (*Vitex agnus castus*).[43] Previous studies have also shown a positive effect of chasteberry extract on PMS,[44] including in women with known luteal phase deficiency.[45]

If you wish to try chasteberry to overcome PMS, I suggest that you use it as part of a product called Fertility Blend. This supplement contains chasteberry extract, but it also contains other antioxidants: green tea extract, vitamin E (150 mg), folic acid (400 mcg), iron (18 mg in the preferred chelated form), magnesium (400 mg), and selenium (70 mcg). A study in 2006 examined the use of Fertility Blend for the achievement of pregnancy among infertile women. The researchers reported that chasteberry extract was safe and effective for use among women seeking pregnancy. Importantly, this study noted that chasteberry can increase progesterone levels and decrease prolactin levels.[46] Fertility Blend's complete contents are listed in Appendix A. (See "Resources.")

CALCIUM SUPPLEMENTS. Calcium is an essential nutrient which is best known for its bone-building effect. It is critical to nerve function as well, and it performs a variety of regulatory roles in the body. It cannot be absorbed without vitamin D, and the mineral magnesium enables it to work properly. Its levels fluctuate throughout the menstrual cycle.[47] (In fact, when I was a student in graduate school, I served as a subject in a study in which women took their basal temperatures daily, and then had their blood calcium levels measured before and after ovulation.) Women who get calcium and vitamin D from their diet are less likely to have PMS.[48]

Two large double-blind studies have shown that calcium supplements alone, in the antacid form of calcium carbonate, are effective against the symptoms of PMS.[49] Since calcium without vitamin D is poorly absorbed, I suspect that calcium in this form works at least in part by slightly increasing the blood pH, which some authorities believe results in improvement of mood and energy levels.[50]

However, I do not recommend calcium supplements alone as the remedy for PMS. You can obtain at least some of your calcium through use of dairy foods. If you do not use dairy products, supplements of calcium citrate, calcium malate, or other "chelated" forms of calcium, along with vitamin D$_3$ and magnesium, may be most helpful. Try for total calcium (diet plus supplements) of about 1,000 mg per day. For example, since typical servings of dairy foods (milk, yogurt, cheese) average about 250 mg of calcium, if you have two servings of dairy products daily, supplement about 500 mg of calcium. A total of 500 to 1,000 mg of magnesium, ideally in a chelated form, can be supplemented to balance the calcium. Of course, it is prudent to improve your diet and to supplement comprehensively, as nutrients work together.

PROGESTERONE SKIN CREAM. If a serious attempt to improve your daily diet and vitamin, mineral, and essential fatty acid status is not effective after three months, you may wish to consider over-the-counter natural progesterone cream for PMS, in addition to continuing your improved nutrition.

The goal in using natural ("bio-identical") progesterone cream is to raise progesterone to normal levels during the luteal phase of the cycle. The cream is rubbed onto thin skin, such as on the abdomen, neck, or inner arms. The suggested amounts to be used are noted on the product label. While progesterone is absorbed easily through the skin, the amount of it absorbed varies with the thickness of the skin, the skin temperature, and the blood flow to the skin.

If you choose to use progesterone cream, it is important to wait until a temperature rise of three days confirms that you have ovulated. Women who do not chart their temperatures may inadvertently use progesterone cream before ovulation and interfere with the cycle, as it is not natural for the ovaries to produce progesterone until after ovulation. Even though progesterone cream is a readily-available, nonprescription product, it is advisable to discuss its use with your physician, especially if you may become pregnant. If you have severe PMS, you may wish to try it immediately while you also implement better nutrition, but if you do so, aim to decrease the progesterone gradually as you improve your nutrition.[51]

For detailed information on the use of progesterone skin cream, see the chapter on PMS in *What Your Doctor May Not Tell You about Premenopause* by John Lee, M.D., and colleagues. (See "Further Reading.")

ORAL MICRONIZED NATURAL PROGESTERONE. If you have PMS that needs treatment beyond better nutrition and over-the-counter progesterone, Women's Health America (WHA) can help you in a systematic way. The founder, pharmacist Marla Ahlgrimm, R.Ph., has been a pioneer in holistic treatment of PMS since 1982. Her organization is a group of like-minded pharmacists and other professionals who emphasize diet, exercise, vitamin and mineral supplements (ProCycle or Optivite), stress management, and education for PMS first. If PMS symptoms have not improved after three months with such self-care, WHA recommends complete hormonal testing via nonprescription saliva tests.[52] Based on the test results, they may recommend replacement of natural progesterone (and possibly other hormones). They prefer oral "micronized" natural progesterone rather than skin creams, because they consider the oral form easier to dose accurately. However, oral progesterone is available by prescription only.

If you are interested in WHA's approach, you do not have to visit them in person. Their staff can guide your own health care practitioner, or they can help you find a local doctor who is both nutritionally-oriented and familiar with the use of prescription progesterone in this form. Women's Health America, which is located in Madison, Wisconsin, can be contacted via their website, ***www.womenshealth.com***. (See "Resources.")

BACK TO BASICS: NON-NUTRITIONAL ANTI-PMS STRATEGIES

REGULAR OUTDOOR EXERCISE. Exercise is good for just about everything, and it is wonderful for improving the symptoms of PMS. It elevates your mood and reduces your stress. It helps you to sleep better. Exercise that is done outdoors with plenty of natural sunlight is better yet, and there is even scientific evidence to support the common experience that bright light elevates your mood.[53] Who does not agree that there is nothing like a brisk walk on a beautiful day to make you feel great? Even walks in the bright snow may be helpful, but exercise in itself should be the goal, indoors or out, sunny or cloudy. Just do not overdo it, because it can increase your stress and be counterproductive. Start slowly if you are not accustomed to vigorous exercise.

REASONABLE BODY WEIGHT. Having your body weight at a comfortable level for you — not necessarily at some theoretical ideal weight — is helpful to preventing PMS,[54] and it tends to normalize the levels of estrogen.[55] Especially if you are overweight, just a small decrease in weight may help you to feel better. See Chapter 8 for some recommendations for modest weight loss.

STRESS MANAGEMENT. Worrying about how to reduce stress can be a major stress! Here is some good news: improved diet and supplementing vitamins and minerals helps decrease the hormonal response to stress, so that you "roll with the punches" better. That is, you reduce stress just by being well-nourished, because poor nutrition is a physical stress. Exercise also reduces stress, provided you do something you enjoy at a level that does not leave you physically exhausted. See Chapter 14 for more information on stress.

ADEQUATE SLEEP. I am convinced that increasing your sleep is even more important than good diet, supplements, and exercise for decreasing stress. Putting good nutrition together with enough sleep may be all you need to "decompress." When you sleep, the levels of the stress hormones cortisol and adrenaline drop, and that is very beneficial. If more sleep means less work, or less chauffeuring, or fewer volunteer activities, try your best to say "no" to the extras that so many women try to fit into already full schedules. In addition, sleeping in a very dark room may increase your progesterone levels, as explained in Chapter 9 under the heading, "Sensitivity to Night Lighting."

CHARTING. Simply knowing when to expect PMS by using an NFP chart is useful, and including notes on the type, severity, and duration of PMS symptoms is an excellent self-help practice to chart your progress. Using NFP may help you avoid PMS in another way; oral contraceptives worsen PMS in some women,[56] and PMS may become severe after a tubal ligation because the surgery damages the blood supply to the ovary, causing the ovary to function less well after the procedure is done.[57] Hysterectomy may also worsen PMS.[58]

OTHER POSSIBILITIES. If the guidelines given here are not helpful to you, you should consider factors other than PMS. Thyroid dysfunction, yeast overgrowth, and adrenal exhaustion are all possibilities to investigate, ideally with your physician's help. (See "Low Thyroid Function" and "Hyperthyroidism" in Chapter 7; "Yeast Overgrowth" in Chapter 9; and Chapter 14.)

PMS DIET AND SUPPLEMENTS FOR OTHER CYCLE PROBLEMS

As noted in the opening paragraphs of this chapter, I recommend improved diet and Dr. Abraham's PMS supplement plan for several other female reproductive disorders, since it provides excellent overall nutrition and tends to normalize the levels of estrogen and progesterone. Some women have reported longer luteal phases, which are a sign of better progesterone levels, and others have noticed clearer mucus patterns. Some women believe that it has helped them to achieve a pregnancy after infertility or miscarriage. The following anecdote illustrates several of these points:

A married couple who had never had children visited my husband and me to discuss their inability to conceive. They had taken our natural family planning classes as an engaged couple and had initially used the method to avoid a pregnancy. However, for over two years they had been trying to conceive, and the wife, whom I'll call Lana, was now 30. They had already undergone medical testing which confirmed that the husband's sperm count was normal and that Lana's fallopian tubes were unblocked.

I noticed that the post-ovulatory temperatures on Lana's charts were elevated for a shorter than normal number of days — evidence of possible luteal phase deficiency. "Does she have PMS?" I asked her husband. He nodded vigorously while she giggled. I explained the PMS nutritional plan to them, and we also discussed medical intervention as an immediate option, since the infertility had persisted for so long a time. Lana decided to take the recommended six tablets of Optivite and 500 mg of magnesium daily. Her day-to-day diet was already quite good, so she made no other changes.

"They helped everything!" Lana said of the vitamins. The supplements worked so well in reducing her PMS irritability that she and her husband jokingly called them her "nice" pills. The duration of her post-ovulatory temperatures increased by "at least two or three days." And she was pleasantly surprised to find that within a cycle or two, her painful menstrual cramps, which had been worsening for two years, also disappeared completely. Best of all, four months after she started the vitamins, she became pregnant. The baby, a girl, was born after a healthy pregnancy.

Incidentally, with her doctor's approval, Lana used six tablets of Optivite daily as her prenatal vitamin supplement, a practice approved by Dr. Abraham.[59] A recent study has confirmed that large doses of vitamin B6 during pregnancy, when it is often recommended to overcome nausea, do not harm the unborn child.[60] If you do use Optivite as a prenatal vitamin supplement, however, increase the folic acid to a total of at least 400 mcg, and up to 4,000 mcg if you are an older mother or have had problems conceiving. ProCycle (4 tablets) contains 800 mcg of folic acid, and is also safe for use during pregnancy.[61]

Despite any confusion caused by the labeling, neither Optivite nor ProCycle exceeds a safe limit of vitamin A. Each contains only 5,000 IU of true vitamin A (retinyl palmitate) per full dose; the other "vitamin A" is actually beta-carotene (7,500 IU), which has never been implicated in birth defects.

Summary — Chapter 5

➤ Premenstrual syndrome (PMS) refers to a group of troublesome symptoms (including anxiety, irritability, bloating, and breast tenderness) that may occur during the second half of the cycle in some women.

➤ One important cause of PMS is luteal phase deficiency, which means that estrogen is too high and progesterone is too low during the luteal phase. This hormonal imbalance is often termed "estrogen dominance."

➤ Research by gynecologist Guy Abraham, M.D., showed that improved diet and vitamin/mineral supplements rich in vitamin B6, other B vitamins, vitamin C, zinc, and magnesium can improve the symptoms of PMS, even under double-blind conditions.

➤ There are also other approaches to overcoming the symptoms of PMS, including supplements of the herb Vitex agnus castus or supplements of calcium.

➤ Improved diet and PMS vitamins and minerals may also be helpful to short luteal phase, some types of infertility, recurrent miscarriage, endometriosis, and other problems related to estrogen dominance.

➤ While no cases of vitamin B6 toxicity were reported in over 100,000 women using Optivite for several years, it is prudent to discuss vitamin supplements with your health care practitioner. The vitamin A in the supplements suggested (Optivite, ProCycle, and Professional Prenatal) does not exceed a safe dose for women who may become pregnant.

6

Shorter, Lighter, & Pain-free Periods

A woman with a hemorrhage of twelve years' duration, incurable at any doctor's hands, came up behind him and touched the tassel on his cloak. Immediately her bleeding stopped. — Luke 8:43-44

Some cycle problems are easier to solve than others. In counseling women with various cycle irregularities, I have found that heavy and prolonged bleeding almost always can be improved with better nutrition. Cramps and menstrual pain will often improve once the menstrual period is lightened up, but there are also additional nutritional strategies aimed at decreasing menstrual pain. Because there is some relationship between heavy or long periods and menstrual pain, I would like to deal with bleeding problems first.

—— HEAVY OR PROLONGED MENSES ——

The typical period lasts about five days, with two or three days of moderate flow and two or three days of light flow or spotting. If you are experiencing heavy or long periods and are in doubt as to whether or not it is normal, make sure your doctor is aware of your concern. If you have episodes of spotting or bleeding at times other than your expected period, let your doctor know. The vast majority of such episodes are explainable, especially with the information that you gain from your NFP charts, and in most cases your doctor will reassure you. Still, you need to know if fibroid tumors, endometriosis, low thyroid function, or some other condition is contributing to the problem. If heavy or prolonged bleeding has been ongoing, you should also ask for a test for anemia.

Even if your doctor assures you that you are in good health, why not try the nutritional measures outlined in this chapter to make your periods lighter and shorter as a matter of convenience? While up to a full week of menstrual bleeding or spotting is considered normal, a long or heavy period is not necessary to shed the lining of the uterus. Better nutrition can noticeably shorten the length of the menses as well as the amount of blood loss. As a side benefit, the better health of your mucus membranes may also make your mucus signs clearer and easier to read.

CAUSES OF HEAVY OR PROLONGED BLEEDING

Certain patterns of heavy or prolonged menses may indicate other problems, and charting can give you very good insight into what the underlying cause might be. If one of the following possibilities seems to fit, please also refer to the follow-up information, as noted.

ENDOMETRIOSIS. Severe menstrual pain is the foremost symptom of endometriosis, though prolonged or heavy bleeding may occur with it. Endometriosis is the final topic of this chapter, and that section offers some specific self-care options for you, but working closely with a compassionate physician who is an expert at helping you to manage your endometriosis is essential.

COMING OFF THE PILL. Elevated levels of vitamin A, which are caused by oral contraceptive use, along with the synthetic hormones themselves, contribute to the very light bleeding typical of birth control pill users. Conversely, discontinuing the Pill lowers vitamin A, sometimes resulting in heavy or prolonged periods. Refer to the section in Chapter 9, "Discontinuing Birth Control Pills," for a discussion of nutrition aimed at normal cycles following Pill use.

LUTEAL PHASE DEFICIENCY. If your period starts with one to three days of light spotting while your temperatures are still elevated and then becomes a normal, full flow as your basal temperature drops, or if your period ends with a discharge which is brownish rather than the usual pink or honey color, suspect luteal phase deficiency. This term refers to a luteal (post-ovulatory) phase in which progesterone is too low. Often the premenstrual spotting, called "irregular shedding," begins soon — too soon — after your temperature and mucus patterns have confirmed that you have ovulated. In addition to this chapter, see the section in Chapter 7 titled "Luteal Phase Deficiency."

"BREAK-THROUGH" BLEEDING (MID-CYCLE SPOTTING). In this pattern your temperature confirms that you have ovulated, but some time around ovulation several days of spotting may occur. This may simply be from excess buildup of endometrium that is shed after the hormonal readjustment that follows ovulation. In addition to the nutritional information of this chapter, see Chapter 5, as the self-care for PMS may also help breakthrough bleeding.

LOW THYROID FUNCTION. Low thyroid function is a common cause of heavy or prolonged menses. Suspect low thyroid function if your basal temperatures are low, in the range of 97.2 or below, during the pre-ovulatory phase. You may or may not experience long cycle lengths. Your mucus pattern may be unclear with an ongoing less-fertile type mucus pattern. Even if you have had a test for your thyroid hormones that came back normal, you should still consider this possibility. See "Low Thyroid Function" in Chapter 7, in addition to the nutritional suggestions later in this chapter.

UNDERWEIGHT, LOW BODY FAT, AND/OR VIGOROUS ATHLETIC ACTIVITY. Along with heavy or long periods, you may have long cycles with a delay in ovulation, or you may have anovulatory cycles followed by periods, with your temperatures showing that you have not ovulated. If you are not charting, you may be puzzled to have some light and some heavy or prolonged periods which occur irregularly.

Your low body fat is the probable explanation. A marginal lack of body fat will cause a delay in ovulation at first, but as more body fat is lost, cycles without ovulation (anovulatory cycles) may occur. Just a small gain in weight, perhaps three to five pounds, can improve the entire cycle. When the hormones that trigger ovulation kick in sooner, the endometrium repairs itself faster, meaning that the length of the period may shorten and lighten. When you gain enough weight, you are not likely to have anovulatory cycles with their unpredictable timing and bleeding pattern. If, on the other hand, more regular cycles cause heavier bleeding when before it was very light, try the nutritional strategies discussed below. Also refer to "Underweight or Inadequate Body Fat" in Chapter 7.

POLYCYSTIC OVARY SYNDROME (PCOS). If your cycles are long, and you have prolonged or heavy episodes of bleeding at irregular intervals with or without the temperature rise that confirms ovulation, it may be PCOS that underlies your problem. In this case, your pre-ovulatory temperature levels are usually normal (around 97.6°F.), and often your mucus pattern consists of on-and-off more-fertile mucus. If PCOS is contributing to heavy or prolonged bleeding, you may also tend to have abdominal weight gain and perhaps other signs of "male" hormones. See this topic in Chapter 8, as well as the information on basic nutrition for heavy or prolonged bleeding discussed later in this chapter.

FIBROID TUMORS. These abnormal but benign growths, which originate in the muscular layer of the uterus, are most likely to occur as you enter your late thirties or forties. Fibroids thrive on estrogen, so obesity is a risk factor, as well as the "estrogen dominance" pattern of hormones that is common in the forties. Sometimes fibroid tumors cause no problems, but because they can interfere with the healing of the endometrium, they may contribute to heavy or prolonged bleeding at irregular times in the cycle. They frequently cause pain as well and can lead to the need for surgery. The basic nutritional information that is the focus of this chapter can help you to limit extra blood loss while you decide what course of action to take with the fibroids.

MISCARRIAGE. First, if you have experienced a miscarriage, I would like to express my sympathy for your loss. While I know that it is a difficult experience to deal with emotionally, it is important to care for yourself physically as well as emotionally as you recover. Bleeding after a miscarriage can be quite heavy and may be prolonged, depending on a number of factors. The nutrition suggested below can make the blood loss after a miscarriage considerably shorter and lighter, and nutrition for overcoming anemia can help you get your energy back sooner. It is likely that you will ovulate two to four weeks after the loss of your child, and if you avoid a pregnancy as you recover, you should expect a normal period.

Sometimes you may suspect that an early miscarriage has caused heavy or prolonged bleeding, but you may not be sure. Having a long cycle, even if followed by heavy bleeding, is not a sign of miscarriage in itself. In most cases it simply means that you have ovulated late — or maybe not at all — perhaps for one of the reasons listed above. On the other hand, if you have had at least 21 days of elevated temperatures without a period as part of your luteal phase, and then experience heavy or prolonged bleeding, particularly with unusual cramping, an early miscarriage unfortunately is the most likely cause.

CHILDBIRTH (POSTPARTUM LOCHIA). After childbirth, your estrogen and progesterone levels will be quite low, especially if you are breastfeeding your baby, and considerable healing of the endometrium must take place. The nutrition suggested below in this chapter will lighten and shorten the "lochia," as the normal postpartum discharge is called. You will probably notice soon after the birth that when your baby latches on to nurse, you may have a brief increase in bleeding as the uterus contracts. That is good, because despite the slight increase in flow, the contraction of the uterus helps to limit the amount of blood loss overall. If you have had heavy postpartum bleeding in the past, I think you will be pleasantly surprised at the improvement that nutritional strategies make.

DIET FOR BETTER HEALING AND NORMAL BLOOD CLOTTING

Loss of much bright red blood that runs easily, as opposed to a discharge with mucus that lightens in color after three or four days, is a sign that the clotting and healing mechanisms are not working as well as they might. Proper clotting and the healing of the mucus membranes depends on sufficient amounts of many nutrients — vitamin A, B-complex vitamins, vitamin C, related phytochemicals called bioflavinoids, vitamin K, iron, and the essential fatty acids. Vitamin E prevents destruction of the essential fatty acids.[1] Calcium is necessary to proper blood clotting, and vitamin D is necessary for absorption of calcium. Zinc works along with vitamin A to maximize healing.

GOOD FOODS FOR BETTER HEALING AND NORMAL CLOTTING. Eggs are a good natural source of true vitamin A. Plenty of orange or yellow vegetables and fruits will provide beta-carotene, the precursor of vitamin A. Carrots, sweet potatoes, squash, and apricots are examples. Many whole plant and animal foods provide B-complex vitamins. Citrus fruits are the best source of vitamin C, and if you eat the white parts inside the rind, you will get bioflavinoids, which work together with vitamin C to promote tissue healing and stronger blood capillaries. Milk products, of course, provide abundant calcium, and the fat in whole milk products assists in the absorption of the fat-soluble vitamins A, D, E, and K. Raw pumpkin seeds and freshly ground flax seeds are the best food sources of the essential fatty acids. Expeller-pressed canola oil provides some of both of the two essential fatty acids.

VITAMIN K SOURCE. Vitamin K is involved in the production of several clotting proteins. It is frequently assumed to be plentiful in the body since "friendly" bacteria within the large intestine synthesize it, and it is available in the diet if dark green leafy vegetables are eaten. However, antibiotics harm the intestinal bacteria, and typical Americans eat far too little of the vitamin K-rich foods. Emphasis on these foods and regular intake of bacteria-containing yogurt or capsules of friendly bacteria (probiotics) will help provide vitamin K, especially if nonessential antibiotics and aspirin, which deplete this vitamin, are avoided.

IRON FOR HEAVY BLEEDING. While you might think of iron only in terms of overcoming anemia, it actually helps to prevent heavy bleeding as well.[2] Good sources of iron are red meat, organic liver, blackstrap molasses, beans, eggs, and spinach.

SUPPLEMENTS FOR BETTER HEALING AND NORMAL BLOOD CLOTTING

MULTIVITAMINS/MULTIMINERALS. A multivitamin/multimineral supplement which supplies a balance of the vitamins and minerals mentioned in the preceding section is important to ensure that the endometrium has the raw materials it needs for rapid healing. Professional Prenatal Formula by Lifetime provides most of these specific nutrients in the amounts needed. It also provides the many nutrients, including iron, that are necessary to overcoming anemia, should blood loss be severe. (See "Resources.")

FLAX OIL. The two essential fatty acids (linoleic acid and alpha-linolenic acid) are neither vitamins nor minerals, so they are not found in vitamin/mineral supplements. Because alpha-linolenic acid is difficult to get in the Western diet — it is found in some seed oils, but is destroyed by exposure to light, heat, and oxygen — I strongly recommend that you supplement it. Flax oil contains a high percentage of alpha-linolenic acid, and five to 10 1 g capsules daily makes a noticeable difference to a number of reproductive health problems, including heavy or prolonged bleeding. Vitamin E prevents destruction of the essential fatty acids, an example of one more reason why a comprehensive multivitamin/multimineral supplement is best.

FISH OIL. Instead of, or in addition to flax oil, you can use fish liver oil, which is rich in the fatty acids EPA and DHA. Fish oil is not essential; the healthy DHA and EPA can be made from the alpha-linolenic acid, as long as B vitamins, vitamin C, zinc, and magnesium are available. If you prefer fish oil, one teaspoon daily of good tasting, toxin-free, concentrated fish oil will provide what you need. Cod liver oil provides vitamin A and vitamin D, both beneficial to healing. Just be sure to get some vitamin E with it, about 400 IU daily.

VITAMIN A. Vitamin A can greatly reduce heavy or prolonged periods, especially if used in large amounts. If you are attempting to conceive, however, do not take more than 8,000 IU daily without consulting your doctor — at levels over 10,000 IU it has been associated with birth defects.[3] Reading labels can be confusing, though, as the listing "vitamin A" will be subdivided into retinyl palmitate or retinyl acetate, which are true vitamin A, and beta-carotene, which is not the same and has never been related to birth defects. Vitamin A is a necessary nutrient, and you should not fear healthy amounts of it, including the amounts found in fish oil supplements. If there is no chance of conception, 20,000-25,000 IU of true vitamin A daily is acceptable.

BIOFLAVINOIDS. The bioflavinoids, found abundantly in the white rind and sectional membranes of citrus fruits, strengthen capillary walls and therefore are useful to moderate the tendency to heavy bleeding. They are also available as supplements, and 1,000 mg tablets twice daily is the recommended dose.[4]

FAST ACTION FOR HEAVY BLEEDING

Sometimes heavy bleeding may catch you by surprise, whether it relates to your cycle, a miscarriage, or a postpartum problem. There are steps that you can take right away which are very helpful and fast-acting. Capsules of chlorophyll, which is rich in vitamin K, work rapidly to reduce heavy bleeding, often within a couple of hours. They are available in health food shops in amounts of approximately 30 or 60 mg, and taking four or five capsules throughout the days of heavy flow is quite effective in reducing blood loss. While the other supplements mentioned above should be taken all month, chlorophyll capsules only need to be taken shortly before or during the bleeding episode.

Chlorophyll in liquid form also rapidly controls postpartum bleeding, according to midwives familiar with its use. Like chlorophyll, cayenne pepper in tablets (also called capsicum) quickly slows any type of bleeding. Extra flax oil (ten 1 g capsules or 2 teaspoons) taken before and during the period will often lighten bleeding also, so much so that it may make chlorophyll or cayenne pepper unnecessary.

A SPECIAL CAUTION ABOUT MISCARRIAGE

I have spoken to several women who have lost frightening amounts of blood during an early miscarriage. In addition to the loss of their child, they have had to deal with the prolonged and unexpected physical weakness that such blood loss brings. The section above, "Fast Action for Heavy Bleeding" can moderate the bleeding caused by a miscarriage.

However, if you ever believe you are losing too much blood, especially with a miscarriage, make sure that you contact a doctor. Yet I know women who have phoned their doctor's office in the face of extremely heavy bleeding, only to be told to "wait and see." Such long-distance diagnosis of bleeding resulted in one friend of mine receiving several pints of blood after a harrowing ambulance run.

Better advice: Heavy bleeding and dangerously heavy bleeding cannot be distinguished over the phone. You are the ultimate judge. If in doubt, go to a hospital emergency room.

DEALING WITH SEVERE BLOOD LOSS

The following anecdote illustrates how appropriate medical intervention and nutritional counseling enabled a young girl with severe menorrhagia (heavy menstrual bleeding) to recover from a frightening incident. Only 12 years old, this girl lost a large amount of blood during a heavy, prolonged period of which her parents were at first unaware. When they realized it, her hemoglobin was an extremely anemic 6.5 (normal is 12-16 mg/dl) and she was still bleeding. The attending gynecologist prescribed Provera (synthetic progesterone), but the little of it she did not vomit did no good.

At the parents' request, a transfusion of two pints of relatives' blood was arranged. It did not stop the bleeding, but it did bring her hemoglobin to an improved though still anemic 10. The gynecologist warned the parents that because of the severity of the situation, birth control pills were the probable next step, but he was willing to take a "wait-and-see" attitude for a short while.

The parents, concerned about the side effects of the Pill, turned to nutritional counseling. Cayenne pepper tablets (520 mg, five times daily) helped slow the bleeding significantly. The girl also began taking a balanced non-prescription multivitamin/multimineral which supplied 10,000 IU of true vitamin A, 75 mg/mcg of B-complex vitamins, 60 mg of chelated iron, and generous amounts of vitamin C, zinc, and the other micronutrients. The goal was to enable her body to produce its own clotting elements and more of its own hormones, and to overcome the anemia.

Her next period was very heavy but manageable. Two months later, she was no longer anemic and had a normal menses. Nine months later, her mother reported that she still tended toward heavy periods but was "definitely helped" by the cayenne pepper during her menses. Aside from the transfusion, her mother credits her daughter's faithfulness in taking the vitamins, cayenne pepper, and plenty of rest as the factors that enabled the girl to recover rapidly from this frightening incident.

I would add that flax oil would also be helpful in a case like this, or in any case in which a woman is trying to overcome post-hemorrhagic anemia. Additionally, chlorophyll capsules can enable the levels of fibrinogen (a key clotting protein) in the blood to return to normal, even within a few days.

OVERCOMING ANEMIA
If menorrhagia has been severe enough to cause anemia, as in the above anecdote, do not make the mistake of supplementing only iron to overcome it. The B vitamins, including folic acid, B6, and B12, vitamins C and E, zinc, copper, and adequate protein are among the nutrients which are also necessary to produce new red blood cells. Good foods for overcoming anemia are liver, spinach, citrus fruits, and cod liver oil. Professional Prenatal Formula by Life Time is an excellent supplement for overcoming anemia. (See "Resources.")

— PAINFUL PERIODS

Pain is a symptom of a problem; severe pain the more so. Menstrual cramps and pain may simply reflect common dietary or hormonal imbalances, or they may be a sign of endometriosis, uterine fibroids, infection, or other abnormalities. It is important to alert your doctor if your menstrual pain is worse than the moderate discomfort that is so common, especially among younger women who have never borne children. In most cases, the diagnosis will be "primary dysmenorrhea"; that is, pain during the period without any other problem such as endometriosis or fibroid tumors being involved. Primary dysmenorrhea is the main focus of the nutritional information that follows, though the chapter ends with a discussion of endometriosis.

CAUSES OF PAIN DURING MENSES

When painful menstruation occurs, it almost always is part of a period that follows ovulation, as opposed to an anovulatory cycle. The interplay of estrogen and progesterone, especially the drop in progesterone shortly before the period begins, is involved in the pain. The main culprits responsible for primary dysmenorrhea are inflammation-promoting prostaglandins, named $PGF_2\alpha$ and PGE_2, which are released from the endometrium during the menses. Not surprisingly, women with dysmenorrhea release many times more of these "bad" prostaglandins than do women without painful periods. These prostaglandins, which are actually found in the menstrual discharge, increase contractions of the uterus, decrease the blood supply to it, and increase inflammation. The result is pelvic pain that may feel crampy, achy, or congested. It is common for the ache to seem to originate from the back or from between the thighs. Some women experience nausea, vomiting, diarrhea, or headache along with their period.[5]

There are several risk factors for dysmenorrhea. Girls who begin their periods at a younger-than-average age have a higher risk of dysmenorrhea. Having long or heavy periods is also a factor in painful periods. Obesity is involved, as is stress, smoking, and alcohol use.[6] Tubal ligation is a risk factor, because it may disrupt the blood flow to the ovaries.[7]

DIET FOR PAINFUL PERIODS WITH HEAVY BLEEDING

Since heavy bleeding is a risk factor for painful menses, if you are having heavy periods along with pain, review the first part of this chapter and implement the nutritional strategies, especially the multivitamins and flax oil, to overcome the heavy bleeding. Doing so will very likely decrease your menstrual pain as well. Interestingly, the same prostaglandins that cause menstrual pain are also involved in heavy bleeding.[8]

PMS NUTRITION FOR MENSTRUAL PAIN

Even though dysmenorrhea is not part of premenstrual syndrome (PMS), these two cycle problems share some common ground. In some cases, they may occur together. For example, dysmenorrhea is often thought to be a problem of teenage girls and young women that disappears after the birth of the first child, or gradually decreases with age. PMS, alternatively, is often considered to increase in incidence with age, up to the age of menopause. However, while painful periods are common in adolescents, so is PMS. In one study of girls with dysmenorrhea, over 70 percent also had PMS.[9]

The understanding that inflammatory prostaglandins cause menstrual pain is another link between dysmenorrhea and PMS. This understanding has fueled interest in new nutritional research designed to reduce levels of the "bad" prostaglandins. Yet older nutritional research on PMS was also directed at reducing the very same prostaglandins, PGE2 and PGF2α. Dr. Guy Abraham's research on PMS, described in Chapter 5, specifically mentioned these prostaglandins as being involved in some of the causes of PMS. Newer research also provides interesting evidence that PMS mood symptoms occur at times when inflammatory chemicals are high.[10]

This is not to overstate the relationship between PMS and dysmenorrhea, because there are significant differences. While the "nonsteroidal anti-inflammatory drugs" (NSAIDs: aspirin, ibuprofen) are quite effective for menstrual pain, they are not helpful for PMS. Taken in the luteal phase, they may make PMS worse by blocking the production of helpful prostaglandins.[11]

Nevertheless, the PMS nutritional plan in Chapter 5, which is interchangeable with the "Twelve Rules for Better Nutrition" in Chapter 1, is aimed at decreasing the inflammation-producing prostaglandins and stimulating the production of healthy prostaglandins. For this reason, I recommend the PMS diet for menstrual pain that occurs without heavy bleeding.

WATER FOR MENSTRUAL PAIN

What does the best drink of all — water — have to do with painful menses? The hormone vasopressin, also called antidiuretic hormone (ADH), is a factor in dysmenorrhea. Vasopressin stimulates contraction of smooth muscle, and when the smooth muscle of the uterus contracts excessively, you feel it as cramps. Medications have been used to decrease vasopressin in women with menstrual pain, who are known to overproduce this hormone.[12] However, there is a simple and natural way to decrease vasopressin — drink more water. Drinking more water beginning about three days or so before you expect your period is worth a try. You do not need huge amounts, but perhaps the eight glasses daily that many authorities recommend (but few women actually drink!).

SUPPLEMENTS FOR MENSTRUAL PAIN

FISH OIL. Fish oil, which is rich in the fatty acids EPA and DHA, has a strong anti-inflammatory effect. The "omega-3" fatty acid EPA is used by the cells to form the beneficial "series-3" prostaglandins that block the production of inflammatory prostaglandins. Several studies confirm the value of fish oil for menstrual pain.[13] In one study, Catholic high school girls in Cincinnati, all with dysmenorrhea, were given fish oil in capsules (1080 mg of EPA and 720 mg of DHA, the amount in about two teaspoons of cod liver oil) or a placebo. During the study, which was carried out in single-blinded, cross-over fashion, the girls were instructed to take ibuprofen for pain as needed. On average they took half as many ibuprofen pills for menstrual pain when they were using fish oil compared to the placebo.[14]

In a study involving Danish women, fish oil along with vitamin B12 (7.5 mcg/day) was used successfully to reduce menstrual pain. The authors noted that vitamin B12 strengthened the effect of the fish oil.[15] Natural fish oil (1-2 teaspoons daily), along with non-steroidal anti-inflammatory drugs if needed, is commonly used in Sweden by women with dysmenorrhea.[16]

VITAMIN E. In addition to lightening the period, vitamin E is also helpful for reducing menstrual pain.[17] It is an antioxidant that protects the beneficial fatty acids from destruction, which promotes an anti-inflammatory effect. Try a total of 400 IU of natural vitamin E daily, along with the other recommendations here, to help with menstrual cramping and pain.

MAGNESIUM, CALCIUM, AND VITAMIN D. Magnesium is a natural muscle relaxer, and is helpful to menstrual cramps.[18] About 800-1,000 mg/day is beneficial. Calcium also enables muscle relaxation. If you do not use dairy products, be sure to supplement about 800 mg daily. Calcium absorption requires vitamin D, so both are needed.

MULTIVITAMIN/MULTIMINERALS. Professional Prenatal Formula comes closest to "covering all the bases" for dysmenorrhea, but Optivite has also helped relieve menstrual pain, perhaps by increasing progesterone. (See "Resources.") Use either along with fish oil, or flax oil if you prefer. While flax oil has not been tested for dysmenorrhea, its omega-3 essential fatty acid can be converted to EPA and DHA if various vitamins and minerals are present, and it is wonderfully helpful for lightening heavy periods that contribute to menstrual pain.

—— ENDOMETRIOSIS ——

Endometriosis is one of the most common causes of very severe pain during menstruation, pain during intercourse, and heavy or irregular bleeding. The disease apparently begins when endometrial tissue moves backward through the fallopian tubes during the menses and is deposited within the abdominal cavity. Living cells in this tissue can proliferate within the abdomen, and when these abnormal "implants" are stimulated by cyclic hormonal changes, they build up and then bleed, causing inflammation and intense pain. However, as much as the pain must be managed, it is the high rate of infertility that concerns many women with endometriosis, as about one third of women with endometriosis have fertility problems.

The reasons for the high risk of infertility have not been well explained. If endometriosis is left untreated, infertility can be explained by scarring and inflammation from the endometrial implants. Yet the question remains: Why does infertility occur in women with milder degrees of the disease? Some possibilities may be problems with the endometrium that prevent implantation, ovarian hormone problems, ovulatory dysfunctions such as luteinized unruptured follicle (See Chapter 16, "Questions & Answers, Part II"), anti-sperm chemicals in the abdominal fluid, and luteal phase deficiency.[19] Resistance to the effects of progesterone because of inability of the receptors to respond to progesterone is one of several other areas of research.[20]

If you have endometriosis, you should make every effort to find a doctor who is an expert in this disease, and who is committed to doing his or her best to help you preserve your fertility if at all possible. However, your own self-care in the form of excellent nutrition can help with healing, reduce inflammation, reduce pain, and perhaps help prevent or overcome infertility.

LUTEAL PHASE DEFICIENCY AND ENDOMETRIOSIS
A possible link between luteal phase deficiency and endometriosis is worth considering. Luteal phase deficiency refers to low progesterone levels in the post-ovulatory (luteal) phase of the cycle. When a cycle is charted, it can be seen as poor temperature rise and fewer than normal elevated temperatures following ovulation. A study that compared women with endometriosis who were fertile to women with endometriosis who were infertile showed that the infertile group had low progesterone levels as well as elevated prolactin levels. The low progesterone seemed to be related to the elevated levels of the hormone prolactin; that is, high prolactin can affect the corpus luteum and decrease progesterone levels.[21]

Luteal phase deficiency may explain the high prevalence of endometriosis among women with PMS. As described in Chapter 5, abnormal luteal function is one cause of PMS. Doctors Joel Hargrove and Guy Abraham found that half of 137 PMS patients who underwent exploratory surgery for menstrual pain and/or infertility also had endometriosis.[22] These researchers have also found abnormal luteal function in women with endometriosis.[23]

Dr. Hargrove, a gynecologist in Vanderbilt, Tennessee, reports that 80 to 90 percent of women with endometriosis also have PMS. He has found that vitamin B6, which is a key vitamin for nutritional management of PMS, is also useful for symptomatic self-help treatment of endometriosis.[24]

PMS NUTRITIONAL STRATEGY FOR ENDOMETRIOSIS
Based on the research that supports the possibility of luteal phase deficiency as one of the causes of endometriosis, I recommend that you implement the complete PMS nutritional strategy, diet and supplements detailed in Chapter 5 as your basic nutritional self-care for endometriosis.

This diet and supplement program has been shown to improve luteal function by decreasing estrogen and increasing progesterone levels, as referenced in Chapter 5. Progesterone secreted by the corpus luteum prevents contractions of the uterus, which may be one link between luteal function and endometriosis. I am not aware of any studies in which the PMS nutritional plan has overcome infertility specifically related to endometriosis. However, if you are experiencing difficulty in conceiving because of this disease, I encourage you to implement the complete PMS program vigorously. Be sure to include supplemental flax oil and fish oil in amounts suggested in Chapter 3 for their anti-inflammatory effect. I also recommend this nutritional plan to help prevent recurrence of the disease following surgery to remove the abnormal endometrial tissue.

A large new study has shown that comprehensive nutritional supplements were as effective as oral contraceptives or gonadotropin releasing hormone analogues (GnRH-a) in reducing the pain of women who had undergone surgery for severe endometriosis. (The latter drug, in particular, has significant side effects similar to severe menopausal symptoms.) In this study, the women were given vitamins A, B6, C, and E; the minerals calcium, magnesium, selenium, zinc, and iron; a mix of "friendly" bacterial supplements; and omega-3 and omega-6 fatty acids for six months. The authors noted that nutritional therapy can be used indefinitely, and the patients in the study not only reported less pain, but also significantly better overall health and vitality.[25] Obviously, if a woman with endometriosis is attempting to become pregnant or to use NFP, nutritional therapy offers additional benefits compared to drug therapies which suppress her own hormones. Though the amounts of the supplements were unspecified, all of them, except for the "friendly" bacterial supplements, have been part of Dr. Guy Abraham's PMS diet plan since the 1980s.

OTHER HELPS FOR ENDOMETRIOSIS

ENZYMES, HERBAL REMEDIES, AND HORMONAL SUPPLEMENTS. Susan Lark, M.D., who is a nutritionally-oriented women's medical doctor, recommends a comprehensive multivitamin/multimineral supplement, as well as supplements containing the omega-3 fatty acid, EPA, found in fish oil (600 mg EPA daily, the amount in approximately 1½–2 teaspoons of cod liver oil). In addition, however, Dr. Lark recommends taking the digestive enzymes bromelain (500 mg) and papain (200-300 mg) between meals. She also recommends the herb pycnogenol (60 mg/day).[26] Pycnogenol, which is available at many health food shops, has been shown to reduce menstrual and pelvic pain more effectively than medications that work through repressing the entire cycle.[27] Based on animal studies, Dr. Lark also recommends 300 mcg to 1 mg of melatonin before bedtime.[28] If you are hoping to become pregnant, get your doctor's approval to use pycnogenol or melatonin supplements.

YEAST OVERGROWTH. Candidiasis, also called yeast overgrowth, is discussed in Chapter 9. It has been linked to a number of reproductive problems, including endometriosis. *The Yeast Connection and Women's Health*, by the late William Crook, M.D., contains a chapter on this "connection." In this chapter he also notes the close association between PMS, menstrual cramps, and endometriosis.[29] (See "Further Reading.")

NUTRITION, FERTILITY, AND ENDOMETRIOSIS. *Endometriosis: A Key to Healing through Nutrition*, is a very complete resource for all aspects of endometriosis, but especially for the role of nutrition in maintaining health and promoting fertility. It is a reference, not a page-by-page read, but the compassion of the authors and their encouragement permeate the book. (See "Further Reading.")

THE ENDOMETRIOSIS ASSOCIATION. Founded by Mary Lou Ballweg, who herself has endometriosis, and Carolyn Keith, its purpose is to assist women with endometriosis to find the best answers to their particular situation. (See "Resources.")

THE PMS DIET AND SUPPLEMENTS FOR SEVERE MENSTRUAL PAIN

The diet and supplements suggested in this chapter phenomenally helped a 24-year-old single woman with the worst dysmenorrhea I have ever encountered; in truth, I wonder if she actually had undiagnosed endometriosis. Her concerned older sister asked if she could bring her to me to discuss this problem. During our visit she described abdominal and back pain so wrenching she could hardly walk. She would be so ill that she spent three to five days in bed each month. I suggested that she consider Dr. Abraham's diet and nutritional supplements as explained in Chapter 5, including about 1,000 mg magnesium in a 2:1 ratio to calcium. She took the list of supplements and selected her own brands of vitamins from a health food shop. She felt "1,000 percent" better during her next period, and by the third cycle was "5,000 percent" better. Her sister and I chatted ten months later; she reported that the younger woman no longer misses any work, her PMS has also improved, and she is "5,000 percent better — at least!"

➤ Heavy, prolonged, and painful menstrual bleeding are common problems that usually respond quite well to improved nutrition.

➤ Diet and supplements aimed at improving the healing of the endometrium are helpful for prolonged or heavy bleeding, and less bleeding often reduces menstrual pain. Underlying causes such as fibroid tumors, endometriosis, and low thyroid function should also be considered.

➤ Besides improved diet, drinking more water, beginning two or three days before the period is expected, may help prevent menstrual cramps.

➤ Menstrual pain has been helped by supplements of fish oil, and since the same "bad" prostaglandins are involved in menstrual pain and PMS, the PMS nutritional plan described in Chapter 5 may be helpful.

➤ New research into the causes of endometriosis has led to studies involving supplements that decrease inflammation.

➤ Nutrition directed at overcoming PMS and short luteal phase is also helpful to endometriosis, since women with endometriosis often experience both of those symptoms.

7

Four Common Causes of Cycle Irregularities & Female Infertility

There is an appointed time for everything, and a time for every affair under the heavens. — Ecclesiastes 3:1

It is paradoxical that the same information that allows couples to use natural family planning (NFP) to avoid becoming pregnant is also extremely helpful to couples who are hoping to become pregnant, but are having difficulty doing so. In both cases, the NFP chart reveals the potentially fertile time. Couples wishing to postpone a pregnancy avoid relations during the fertile time, while couples having difficulty conceiving identify the fertile time and then specifically use that time in order to increase their chances of conceiving.

Attempting to make the menstrual cycle more regular also helps women, whether they are postponing a pregnancy or are actively trying to conceive. For women using NFP in order to avoid conceiving, a more regular cycle makes it easier to identify the potentially fertile versus infertile times, and so it often shortens the time of abstinence. This is true even though high effectiveness can be achieved despite irregular cycles, since modern NFP relies on ongoing signs of fertility and infertility. For women trying to increase their chances of becoming pregnant, a more regular cycle is often a healthier, more fertile cycle with more chances of ovulating a mature ovum. Improving cycle irregularities with better nutrition is a basic self-help tool for those experiencing infertility.

If you are hoping to increase your fertility through self-care, improved nutrition may help you to conceive, as it has other couples in the studies cited in this chapter. However, even if your focus on nutrition does not help you directly, you will be in much better physical condition to respond to hormonal or medical therapy, if that is what it takes to help you to achieve your desire for a child.

FERTILITY AND INFERTILITY: A CONTINUUM
Your fertility depends on a complex interaction among several hormones which stimulate ovulation and maintain the cycle afterwards. As a review, please reread the information on the normal fertility-menstrual cycle which

appears at the beginning of Part II. It is also useful to realize that female fertility is not an "all-or-nothing" phenomenon. Instead, a continuum exists between normal high fertility, cycle irregularities, and complete infertility. This is not to imply that irregular cycles generally indicate infertility, although in some women some types of recurring cycle irregularities do signal decreased fertility. Cycle irregularity differs from infertility by a matter of degree, as sprinkles differ from a rainstorm. That is why the same nutritional guidelines apply to the fertile woman with troublesome cycle characteristics as to the woman having difficulty in conceiving.

THE CONTINUUM OF FERTILITY: BREASTFEEDING. The experience of a nursing mother — as she follows a continuum from complete infertility to normal fertility — is instructive for non-nursing women with irregular cycles or unexplained infertility.

When the hormones of ovulation — FSH and LH — are consistently low, as in a nursing mother with extended amenorrhea (the absence of periods), follicle development does not occur and the endometrium does not develop. The result is that neither ovulation nor menstruation occurs. As she begins to produce more of the reproductive hormones, cervical mucus appears and the endometrium develops. If the nursing mother does not ovulate, eventually the endometrium will be shed anyway, causing spotting or a full, sometimes prolonged episode of bleeding. Such a "period" without previous ovulation indicates that an infertile, "anovulatory cycle" has occurred. It is common for a breastfeeding mother to have one or several such anovulatory cycles and periods.

As the inhibition of fertility caused by the hormones of breastfeeding continues to subside, increased FSH and LH may stimulate an ovarian follicle to develop to some extent, and an immature egg, probably incapable of fertilization, may be ovulated. If so, a basal temperature shift occurs, although it may be less than the usual shift of 0.4° F. Since the levels of FSH and LH in the pre-ovulatory phase set the stage for the function of the corpus luteum after ovulation, luteal function may be reduced. A sympto-thermal chart, on which the signs of fertility are recorded, may show this with a luteal (post-ovulatory) phase which is quite a bit shorter than the normal twelve to sixteen days of elevated basal temperatures. Pregnancy is less likely to occur if the duration of elevated temperatures in the luteal phase is less than nine to twelve days. Spotting may also occur before the actual period begins, while the temperatures are still elevated. Such "irregular shedding" may be yet another manifestation of luteal insufficiency. The entire pattern at this stage of the nursing mother's return to fertility commonly includes an extended patch of "more fertile" mucus prior to ovulation, as well as a delay in ovulation that may cause a long cycle.

Finally, the fertility pattern of the nursing mother returns to its familiar norms, and she may continue to nurse for many months while having fertile ovulatory cycles, and she may even conceive again while doing so.

THE CONTINUUM OF FERTILITY: WEIGHT LOSS. Another example of the continuum between fertility and infertility is the change that takes place in a woman who exercises vigorously, but does not eat enough food to maintain her body fat. If she would eat enough calories for the exercise and to maintain body fat, she could expect to have normal, regular cycles. However, if she loses too much body fat, she may experience a delay in ovulation, resulting in a long cycle. Or, she may seem to have no change in her overall cycle length, but charting will reveal that she is ovulating later in the cycle than before, and that she has developed a short luteal phase. If she continues to exercise vigorously and to lose more body fat, she will experience anovulatory cycles. Further loss of body fat will put her into complete amenorrhea.[1] Such a pattern is quite reversible if she can consume sufficient calories, or if she cuts down on the amount of strenuous exercise.

THE CONTINUUM OF FERTILITY: PERIMENOPAUSE. Yet another example of this continuum occurs as women approach menopause. During this time, the menstrual cycles often become shorter, with short pre-ovulatory phases along with short luteal phases. As more time passes, though, longer cycles with delayed ovulation become common. The last few episodes of bleeding are likely to follow anovulatory cycles, and by definition menopause is followed by complete — and final — amenorrhea.

There are many causes of cycle irregularity in women. Sometimes the cause is not known for certain, but often the NFP chart provides excellent clues as to what is actually occurring. What follows are cycle irregularities that can be seen by charting, along with strategies to improve them. Even though you may never be absolutely certain of the cause of your cycle irregularity or infertility, you can take heart from the fact that nutrition by itself can often improve cycle irregularity and sometimes lead to long-awaited pregnancies.

—— LUTEAL PHASE DEFICIENCY ——

CHARTED SIGNS OF LUTEAL PHASE DEFICIENCY, also called "luteal phase defect" or "luteal phase inadequacy": *Short luteal phase (fewer than nine to twelve days of elevated post-ovulatory temperatures, or fewer than nine days of post-peak mucus days[2]), premenstrual spotting, postmenstrual brown bleeding or spotting, poor temperature rise after ovulation, extended mucus, poor mucus quality, amenorrhea, early miscarriage, infertility.* In some women, the periods occur at quite regular intervals, and the entire cycle is short in length. In other women the entire cycle may be prolonged, as ovulation is delayed. In either case, when the cycle is charted it is obvious that the post-ovulatory phase is short. PMS may also be related to this pattern.

It is entirely possible for any woman to have a short luteal phase cycle occasionally, but more often such cycles recur month after month. The hormone levels of the previous cycle set the stage for the next cycle, so that one cycle is intimately connected to the next. If your pattern of short luteal phase is occurring regularly, there are steps you can take to improve it. Improving the short luteal phase will increase the post-ovulatory infertile time for couples avoiding a pregnancy, reducing abstinence, and it will increase the chance of conception among couples attempting to overcome infertility.

UNDERLYING CAUSES

Luteal phase deficiency results from low levels of progesterone during the post-ovulatory phase of the cycle. The corpus luteum, which produces the progesterone after the ovum is released from the follicle, does not do its job as well or as long as it ought. Since progesterone is the cause of the basal body temperature elevation during this time, low levels of progesterone cause the poor upward shift of temperatures and the short luteal phase. Progesterone distinctly affects the characteristics of the mucus, explaining why a poor mucus pattern may result. Progesterone causes growth in the thickness of the endometrium and prevents menstruation. When it is too low, spotting may occur before the full period, and brown spotting may follow or end the period.

What causes progesterone to be too low? Or more specifically, what causes the corpus luteum to secrete inadequate amounts of this hormone? One possibility is high levels of estrogen, caused by poor diet or by overweight. High estrogen levels decrease progesterone. "Bad" local hormones, called prostaglandins, are another cause, since they interfere with the function of the corpus luteum. High levels of the hormone prolactin may be involved;[3] it is known that in breastfeeding women, high prolactin, which is normal while nursing, inhibits the FSH and LH and so inhibits the development of the follicle and corpus luteum.

Low thyroid function can also underlie short luteal phase. If you are experiencing very low pre-ovulatory temperatures, in the range of 97.2° F or below, please refer to "Low Thyroid Function" later in this chapter. Vigorous exercise that causes you to lose body fat can also cause short luteal phases, and the topic "Underweight or Inadequate Body Fat" in this chapter is intended to help you get started on the goal of restoring normal cycles. Of course, if you are currently breastfeeding a baby, short luteal phases can be a natural part of the transition from infertility to fertility, as explained in the introductory example of this chapter.

INFERTILITY AND RECURRENT MISCARRIAGE

Luteal phase deficiency results in an increased risk of infertility and miscarriage.[4] Many researchers attribute this to the poor development of the endometrium, which results in poor implantation of the embryo if conception occurs.

However, what happens before ovulation affects the luteal phase, and also affects fertility even before the time of implantation. If the follicle does not develop well before ovulation, the corpus luteum will also be inadequate, and will produce inadequate progesterone.[5] But equally important, immediately before ovulation, the unfertilized ovum must complete the cell division called meiosis I, as explained in the Introduction to Part II. The same hormones responsible for development of the follicle and its secretion of estrogen before ovulation — FSH and LH — are also responsible for stimulating the cell division of the ovum, which is called the maturation of the ovum. If the hormonal "push" early in the cycle is insufficient to cause the all-important meiosis I to occur properly, then the ovum will not be genetically normal. Most often it will not be able to be fertilized, so that conception will not occur. If conception does occur with such an abnormal ovum, the newly conceived child cannot develop properly, and an early miscarriage will result.[6]

NUTRITION FOR LUTEAL PHASE DEFICIENCY

Can nutrition help you to overcome a short luteal phase and its related manifestations? The nutritional research says "yes."

OVERALL DIET. Most of the underlying causes of luteal phase deficiency are also involved in premenstrual syndrome (PMS), which has been related to poor luteal function. The nutritional plan developed by Dr. Guy Abraham and explained in Chapter 5 is intended to correct these problems and to raise progesterone. For this reason, the overall nutritional strategy for improving luteal phase deficiency is to implement the PMS dietary guidelines of Chapter 5. The dietary recommendations of the PMS diet plan are similar to "Twelve Rules for Improved Nutrition" in Chapter 1, and can be used interchangeably.

VITAMIN B6. Vitamin B6 alone (200-600 mg/day) has lowered prolactin levels and restored regular cycles to women with the severe overproduction of prolactin that causes both amenorrhea and galactorrhea (milk in the breasts of non-nursing women).[7]

In a truly remarkable study, vitamin B6, a critical nutrient for PMS sufferers, was given in 100-800 mg/day doses to fourteen women who had normal menstrual cycles but also had PMS and infertility of eighteen months to seven years' duration. Ten of the fourteen had never borne a child, while the other four were experiencing secondary infertility. Twelve of the women conceived, eleven within six months of the vitamin B6 therapy. In this study, prolactin levels were not found to change, but progesterone levels were significantly increased in several of the women, indicating that the vitamin B6 had improved their luteal function.[8]

Please note that these amounts of vitamin B6 are not recommended by themselves. Instead, B6 should be taken in amounts not exceeding 300 mg daily, and along with other B vitamins and magnesium, as explained in Chapter 5.

VITAMIN C. Another study has shown that vitamin C can increase progesterone levels to normal in some women with luteal phase deficiency, enabling some of them to conceive. Japanese researchers hypothesized that oxidative stress decreases the activity of the corpus luteum and causes it to secrete insufficient progesterone. They provided the antioxidant vitamin C or a placebo pill to 150 women with carefully diagnosed luteal phase deficiency as well as infertility. Of the women who took vitamin C (750 mg daily), 53 percent had a significant increase in their mid-luteal phase progesterone, from an average of 7.51 to 13.27 ng/ml (greater than 10 ng/ml was considered normal). Twenty-five percent of the women taking vitamin C conceived within six months. Of the placebo group, 22 percent had improvement in their progesterone level spontaneously, and 11 percent conceived. The miscarriage rate was 16 percent in those taking vitamin C and 20 percent in those taking the placebo (though this difference was not statistically significant).[9]

It is worthwhile to note that in this study the vitamin C was discontinued as soon as pregnancy was confirmed, which I believe was an imprudent aspect of the experimental design. I suspect that the miscarriage rate would have been significantly lower if the vitamin C, which is safe and beneficial during pregnancy, had been continued. The women in the study had previously experienced low levels of progesterone that were normalized by the supplementation of vitamin C, and continued vitamin C very likely would have continued to support their progesterone levels.

OPTIVITE PMT. The PMS nutritional supplement Optivite PMT, developed by Dr. Guy Abraham and recommended in Chapter 5, contains several nutrients (vitamin B6, magnesium, and zinc) that help to reduce prolactin. In reality, the supplement is designed to overcome the luteal phase inadequacy that may contribute to PMS.[10] Optivite's 300 mg of B6 and 1,500 mg of vitamin C are most likely responsible for the finding that Optivite, plus dietary improvement, has restored low luteal phase progesterone and high luteal phase estrogen to normal levels.[11] Mucus and temperature patterns returned to normal within three to six months in some women who followed Abraham's PMS nutritional plan as well as exercise and stress reduction.[12] Improvement in the length of the luteal phase as well as improved mucus pattern have been commonly reported to the Couple to Couple League by women who have taken Optivite.

PROCYCLE PMS is a supplement which is very similar to Optivite, but contains no iron and is formulated for only four tablets daily. You may prefer to use it instead. (See Appendix A for complete contents of Optivite PMT and ProCycle PMS.)

FERTILITY BLEND. A nutritional supplement called Fertility Blend has also improved the rate of conception in women with infertility, while significantly raising the mid-luteal levels of progesterone in women with low progesterone before treatment. Fertility Blend contains green tea, which has antioxidant capabilities higher than that of vitamin C. It also contains the herb *Vitex agnus castus*, or chasteberry extract, which previous studies have shown to increase progesterone levels.[13] In addition, it contains the antioxidant vitamin E (150 IU), folic acid (400 mcg), magnesium (400 mg), selenium (70 mcg), zinc (15 mg), as well as other nutrients. (See Appendix A.) Of 53 infertile women taking Fertility Blend in a double-blind study, 26 percent conceived within three months, compared to 10 percent of women taking the placebo. Also of interest to NFP users was the effect on charted basal body temperature: Women taking Fertility Blend in non-conception cycles averaged two more days per cycle of temperatures over 98.6° F compared to controls.[14]

A double-blind study using chasteberry extract alone produced similar results; 20 mg daily of Vitex extract given to 52 women with luteal phase deficiency due to elevated levels of prolactin resulted in a reduction of their prolactin levels. Levels of progesterone returned to normal, as did the length of the luteal phase.[15]

SUMMARY OF RECOMMENDATIONS FOR LUTEAL PHASE DEFICIENCY. Improve your diet as recommended in Part I of this book. Review Chapter 5, "Premenstrual Syndrome (PMS)," even if you do not have PMS. PMS has been related to luteal phase deficiency, and the details of diet and vitamins, minerals, and essential fatty acids for PMS have been studied, and are also helpful for luteal phase problems.

With your doctor's approval, supplement Optivite PMT, ProCycle PMS, or Fertility Blend, along with flax oil and/or fish oil in the amounts recommended in Table 7 (Chapter 3). Chapter 5 compares Optivite PMT to ProCycle, and also explains that any other brand of vitamin and mineral supplements can be used instead, as long as the amounts of the nutrients are similar. Strenuous exercise and low thyroid function can result in poor luteal phases. See the sections in this chapter, "Low Thyroid Function," and "Underweight or Inadequate Body Fat" for a discussion of these topics. Finally, if you are hoping to achieve pregnancy at an older age, or if you have had recurrent miscarriages, see the section on "Age-Related Infertility" in Chapter 9, or "Repeated Miscarriage & Birth Defects" in Chapter 11.

—— LOW THYROID FUNCTION ——

CHARTED SIGNS OF LOW THYROID FUNCTION: *Unusually low basal temperatures, long cycles, prolonged "less fertile" mucus, short luteal phase, anovulatory cycles, heavy menses, prolonged menses, unexplained infertility or miscarriage.* In addition, low thyroid function can also cause or contribute to reproductive problems not seen on the chart, notably low sexual desire, PMS, painful periods, and galactorrhea (milk in the breasts of non-nursing women). It is also responsible for a number of non-reproductive problems — anxiety, mental confusion, intolerance to cold, weight gain, dry skin, hair loss, and ongoing fatigue.

If you have suffered from some of the reproductive symptoms of low thyroid function listed above, there is a good chance that your physician has already tested your thyroid hormones. It is well known that thyroid dysfunction can cause problems with a woman's cycle and fertility. For reasons that are not always clear, however, low thyroid function may not be detected by blood tests for the various thyroid hormones. This problem of diagnosis has led to the term "subclinical hypothyroidism." Or, you may have had a diagnosis of hypothyroidism and are taking thyroid medication, yet you are still experiencing cycle irregularities. Insufficient thyroid hormone replacement could be involved.

THYROID HORMONES

The thyroid gland, situated like a small bow tie right at the base of the neck, secretes several hormones. The two most important ones are abbreviated "T₄" for thyroxine and "T₃" for tri-iodothyronine. Thyroid hormones contain iodine; T₄ refers to the hormone with four iodine molecules, and T₃ contains three attached iodines. About four-fifths of the hormone secreted into the blood is T₄; the rest is T₃. However, T₄ is much less active than T₃, so the body must convert the T₄ into T₃, a process that depends on several nutrients. The thyroid hormones affect virtually all cells in the body by stimulating their various activities, which explains why low thyroid function can have such seemingly diverse symptoms as hair loss, infertility, and mental confusion.

THYROID FUNCTION AND THE CYCLE. The major effects on the menstrual cycle and fertility occur because thyroid hormones affect or are affected by several other hormones, including estrogen, progesterone, prolactin, and cortisol. Low thyroid hormone can indirectly cause elevated prolactin, which in turn can be responsible for short luteal phase, infertility, miscarriage, and galactorrhea. Thyroid hormones enable body cells to use more fuel and to produce more heat. When thyroid function is low, the basal body temperature is often lower than normal. That is the link between easy weight gain and hypothyroidism; without normal thyroid function, the cells burn their fuel more slowly than normal. Thyroid hormones also affect blood clotting; low levels decrease the production of coagulation factors needed by the blood, explaining at least in part the heavy menses that often occur with low thyroid function.[16]

UNDERLYING CAUSES OF LOW THYROID FUNCTION

There are a number of factors that may cause thyroid function to be abnormally low, resulting in either subclinical or full-blown hypothyroidism. Nutritional deficiencies can prevent the thyroid gland from doing its job. Iodine is well known to be essential for the production of thyroid hormones, but a number of other vitamins, minerals, and the essential fatty acids are also necessary for the production and activation of thyroid hormones.

One of the most common causes of hypothyroidism is Hashimoto's thyroiditis, an autoimmune disease in which one's own antibodies disrupt normal thyroid function. In some women, the thyroid gland may temporarily malfunction for a time after a woman gives birth, but it often corrects itself within a few months. Sometimes, though, persistent hypothyroidism begins after childbirth. (See Chapter 10's section on "Postpartum Thyroiditis" for more information.) Removal or inactivation of the thyroid gland to treat elevated thyroid function (hyperthyroidism) or more rarely, thyroid cancer, also produces hypothyroidism which must be treated medically. Low thyroid function can occur due to insufficient medical replacement of thyroid hormone, or replacement with T₄ alone, instead of a mix of T₄ and T₃, as is more natural.

Hormones from other glands also affect thyroid function. Normal levels of progesterone from the corpus luteum promote thyroid function in several ways. Progesterone enables the body's cells to bind T3, so that the cells can respond to thyroid hormone. Progesterone also decreases the production of a blood protein called thyroxine-binding globulin, an effect that increases the availability of thyroid hormone to the cells. Conversely, high estrogen levels block the function of thyroid hormones within the body cells.[17] The adrenal hormone cortisol, which rises during prolonged stress, also blocks the function of the thyroid hormones within the body's cells.[18]

NUTRITION FOR LOW THYROID FUNCTION

FOODS THAT INTERFERE WITH THYROID FUNCTION. Trans fats found in processed foods such as shortening and margarine interfere with normal cellular function and should be avoided, as pointed out in Rule 3 of Chapter 1. Of course, improving diet generally is helpful to the entire body, and it is basic to glandular health.

However, when it comes to low thyroid function, certain foods should be avoided or eaten in moderation. Unfermented soy foods eaten in significant quantities have anti-thyroid properties that can affect thyroid function.[19] Avoid soy milk, soy powder, tofu, and so forth as part of your self-care for low thyroid function. (Intake of foods which contain soy oil, such as salad dressings, need not be restricted.)

Very high consumption of certain raw vegetables and fruits can also have anti-thyroid effects. These include cabbage, Brussels sprouts, broccoli, kale, radishes, turnips, spinach, mustard greens, peanuts, peaches, and pears. Please do not avoid these healthy foods entirely; if they are cooked, the potentially anti-thyroid enzymes are destroyed. According to thyroid patient advocate Mary Shomon, people who have had their thyroid gland removed and who are receiving thyroid replacement hormones do not need to be concerned at all, but even those who are dealing with low thyroid function can eat these vegetable and fruits, raw or cooked, in moderation.[20]

Finally, if you are fighting low thyroid function, you may wish to drink purified water. Both fluoridated and chlorinated water can interfere with the thyroid gland's use of iodine.[21]

SUPPLEMENTS FOR LOW THYROID FUNCTION. Adding iodized salt (not plain sea salt) to the diet has improved cycle irregularity and irregular mucus patterns in women who were using little or no iodized salt.[22] If you prefer not to consume extra salt, you can get iodine from a multivitamin/multimineral or from tablets of kelp, a type of seaweed (150–225 mcg of iodine is a typical daily dose). Besides iodine, the B vitamins and vitamins C and E aid thyroid function. True vitamin A from fish oil helps the thyroid gland. Some people with low thyroid function cannot turn beta-carotene, the precursor of vitamin A, into true vitamin A. Zinc and selenium are especially important to thyroid function, in part because they enable the conversion of T4 into the active form, T3. Two hundred mcg of selenium daily can also help reduce autoimmune inflammation, as in Hashimoto's thyroiditis.[23] The essential fatty acids found in flax oil stimulate all glands, including the thyroid gland, and the omega-3 essential fatty acid has anti-inflammatory properties.

I usually recommend Professional Prenatal Formula as well as flax oil (five to ten 1 g capsules daily) when I see very low temperatures as well as poor mucus patterns and poor temperature rises on a chart. (See "Resources.") I have seen women's basal temperatures gradually rise to normal, over a period of about two to three weeks, when they supplement as recommended here. I have also had the interesting experience of seeing the reverse — women with low basal temperatures and poor chart patterns whose charts improved substantially once they took a supplement like Professional Prenatal Formula, only to gradually revert back to poor patterns and low temperatures after they discontinued it.

OTHER SELF-CARE

Moderate exercise, especially in cool weather, or cool-temperature activities such as swimming, may stimulate the thyroid gland, as it naturally responds to cold temperatures by increasing its hormonal output. Oppositely, the stress of excessive exercise accompanied by loss of body fat may contribute to a "hypometabolic state" which includes lowered levels of progesterone.[24]

Rose Frisch, Ph.D., who studied Harvard University women athletes throughout her long career, observed the effect of excessive exercise on body temperature. She wrote that "the baseline temperature measurement of most of the well-trained athletes amazed us right from the start. Their evening temperatures ranged around 96.5° F. Practically no one had an evening temperature of 98.6° F."[25]

This effect may well be related to high levels of the stress hormone cortisol, which interferes with thyroid function. Excessive exercise is a stress that can take its toll on the thyroid. Besides engaging in moderate exercise only, other effective ways of lowering your stress hormones include eating a good diet, taking supplements of essential nutrients, and getting enough sleep. Doing so is not just good for your moods and energy; it is good for your thyroid gland, too. (See Chapter 14, "Increasing Your Energy & Decreasing Your Stress.")

MEDICAL TREATMENT

Nutrition and other self-care by themselves can improve the symptoms listed above. However, in some cases thyroid hormone replacement may be necessary. If so, you should be aware that there are more and more doctors who are willing to prescribe natural "Armour" thyroid replacement, because it contains the active T3 form as well as the less active T4 hormone.[26] L-thyroxine (Synthroid, Levoxyl, Levothroid) contains the T4 hormone only. About 25 percent of people with subclinical hypothyroidism are actually taking T4 therapy alone, according to a recent review article.[27]

DIAGNOSING LOW THYROID FUNCTION. During my early years as an NFP teacher, I was often puzzled that women with several of the cycle problems listed above, such as very low basal temperatures, would test normal for blood levels of thyroid hormones. That puzzle was solved for me when I discovered the book *Hypothyroidism: The Unsuspected Illness*, by the late Broda Barnes, M.D. Dr. Barnes was a young physician before World War II. Like other physicians back then, he used physical findings such as heavy bleeding, infertility, and so forth to diagnosis low thyroid function, along with a determination of basal metabolic rate, the oxygen consumption test. He treated patients diagnosed with low thyroid function with natural thyroid hormone, and found that it was effective in helping such women overcome heavy periods, repeated miscarriage, and infertility. When blood tests for thyroid hormone became available in the 1940's, these laboratory blood tests replaced the diagnosis based on the patient's symptoms and physical examination — but many fewer women were diagnosed with hypothyroidism, even if they still had clinical symptoms of it, or even if they had been on thyroid replacement and had been doing well with it.[28]

Instead of relying on blood tests that he considered inaccurate, Dr. Barnes developed the "Barnes basal temperature test" for thyroid function. He studied the relationship between the underarm basal temperature and the "gold standard" oxygen consumption test, and found that the easy-to-take basal temperature correlated very well with the cumbersome but reliable oxygen consumption test. He considered basal temperatures below 97.8° F a possible sign of low thyroid function. For menstruating women, he used pre-ovulatory temperatures taken on days 2 or 3 of the cycle; for other women, men, or children, any day's temperature was usable.[29] His book states that the underarm basal temperature is about the same as the oral basal temperature.[30]

Dr. Barnes died in 1988, but his work is being carried on through the Broda O. Barnes Research Foundation. (See "Resources.") This organization, located in Trumbull, Connecticut, promotes membership of "Barnes-aware" physicians who value the basal temperature chart as a diagnostic tool. The organization also promotes 24-hour urine tests for thyroid hormone as well as other hormones, and recommends natural thyroid hormone replacement instead of synthetic hormones such as Synthroid.[31]

I have looked at many NFP charts over the years, and on one point I disagree with the work of Dr. Barnes. While he states that basal temperatures below 97.8° F may indicate low thyroid function, I have seen many, many charts with pre-ovulatory temperatures in the range of 97.3–97.7° F that seem otherwise completely normal, and the women were experiencing good health. This discrepancy may actually have to do with Dr. Barnes' protocol of using temperatures during Days 2–3 of the cycle, whereas I always consider the six low temperatures right before ovulation occurs and the temperatures rise. When temperatures during the pre-ovulatory time hover around 97.2° F and below, I think low thyroid function should certainly be considered if the chart shows other irregularities or if infertility is an issue. Self-help to improve thyroid function, as described above, should be the first step, and should be tried for about three months.

WHY AREN'T THYROID TESTS COMPLETELY RELIABLE? There are several theories to explain why tests for thyroid function are not always accurate. First, the thyroid hormone in the blood is overwhelmingly the inactive "T4" hormone, which must be converted in the tissues to the active form, "T3." Direct testing of the active T3 hormone in each cell is not possible. The conversion of T4 to T3 depends on a number of nutrients, including the mineral selenium. Second, the standards for "normal" thyroid function may be too broad, even though the range for "normal" has been narrowed in the last few years. Third, high levels of estrogen can block thyroid function within the body cells, as can high levels of stress hormones.

DIFFICULTY IN DIAGNOSIS OF HYPOTHYROIDISM: ONE WOMAN'S EXPERIENCE. A woman I'll call Jane was very much helped by Dr. Barnes' research regarding the value of the basal temperature chart, other charted information, her own persistence, and the assistance of a "Barnes-aware" medical doctor. When she contacted me, her pre-ovulatory temperatures were as low as 96.3° F. Her temperature shift was poor, with only nine elevated temperatures in the luteal phase before the next menses. (Twelve to sixteen elevated temperatures are normal for the luteal phase.) She had brown bleeding at the end of the menstrual period, and then a pattern of less-fertile "tacky" mucus that began immediately and never changed to stretchy, more-fertile mucus.

Jane was in her mid-30's at the time and had four young children, none of them breastfeeding. She made some other notes on her charts, especially about the painful periods. She felt generally unwell, and was avoiding a pregnancy. Because of the chart problems — this was her monthly pattern — the abstinence phase was prolonged. She said she had low libido and bad PMS.

When I reviewed Jane's charts, I felt sure that the problem was low thyroid function, and suggested that she get her thyroid hormones tested. Jane did see her family doctor, who performed standard thyroid tests at her request. All came back normal. I encouraged her to seek further testing. She followed up by seeing a hormone specialist who performed new tests. All were normal. When Jane asked this doctor about a lump she found growing on the front of her neck, the specialist was not at all concerned about it.

Jane persisted and made an appointment with a second specialist. When she met him, he had her test results from the previous doctors in his hand, and he said as he walked into the consultation room: "I'm not going to redo these tests. You've already been tested twice. I'm going to put you on [an anti-anxiety medication]. Ninety percent of the patients who come here are anxious." When Jane called his attention to the lump on her neck, he completely changed. She left with an appointment for a biopsy of her thyroid gland and the fear that it might be cancer.

At this point Jane decided to use the services of a "Barnes-aware" medical doctor in another town. This doctor took her history, reviewed her NFP charts and her previous medical tests, and concluded that she had low thyroid function. He recommended that she first have the abnormal growth on her thyroid evaluated and removed by a surgeon. She did so; it turned out to be a benign hypothyroid goiter.

Afterwards, the "Barnes-aware" doctor prescribed nutritional supplements similar to those in this book to see if he could help her improve her thyroid function. (Jane had already tried the nutrition recommended in my book very conscientiously, but to no avail.) When nutrition failed to make a difference, the doctor started Jane on the natural "Armour" thyroid hormone. He very gradually increased her dose over a period of months.

A year later, Jane was so pleased with her improvement that she surprised me by mailing me a recent NFP chart. While her pre-ovulatory temperatures were still low compared to most women's charts, they were noticeably higher than they had been. More significantly, her luteal phase, which had been nine days, was lengthened to twelve days, which is within the normal range. Her period was shorter and lighter, and her mucus pattern was completely normal. The time of abstinence the new chart required was far less than for her previous charts when her hypothyroidism was undiagnosed and untreated.

Please refer to *The Thyroid Hormone Breakthrough* by Mary Shomon, which exhorts women to fight for accurate diagnosis and effective treatment for thyroid and related hormonal dysfunction. (See "Further Reading.")

—— HYPERTHYROIDISM ——
(ABNORMALLY HIGH THYROID FUNCTION)

CHARTED SIGNS OF HYPERTHYROIDISM: *Unusually high basal temperatures (pre-ovulatory temperatures averaging 98.4° F and above), light menses, short cycles, short luteal phase, infertility.* In addition, hyperthyroidism may cause milk in the breasts of non-nursing women (galactorrhea).

This problem is the reverse of low thyroid function, but it can also contribute to cycle irregularity and infertility. However, it is less common than low thyroid function. Aside from the symptoms listed above, hyperthyroidism can cause symptoms unrelated to reproduction, such as excess sweating, hand tremors, anxiety, elevated resting heart rate, unexplained weight loss, and swelling in the neck (goiter). The cause may be an autoimmune disease called Graves' disease that "tricks" the thyroid gland into producing excess hormone. Excess thyroid medication prescribed to treat hypothyroidism (low thyroid function) is another possible cause of hyperthyroidism.[32] Galactorrhea may occur with hyperthyroidism because the imbalance in the control of the thyroid hormones elevates the hormone prolactin, which is responsible for milk production.

If you suspect that hyperthyroidism may be the cause of your cycle irregularities or infertility, you should first seek accurate medical diagnosis. You should also look into the possibility of iodine overdose. Kelp tablets, multivitamins, excess iodized salt, and ocean fish are sources of iodine that should be considered. Hyperthyroidism increases the need for all nutrients because it raises the body's energy expenditure, so excellent nutrition as outlined in Part I of this book is a basic part of recovering health.

However, nutritional improvement alone cannot correct hyperthyroidism, and medical intervention may be necessary. Treating hyperthyroidism may involve removing all or part of the gland, or interfering with its ability to produce the excess hormones. Unfortunately, such treatment results in hypothyroidism, which becomes the long-term situation that must be managed medically. Mary Shomon, the author of *The Thyroid Hormone Breakthrough*, has also written *Living Well with Graves' Disease or Hyperthyroidism*.

—— UNDERWEIGHT OR INADEQUATE BODY FAT ——

CHARTED SIGNS OF UNDERWEIGHT OR LOW BODY FAT: *Long cycles, often with scant cervical mucus, delayed ovulation which may or may not be followed by short luteal phase, anovulatory cycles, complete amenorrhea, infertility, miscarriage.* If your basal body temperatures are low (pre-ovulatory temperatures averaging 97.2° F or less), please also see "Low Thyroid Function." If your basal body temperatures are abnormally high (pre-ovulatory temperatures averaging about 98.4° F), see "Hyperthyroidism."

UNDERLYING CAUSES OF UNDERWEIGHT-RELATED CYCLE IRREGULARITIES

According to the pioneering studies of Harvard researcher Rose E. Frisch, Ph.D., your body fat must contribute at least 22 percent to your total body weight if you are to have normal menstrual cycles.[33] It was Dr. Frisch who first reported that among slender women, losing or gaining as little as three to five pounds could cause the menstrual cycle to stop or to return again.[34]

Body fat profoundly affects female fertility for a number of reasons. First of all, fatty tissue is an important source of estrogen. It converts androgens (male hormones) to estrogen, and during a woman's fertile years it provides about one third of her total estrogen. Second, lean women make a less potent form of estrogen than do women with more body fat, and the less potent estrogen has less ability to stimulate the various reproductive functions. Third, thin women have higher than average amounts of a blood protein — sex hormone-binding globulin — which binds estrogen; therefore, they have less free estrogen available for stimulation of the reproductive organs.[35]

Fourth, in excessively lean women, the part of the brain that controls the pituitary gland, the hypothalamus, does not properly stimulate the fertility hormones FSH and LH. Normally the hypothalamus secretes a hormone, GnRH, in pulses every ninety minutes or so. GnRH stimulates FSH and LH. When the body lacks sufficient fat, the hypothalamus no longer secretes GnRH in the normal pattern. In response, FSH and LH levels drop and are secreted in patterns similar to that of pre-adolescent girls. The hormone leptin, produced by the fat cells, stimulates the normal release of GnRH. A lack of body fat results in a lack of leptin, and so the GnRH secretion drops.[36] For these and for other reasons which are still under investigation, being too lean adversely affects your cycles.

CAUSES OF LOW BODY FAT. As you can see, cycle irregularities and infertility are more related to low body fat than to low body weight. Understanding why your body fat is low is helpful to making the adjustments necessary to restore your cycle regularity or your fertility. Your low body fat could just be part of your natural body build. Perhaps you come from a family of slender folks, and it is easy for you to remain thin, even without much exercise. In this society, many women are motivated to remain thin, as thinness is considered attractive. Maybe it has never occurred to you that your long, irregular cycles are related to being slender. If you are eating a vegetarian or vegan diet, either of these could possibly be at the root of your cycle or fertility problems. Or perhaps you are the type of person who cannot seem to eat well when stressed, and you are under fairly constant, though not necessarily intense, stress. Smoking cigarettes is yet another contributor to underweight, though there are many other serious reasons to quit.

If you are prone to diarrhea when eating certain foods, intestinal disorders or food allergies could be a factor. An intolerance to gluten, a protein found in wheat, rye, and barley, is called celiac disease, and could be responsible for low body weight and low body fat. (Celiac disease is discussed in Chapter 9.) If recurring bouts of diarrhea are part of your low body weight or low body fat, it is important to discuss it with a doctor.

Your exercise regimen could be the cause of short luteal phases, long cycles, anovulatory cycles, or no cycles at all. Vigorous exercise can decrease your body fat and increase your muscle mass while you maintain a completely normal weight for your height. You may enjoy the challenge of preparing for and running a marathon race, or maybe you are a dedicated dancer, gymnast, swimmer, or basketball player. Or perhaps you had regular cycles but were overweight, and you began dieting. As you have progressed toward your goal, to your surprise your periods have gotten irregular or stopped altogether!

In any case, even though anorexia nervosa, bulimia, and "female athlete triad" (lack of periods, disordered eating, and bone loss in female athletes) have gotten a great deal of media attention, you do not need to have any of these psychological disorders in order to have low body fat. Any situation that causes you to take in or to absorb fewer calories than you need will sooner or later result in low body fat, and it will result in long cycles or no cycles at all. Psychological factors do not need to be involved.

OTHER CONSEQUENCES OF LOW BODY FAT. No matter what the reason, if caloric intake is inadequate, a woman who loses her cycles is at risk for loss of bone mass and eventual osteoporosis. Constant restriction of calories by female athletes in order to attain athletic goals also contributes to fatigue, stress, and depression.[37] Correcting your cycle irregularities through improved nutrition and weight gain will contribute to a better quality of life, both in the short term and in the long term.

ARE YOU UNDERWEIGHT? The popular Body Mass Index (BMI), which uses only height and weight to determine normal body weight for all ages and both sexes, has a number of limitations. First, it does not take into account bone structure; that is, whether you are big-boned, medium-boned, or small-boned. Second, it does not take into account the source of the weight — fat versus muscle. Muscle is heavier than fat, so if you are a trained athlete, your BMI may be normal but you may be "underfat."[38] Third, it does not take into account the natural changes that occur with age, as muscle is lost and body fat is gained.

Your chart gives you better information than your BMI as to whether or not you have adequate body fat for optimum fertility. If you have normal temperature levels, normal mucus patterns, ovulations that occur somewhere around Days 14 to 18, and normal luteal phase lengths, you probably have adequate body fat, even though you may be quite slender and active. A small-boned woman may have a rather low BMI, but her chart will reveal whether or not her cycles are normal. If, on the other hand, your ovulations are usually delayed, perhaps to Day 20 or more, you may be somewhat "underfat" despite a BMI in the normal range. My experience has been that when this occurs with a normal luteal phase length (twelve to sixteen days), just gaining three to five pounds will cause ovulation to occur sooner.

If your charts are showing a short luteal phase, especially after delayed ovulation, the cause could be underweight from lack of enough calories, but it could also be from vigorous exercise, too.[39] Cutting back on exercise and improving your nutrition in order to reduce the stress on your body will almost certainly improve your cycle. Of course, no cycles at all when you are underweight or "underfat" is also good evidence that you need to make changes in your exercise level and your overall food intake to bring your body fat up to normal.

DIETING AND LOSS OF CYCLES. Sometimes women of supposedly "ideal" weight, or even considerably higher than "ideal" weight, may experience loss of menses or greatly delayed ovulation because they, too, are underweight! I have personally counseled several women with total amenorrhea for months after seemingly sensible weight loss. These women were emphatically not over-dieting. Yet regaining just a few pounds restored the cycle. For example, a young woman who had previously conceived easily consulted me after her physician could offer no explanation for her prolonged amenorrhea of eight months' duration. The amenorrhea coincided with her loss of forty pounds through a sensible diet plan, and she was maintaining her "ideal" weight. I advised her to regain just a few of the lost pounds. In less than three months, after she had regained seven pounds, she conceived the child for whom she had been hoping.

NUTRITION AND OTHER STRATEGIES FOR WEIGHT GAIN
Fortunately, cycle irregularities and infertility caused by low body fat are

reversible. One of the most important factors in correcting such cycle problems is simply recognizing the lack of body fat as the cause.

Review Part I of this book and make a true effort to eat enough good food to achieve the proper weight for your height. Be sure to include adequate fat in your diet; for example, whole-fat milk and other whole-fat dairy foods. Do not try to gain needed body fat on a low-fat diet! If you are the right weight but have been exercising vigorously, cut back on your exercise, and let some of your normal body fat return. Your chart will show your progress, as your cycles will become more normal.

At the same time, make sure that you are getting plenty of good vitamins, minerals, and essential fatty acids through supplements as recommended in Chapter 3. Underweight women are prone to deficiencies of vitamins B6 and vitamin B2, folic acid, calcium, magnesium, iron, and zinc; in addition, low-fat diets can result in low levels of vitamin E and the essential fatty acids.[40]

If you tend not to eat if you are stressed, work on getting more sleep or at least more rest. (See the question and answer on this topic in Chapter 4. Consider the section titled, "Mood Swings, Anxiety, and Depression" in Chapter 12, as well as Chapter 14.)

For an excellent review of health issues affecting athletic women, including a table of practical suggestions to combine athletics with adequate nutrition and good health, ask your librarian to obtain a copy of "Nutritional Recommendations and Athletic Menstrual Dysfunction," published in 2004 by Dr. Melinda M. Manore of the Department of Nutrition and Food Management of Oregon State University.[41] If you are not particularly athletic but have serious problems gaining weight, read *Dr. David Reuben's Quick Weight-Gain Program*, an encouraging book which I believe is the only one of its type. (See "Further Reading.") If you have an eating disorder such as anorexia, bulimia, or "female athlete triad," let those who love you and care for you assist you in finding a compassionate, nutritionally-oriented medical doctor or psychologist.

MEDICAL INTERVENTION FOR INFERTILITY RELATED TO LOW BODY WEIGHT. If you are a thin or athletic woman who is experiencing infertility related to very long cycles, short luteal phases, anovulatory cycles, or amenorrhea, I urge you not to undergo medically-induced ovulation (Clomid or similar medications) until you have gained sufficient body fat through more food and less exercise. You are much more likely to conceive on your own when your body weight and body fat content is normal. But even more important, normal weight gain during pregnancy is vital to a healthy outcome for both mother and baby. Starting at a naturally fertile body weight will help you throughout the pregnancy, especially if you are a woman who finds it difficult to gain weight.

➤ Cycle irregularity and infertility are related as a continuum, and therefore the self-care for irregular cycles and infertility is the same.

➤ There are several common causes of cycle irregularity and infertility that may be seen on the chart. Short luteal phase, thyroid problems, and underweight or low body fat all affect the charted signs. It is possible for these to occur at the same time.

➤ Short luteal phase may be improved by the same strategies that are helpful to PMS. Consider the use of Optivite PMT, ProCycle PMS, or Fertility Blend.

➤ Low thyroid function (hypothyroidism) can sometimes be improved through better nutrition and supplements (see Chapter 3). If improvement occurs, the levels of temperatures may rise, and better mucus and bleeding patterns will occur. In other cases, medical intervention is necessary, and thyroid hormone replacement can restore normal cycles and fertility.

➤ Hyperthyroidism is less common than low thyroid function. It is seen on the chart through higher-than-normal basal temperatures. Hyperthyroid is not likely to respond to nutrition, and medical care is necessary.

➤ Underweight or low body fat can delay ovulation or cause the complete absence of cycles. Often just gaining a few pounds with good diet is enough to improve the cycle. Reducing excessive exercise may be necessary in some cases.

8

Polycystic Ovary Syndrome (PCOS) & Overweight without PCOS

He fills your days with good things; your youth is renewed like the eagle's.
— Psalms 103:5

We are currently in the midst of an explosion of interest in and research regarding polycystic ovary syndrome (PCOS). Diet, exercise, vitamins, and minerals are now being studied in relationship to this common hormonal disorder, and finally there is research that offers real direction and self-help strategies for cycle irregularity and infertility related to PCOS.

PCOS often occurs with overweight, and I will discuss it first. However, you can be overweight or obese without PCOS. Being overweight, even without any tendency to PCOS, can also disrupt the cycle in some but by no means all women, as the second part of this chapter explains.

— *PCOS*

CHART MANIFESTATIONS OF PCOS: *Long to very long cycles, often with less-fertile mucus patches interspersed with more-fertile mucus; short luteal phases (when ovulation does occur); anovulatory cycles; complete lack of cycles; miscarriage; infertility.* If the basal temperatures are very low (pre-ovulatory temperatures averaging 97.2° F or less), see also "Low Thyroid Function" in Chapter 7.

TABLE 9, POSSIBLE SYMPTOMS OF PCOS AND RELATED HEALTH RISKS		
Symptoms of PCOS (Reproductive)	Symptoms of PCOS (Other)	Related Risk Factors
		Depression
Long cycles	Acne	Non-insulin-dependent diabetes
Anovulatory cycles	Obesity	Cardiovascular disease
Amenorrhea	Hirsutism (excess body hair)	Elevated blood cholesterol
Enlarged ovaries		Autoimmune thyroid disease
Infertility	Carbohydrate intolerance	

UNDERSTANDING PCOS

DEFINING PCOS. The simplest way to define polycystic ovary syndrome is to call it a reproductive dysfunction in which a woman ovulates infrequently or not at all because her ovarian follicles become arrested in their growth and secrete "male" hormones. Many small follicles accumulate on her ovaries — hence the name. Besides the menstrual cycle disruption due to the arrested follicles, abdominal obesity and hirsutism (a masculine pattern of body hair) are often part of the symptoms. PCOS tends to begin early in a woman's reproductive years and continues chronically.

However, PCOS is a complex problem, not an "all or nothing" condition. It may be mild, or it may be severe. A woman can have PCOS and ovulate more or less regularly. She can have PCOS and not be obese or have hirsutism. She can also have PCOS with or without infertility. It may begin later in her reproductive years rather than earlier. The variation in the severity of the disorder partly explains the variation in the symptoms. Equally as important, a woman can have irregular cycles without PCOS; she can be overweight without PCOS; and she can have hirsutism without PCOS. She can even have cysts on her ovaries due to factors other than this syndrome! For example, PCOS is not at all the same as the single large "follicular cysts" that women of childbearing age occasionally experience.

It is no wonder that PCOS is often unrecognized. However, despite controversy regarding what actually constitutes the syndrome, in 2003 a medical consensus statement on the diagnosis of PCOS was created by doctors with expertise in the disease. The diagnosis of PCOS now depends on a woman having at least two of the following three conditions: Chronic anovulation (cycles without ovulation, infrequent ovulation, or no cycles); evidence of elevated "male" hormones, whether through clinical signs such as hirsutism or through blood tests; and multiple small cysts on the ovaries, as confirmed by ultrasound.[1]

UNDERLYING CAUSES OF PCOS. PCOS is a complex hormonal disorder most often characterized by elevated levels of insulin, LH, and androgens ("male" hormones), all of which contribute to the dysfunction of the ovaries. LH is necessary to mature the follicle, but abnormal secretion of this hormone, along with and possibly stimulated by elevated insulin, causes the follicles to stop growing prematurely. At the stage of arrested growth, the follicles secrete androgens that disrupt normal cycle events further, and which cause some women to develop a masculine pattern of hair growth. A condition called "insulin resistance," which leads to high insulin levels, is a major contributor to this disorder.[2]

INSULIN RESISTANCE. Insulin resistance refers to an abnormality in which many of the body's cells decrease in their ability to respond to insulin. The receptors for insulin on these cells fail to transmit the vital message that insulin normally signals, which is to allow the cells to admit glucose. To compensate, the pancreas secretes extra insulin so that the cells get their glucose. Some cells still have trouble getting enough glucose, but there is another complicating factor — the elevated levels of insulin cause other problems, because not all cells are insulin resistant.

Here is an analogy to explain this: Imagine that you have to raise your voice to give directions to people who are hard of hearing. While that may help those people to respond, your shouting may cause misunderstandings among others around you with normal hearing. Is there an emergency? Should they work harder? Your voice is like the insulin giving directions to the cells. Skeletal muscle cells are known to become insulin resistant, so they may benefit from the high insulin "shouting." But some cells in the ovary do not become insulin resistant, and they respond abnormally to the high insulin levels.[3] This analogy also explains the tendency to weight gain, because fat cells which do not become insulin resistant respond to the high insulin levels by "working harder" — taking in glucose excessively and storing it as fat. And when that happens, the brain cells (which do not need insulin's signal) get deprived of their share of glucose, leading to hypoglycemic symptoms of fatigue, brain fog, and craving for carbohydrates.

RISK FACTORS ASSOCIATED WITH PCOS. High insulin levels and insulin resistance are risk factors for a number of other conditions, including abdominal obesity, non-insulin-dependent diabetes (type 2 or "adult-onset" diabetes), and high cholesterol levels which predispose to heart disease. These are exactly the risk factors which affect women with PCOS, and these risk factors relate more to the insulin resistance and high insulin levels than to the problems within the ovaries themselves. Many researchers now consider PCOS to be one more manifestation of a constellation of conditions such as those just mentioned, all caused by insulin resistance.[4] These conditions are collectively called "metabolic syndrome."

SELF-HELP STRATEGIES FOR PCOS

There is good news, though, when it comes to PCOS. It responds to lifestyle changes aimed at improving "insulin sensitivity," which is the opposite of insulin resistance. Insulin sensitivity is the normal condition, meaning that the body's cells sense and respond to insulin as they should. When insulin sensitivity improves, the cells get the glucose they need, and the damaging high levels of insulin naturally drop. It is a "win-win" situation for the entire body.

To understand insulin sensitivity, consider the previous analogy of the hard-of-hearing people. If those hard-of-hearing people could somehow hear better, they will respond to your directions much better. In turn, you will naturally lower your voice. And the others around you with normal hearing will no longer be confused and overstimulated by your shouting. When insulin sensitivity improves, insulin levels drop, and PCOS improves. Here are some guidelines to help you to improve your insulin sensitivity.

1) LOSE WEIGHT IF YOU ARE OVERWEIGHT. The first and most important self-care step for women with PCOS is to lose weight. While losing weight is a struggle for just about everyone who needs to do so, losing only a modest amount of body weight can significantly improve your cycle regularity and

your fertility. For example, a study in Great Britain showed that dropping only 5 percent of their body weight resulted in improved cycle regularity in nine of eleven obese women with PCOS, as well as five pregnancies in seven previously infertile women with PCOS. Women who lost less than 5 percent of their body weight showed no such improvement.[5]

Weight loss in obese women is known to improve insulin sensitivity, and insulin levels in fact dropped in the women in this study who lost weight and regained cycle regularity and fertility.[6] Incidentally, a 5 percent weight loss in a 200-pound individual is only a 10-pound loss. Moreover, dropping just a moderate amount of weight also improves other aspects of PCOS: it lowers androgen levels, cholesterol levels, and the number of ovarian cysts.[7]

While losing a modest amount of weight is recommended by virtually all researchers involved with PCOS, there is no consensus as to what kind of weight-loss diet is best. Some researchers have concluded that a high-fiber, moderate protein, healthy-fats diet is the best,[8] while others recommend a diet that is relatively high in protein, because of the effect of protein on suppressing the appetite.[9] The late Robert Atkins, M.D., anecdotally reported that women with PCOS were very much helped by his famous low-carbohydrate diet. Their cycles returned and even signs of excess androgens, such as hirsutism, subsided after several months on his diet.[10]

Drs. Jorge Chavarro and William Willett, authors of *The Fertility Diet*, recommend that you use a sensible diet plan that works best for you, whether it is low in fat or low in carbohydrates. The diet plan that helps you to be satisfied with fewer calories is the best one for you.[11] These doctors emphasize avoiding trans fats, which increase the risk of ovulatory infertility,[12] including PCOS.[13] They also encourage you to avoid "liquid calories" (soft drinks and juices), which have the same negative effect.[14] They devote an entire chapter of their book to reviewing popular diet books and plans, and offer their own common-sense, nutritionally-sound weight-loss advice.

2) AVOID FOODS THAT RAPIDLY ELEVATE BLOOD GLUCOSE LEVELS. High blood glucose levels are the trigger for the secretion of insulin. Some foods and eating patterns stimulate the release of insulin more than others. In 1981, researcher David Jenkins developed a list of foods, the "Glycemic Index," based on how rapidly they increased blood sugar levels. Since then the list has been modified, but in general simple sugars and refined starches are highest on the list and are therefore to be avoided. Breakfast cereals, bread, rice, potatoes, and corn are foods that are high on the glycemic index. Apples, pears, ice cream, and milk are fairly low in their ability to trigger a release of insulin.[15]

Surprising? In general, refined starches and sugars by themselves will quickly raise the blood glucose levels. On the other hand, fats, proteins, and fiber slow the digestive processes down, which results in a slower release of glucose into the blood, stimulating less insulin. That explains why ice cream, a food containing substantial amounts of sugar, is lower on the Glycemic Index than plain whole wheat bread or brown rice. Its protein and fat slow the release of the glucose into the blood. (Drs. Chavarro and colleagues also found that one or two servings daily of full-fat dairy, such as ice cream, reduced the risk of ovulatory infertility, including PCOS. They attribute this effect to the natural cow estrogens in the fatty portion of milk products, since cows are often pregnant when milking, and pregnancy is a time of high estrogen production. They observed no such effect with skim milk products.[16])

Should you avoid eating healthy but high-glycemic foods? Not necessarily. Instead, cut down on junk foods such as soft drinks, cakes, and candy. Combine healthy whole grains, fruits, and vegetables with foods containing protein and natural fat (for example, cheese, eggs, meat, fish, or nuts). As an example, a white potato has a high glycemic index, but eaten with butter or as part of a meal containing meat, its ability to elevate blood sugar is greatly reduced. Review the "Twelve Rules for Better Nutrition" in Part I for further information on healthy eating. For a practical application of the Glycemic Index, go to *www.glycemicindex.com*.

3) STRICTLY AVOID NUTRASWEET AND OTHER ARTIFICIAL SWEETENERS. Many people were amazed and skeptical when new research, published in 2007 in the prestigious medical journal *Circulation*, showed that drinking only one soft drink daily, whether sugared or diet, significantly increased the rates of obesity, insulin resistance, and cardiovascular problems related to high insulin levels.[17] How could diet drinks, which contain virtually no calories, promote obesity?

That question was answered as long ago as 1990. That year, the distinguished medical consultant H.J. Roberts, M.D., in reviewing the literature and his own clinical experience related to aspartame (NutraSweet), reported that aspartame as well as other artificial sweeteners caused weight gain in some people. He offered several explanations for this paradoxical finding. For example, the very taste of sweetness triggers insulin release by reflex. However, insulin, released in the absence of real, calorie-containing food, abnormally lowers blood glucose levels, which in turn stimulates hunger.[18] Dr. Roberts also referred to research showing that the amino acid phenylalanine, which forms 50 percent of the aspartame molecule, raises the levels of insulin and promotes insulin resistance.[19]

I believe that avoiding diet drinks and all other sources of artificial sweeteners is a vital step in controlling your appetite and your weight, and in lowering high insulin levels. Despite the fact that the American Heart Association and *The Fertility Diet* recommend artificial sweeteners as a way of avoiding calories, I feel certain that the new research published in *Circulation* will stimulate further studies which will continue to link the vast increase in insulin resistance and obesity (and PCOS) to the consumption of artificial sweeteners.

4) CONSIDER COMPREHENSIVE VITAMIN, MINERAL, AND ESSENTIAL FATTY ACID SUPPLEMENTS. Because so many nutrients are involved in PCOS and related health issues, a high-quality, comprehensive multivitamin/multimineral such as Professional Prenatal Formula, ProCycle, or Optivite is a basic starting point.

The B vitamins are important in PCOS. The large Nurses' Study provided evidence that multivitamins containing B vitamins, especially folic acid, reduce the occurrence of ovulatory infertility, including PCOS.[20]

Vitamins B6, B12, and folic acid reduce levels of the amino acid homocysteine, which in excess is harmful to cells. Elevated levels of homocysteine are a risk factor for cardiovascular disease and insulin resistance, and homocysteine levels are elevated in women with PCOS.[21] Administration of B-group vitamins (500 mg vitamin B1, 500 mg B6, and 2,000 mcg B12 daily) or folic acid (348 mcg daily) reduced homocysteine levels in women receiving metformin, a drug that increases insulin sensitivity and the drug of choice for treating PCOS.[22]

In another study, supplementing B vitamins reduced homocysteine levels and improved pregnancy rates more than metformin in women with PCOS.[23] The vitamin brands suggested above contain significant amounts of the B vitamins. See the suggested amounts in Table 7, Chapter 3.

Vitamin D may be especially beneficial to women with PCOS, because low levels of this vitamin correlate with high body weight and with insulin resistance.[24] As an aside, new research indicates that vitamin D may have a powerful anti-cancer effect, and the amounts that are currently recommended may be too low. However, at this writing 2,000 IU/day is considered by the Food and Nutrition Board of the Institute of Medicine to be a safe and beneficial amount to supplement.[25] Getting summer sunshine is wonderful way to get more vitamin D. Light-skinned individuals, though, have to take extra care not to burn, and dark-skinned individuals actually need more sun exposure to make vitamin D. However, because people wear clothes, work indoors, or live in a northern climate, supplementing vitamin D is necessary.

Magnesium (1,000 mg/day), chromium, and vanadium are minerals that are helpful to increasing insulin sensitivity. Using the previous analogy, they can be considered natural "hearing aids," which enable the cells to respond normally to insulin. Dr. Julian Whitaker recommends up to 200–400 mcg/day of chromium, and 30 mg/day of vanadium for help with insulin resistance related to overweight.[26]

As always, discuss these recommendations with a nutritionally-aware health professional, particularly if you are seeking pregnancy.[27] Phyllis Balch, author of *Prescription for Nutritional Healing*, points out that chromium picolinate is so effective at improving insulin sensitivity that individuals with diabetes should check with a nutritionally-aware physician before using it, as it may necessitate a change in their medication.[28]

The essential fatty acids, especially the hard-to-get omega-3 fatty acids, also improve the cells' sensitivity to insulin.[29] The richest source of the omega-3 essential fatty acid, alpha-linolenic acid, is flax oil. Five to ten 1 g capsules a day may be helpful. Flax oil, which is a food, can be taken by the spoonful; 1–2 teaspoons per day (5–10 grams) is sufficient. You may prefer capsules due to the taste of flax oil; though not particularly unpleasant, most Americans are unaccustomed to it. Cod liver oil (1–2 teaspoons daily), which contains omega-3 fatty acids, vitamin A, and vitamin D may also help with infertility related to PCOS.[30] The antioxidant vitamin E is an essential vitamin to take if you supplement the essential fatty acids, as it prevents oxygen damage to these valuable yet fragile molecules.

An additional resource for information on vitamins, minerals, essential fatty acids, and other supplements that are specifically helpful to insulin resistance, weight loss, and indirectly, to PCOS, is Chapter 23 of *Dr. Atkins' New Diet Revolution*, "Nutritional Supplements: Don't Even Think of Getting Along Without Them!" (See "Further Reading.")

5) SERIOUSLY UNDERTAKE A REGULAR EXERCISE PROGRAM. Regular aerobic exercise helps most people to lose weight, but even if exercise does not enable you to lose weight, here is some great news — your insulin sensitivity nevertheless will very likely increase significantly.[31] So do not give up if the weight will not come off as fast or as well as you would like; exercise makes a positive difference even if it does not show on the scales. Brisk walking for half an hour four or five times a week is an example of moderate exercise with beneficial effects on insulin sensitivity. Try combining such brisk walking with taking stairs instead of elevators, parking far away from shop entrances, and other such small but cumulative changes to increase your activity. Higher-intensity exercise, including weight-lifting, may make a greater difference to your weight as well as to your insulin sensitivity and overall health, but a gradual start with a routine that fits into your lifestyle is the best way to begin. Regular exercise has another benefit — it also lowers levels of the harmful homocysteine in women with PCOS. When homocysteine levels decrease, the risk of cardiovascular problems also decreases.[32]

6) READ *The Fertility Diet*. This outstanding new book addresses diet and lifestyle for women with ovulatory disorders, most of whom had PCOS. It has excellent information on the value of exercise, foods that do not stimulate insulin, and the benefit that full fat dairy products such as milk or ice cream may have for you. It reviews a number of popular diet books, saving you the trouble of doing so. It is very opposed to the use of sugary sodas, but instead recommends the use of artificially sweetened drinks. As you have read above, I encourage you to avoid artificial sweeteners totally. Nevertheless, *The Fertility Diet* is an excellent resource for women with PCOS.

7) CONSIDER YEAST OVERGROWTH. Yeast overgrowth refers to health problems that occur when yeast organisms that are normally harmless to the body get out of control within it. They can cause infection, allergic reaction, or inflammation due to the toxins they produce. Carolyn Dean, M.D., authored a chapter in *The Yeast Connection and Women's Health* titled, "Understanding the Weight Connection." She makes the case that yeast overgrowth contributes to overweight, especially belly fat that is hard to lose. If your PCOS includes overweight, especially abdominal fat, you may wish to consider whether yeast

overgrowth is contributing to it. See "Yeast Overgrowth" in Chapter 9 for more information.

AN ENCOURAGING ANECDOTE. The Couple to Couple League received the following letter a few months after I published an article in *Family Foundations* regarding nutrition for PCOS. Not every woman will have the quick and dramatic change that this writer did, but many who try the strategies for PCOS suggested above will be pleased with their improved cycles and fertility.

> After more than a year and a half of infertility after discontinuing the pill, I was finally diagnosed with polycystic ovary syndrome in March of this year. My doctor told me that natural conception would be "highly unlikely." My husband and I were very disappointed, since we had no interest in using fertility drugs and were uncertain about adoption. Then I read Marilyn Shannon's article in *Family Foundations* on the role of sugar in relation to ovarian function. I decided to take her advice of taking flax oil capsules and eliminating sugar from my diet. I purchased the book *Get the Sugar Out!* [See "Further Reading."], and was amazed at how much sugar was in my current diet. The book pointed out not only the pitfalls of foods with high amounts of sugars, but also discussed how to eliminate foods that the body quickly converts to sugar, such as foods made with white flour and starches. Upon reading the book, I was amazed to find out how high in sugar my otherwise healthy, "low-fat" diet truly was.
>
> Within days of beginning my new diet regimen, I ovulated for the first time in years. I was surprised not only that the suggestions were helpful, but also how quickly and dramatically the changes were. I experienced my first thermal shift ever only a matter of days after eliminating sugar from my diet.
>
> My dietary changes not only resulted in ovulation, but also conception as well. My husband and I are both shocked and elated. The baby is due in March and we could not be happier.
>
> Thanks again to CCL for the wonderful nutritional advice for women suffering from PCOS. I am still in disbelief as to how such small changes in my diet made such a dramatic change in my fertility![33]

—— OVERWEIGHT WITHOUT *PCOS* ——

Many women who are significantly overweight have normal cycles and high fertility. In fact, in many cases having several children has contributed to the problem with overweight! On the other hand, overweight, even without the androgens ("male" hormones) and long cycles of PCOS, can be at the root of other cycle problems or infertility.

PCOS OR NOT?

Women who are overweight without PCOS tend to have a "pear-shaped" figure; that is, much of their excess body fat is carried mainly in their hips and thighs. In contrast, overweight women with PCOS usually carry much of their excess body fat around their waist, the so-called "apple" shape. Estrogens are responsible for the pear shape, while androgens promote the apple shape.

PCOS often causes long or very long cycles, and often a masculine pattern of body hair (hirsutism). If you are dealing with a weight problem, body shape, cycle regularity, and whether or not you have a tendency toward hirsutism are all clues as to whether or not PCOS is part of the picture. If you are in doubt, a gynecologist can determine if you have PCOS.

CHART MANIFESTATIONS OF OVERWEIGHT WITHOUT PCOS. Being overweight without having PCOS can cause *short luteal phase, poor mucus patterns, poor temperature rise, amenorrhea, or infertility with or without regular cycles.* You might also wish to consider "Luteal Phase Deficiency" in Chapter 7. If your basal temperatures are very low (pre-ovulatory temperatures averaging about 97.2° F or lower), please refer to "Low Thyroid Function" in Chapter 7.

BODY FAT AND HORMONES. The role of body fat in female fertility is an essential one. Fat is a metabolically active tissue which produces its own hormones. Body fat converts circulating androgens, which are naturally produced by the adrenal glands, into estrogen. In many women, though, too much body fat contributes to elevated levels of estrogen. Elevated estrogen levels interfere with the function of the corpus luteum, decreasing progesterone. Excess estrogen can also interfere with thyroid function by blocking the receptors within the body cells that respond to thyroid hormone.[34] The slowdown of metabolism that occurs when thyroid function decreases encourages storage of more body fat, which in turn increases estrogen levels more. Elevated levels of estrogen are often referred to as "estrogen dominance." The problems of estrogen dominance have been well documented: weight gain, PMS symptoms, uterine fibroid tumors, fibrocystic breasts, and a higher risk of breast cancer.[35] As you can probably guess, losing weight is an important strategy to limit estrogen dominance.

WEIGHT-LOSS DIETS FOR OBESITY. A consensus as to which type of diet plan is best to lose weight is finally developing, after years of debate. That consensus is this: the type of diet that is most helpful to *you* is the best diet for *you.* Almost every informed person agrees that no matter whether you emphasize more animal protein or more vegetables and fiber, whole natural foods are far preferable to sugary foods, refined starches, or foods containing the damaging trans fats.

Even though you may have overweight without PCOS, the weight-loss strategies numbered in the previous topic, "PCOS," are applicable to you as well.

NUTRITIONAL SUPPLEMENTS. Because estrogen dominance is related to overweight without PCOS, look for nutritional supplements that are aimed at increasing progesterone levels and decreasing estrogen levels. The supplements listed for PMS in Chapter 5 may be most helpful to you. These include Optivite PMT, ProCycle PMS, or Fertility Blend. I especially prefer ProCycle PMS, as it contains 200 mcg of chromium. Chromium helps with the problem of insulin resistance, which also affects overweight women without PCOS. For a list of ingredients of all of these, see Appendix A. Add flax oil (about 5–10 g/day) and/or fish oil (1 teaspoon/day).

SOME NOTES ABOUT INFERTILITY. If you are overweight and are having difficulty becoming pregnant, be careful to lose weight slowly with wholesome nutrition and regular exercise. Attempt to overcome hypoglycemia and sugar cravings with small, frequent snacks of good food (see Rule 7, Chapter 1), and appropriate supplements (see Table 7, Chapter 3). As is true of overweight women with PCOS, you should not despair of losing all the weight necessary to attain your "ideal" weight, but should just set a modest goal such as ten pounds. Finally, you and your husband should not overlook less obvious factors that may also contribute to your infertility. Please see Appendix B, "Focus on Infertility," for other self-care suggestions to improve your chances of conceiving.

Summary – Chapter 8

➤ Polycystic ovary syndrome (PCOS) is one manifestation of a constellation of hormonal and metabolic dysfunctions which are related to insulin resistance, the body's inability to respond properly to the hormone insulin.

➤ PCOS affects the reproductive hormones, so it is diagnosed through any two of the following: irregular or absent cycles, evidence of excess "male" hormones, and enlarged or polycystic ovaries. It may be improved by weight loss, dietary modifications, exercise, and vitamin, mineral, and essential fatty acid supplements.

➤ Avoiding artificial sweeteners is a recommended strategy.

➤ While overweight is often associated with PCOS, overweight without PCOS can also disrupt the cycle. In cases in which the excess weight is carried more in the hips and thighs, as opposed to the belly, it may contribute to excess estrogen.

➤ Weight loss on a healthy diet may be very helpful, but women with overweight should look for signs of low thyroid function and short luteal phase on their charts, and address these issues directly as well.

9

Other Factors That May Affect Cycle Regularity or Fertility

But the Lord said to Abraham: "Why did Sarah laugh and say, 'Shall I really bear a child, old as I am?' Is anything too marvelous for the Lord to do?" — Genesis 18:13-14

The two previous chapters dealt with hormonal or other problems that are known to affect cycle regularity or fertility. Luteal phase deficiency, thyroid dysfunction, underweight, PCOS, and overweight may all do so. When they do, it is usually in a predictable way. For example, a slender, athletic woman can expect to see a delay in ovulation if she loses excess body fat. A woman with a tendency to hirsutism and overweight can suspect that PCOS is contributing to her long cycles with irregular mucus patterns. Very low body temperatures with irregular bleeding and mucus patterns lead you to consider whether low thyroid function might be involved. Poor temperature rise with only a few days of elevated temperatures indicate luteal phase deficiency.

However, there are a number of other, perhaps more subtle, factors that may affect your cycles or your fertility, and they are worth considering if you are having problems with either. This is especially true if your chart or body weight does not help you to judge what might be affecting your cycles or fertility. But even if your chart suggests underweight, low thyroid, or so forth, some of the factors described below might also be involved.

—— YEAST OVERGROWTH ——

The late Dr. William Crook, author of *The Yeast Connection*, wrote that several health problems of women may be related to yeast organisms which cause infection, allergic reactions, or toxic reactions. Reproductive problems that he named included PMS, vaginal infections, and vulvodynia (genital pain in women), low thyroid function, endometriosis, low sexual desire, pain with intercourse, overweight, and female infertility, as well as chronic prostatitis in men. Dr. Crook was always careful to state that yeast overgrowth, or candidiasis, as it is more formally called, was not necessarily the actual cause of any of these reproductive problems, but that yeast might very well be an important contributing factor.[1]

A growing number of other doctors have taken interest in yeast overgrowth, and those who deal with this problem generally agree on the diverse symptoms it creates and the diet and medical treatment for its control. But even if yeast is not actually at the root of the problems mentioned above, the diet that Dr. Crook and other "yeast-aware" health professionals recommend will certainly help you to maintain better overall health. It will increase the value of the food you eat, because it eliminates most sugar and emphasizes whole, natural foods. It will help you to discover hidden allergies that might be involved in your health issues. And the recommended nutritional supplements will help you to overcome deficiencies that may or may not be related to yeast overgrowth.

SYMPTOMS. As mentioned, yeast overgrowth may be involved with reproductive problems in both sexes. But the symptoms of yeast overgrowth go well beyond problems of reproduction, and they may also occur in children. They include the symptoms summarized in Table 10.

TABLE 10, SYMPTOMS OF YEAST OVERGROWTH	
Reproductive Symptoms	**Other Symptoms**
Vaginal infections	Extreme fatigue or lethargy (the feeling of being drained)
PMS	
Vulvodynia (genital pain in women)	Depression
	Inability to concentrate
Low thyroid function	Headaches
Endometriosis	Skin problems (such as hives, athlete's foot)
Low sexual desire	Gastrointestinal problems (especially constipation, abdominal pain, diarrhea, gas or bloating)
Pain with intercourse	
Overweight	
Female infertility	Muscular and nervous system symptoms (including aching or swelling in your muscles and joints, numbness, burning or tingling)
Chronic prostatitis in men	
	Respiratory symptoms
	Hyperactivity and recurrent ear problems [in children][2]

In women, repeated vaginal yeast infections are a major sign of this disorder, but it is possible to have yeast overgrowth without such infections. Its symptoms also overlap with those of PMS, though yeast overgrowth is not as closely related to the cycle as is PMS. The strong link to reproductive dysfunction in women makes this disorder worth considering if you feel inexplainably unwell over a prolonged period, or if you are unable to overcome the reproductive problems which have been associated with yeast overgrowth.

If you have enough of the symptoms listed above to believe that yeast might be involved with your health problems, the next step is to get a copy of *The Yeast Connection and Women's Health* by Dr. Crook. Score yourself using the book's questionnaire, which covers these symptoms in detail. If your score puts you in the "probable" or "almost certain" class, you will very likely be helped by an anti-yeast diet and supplements.

UNDERLYING CAUSES OF YEAST OVERGROWTH SYMPTOMS. This disease occurs when the common and usually harmless fungus, *Candida albicans*, reproduces excessively within the body. It may invade body tissues, as it does in vaginal yeast infections and in oral thrush, but it may also make trouble by causing allergic reactions. Toxins that the yeast produce may contribute to inflammation. Yeast overgrowth contributes to "leaky gut syndrome," a descriptive name that refers to intestinal walls inflamed because of yeast or other factors. Whole undigested food molecules can be absorbed through the leaky gut into the blood, triggering allergic reactions. Because of this relationship, controlling yeast overgrowth may benefit individuals with allergies.[3]

LIFESTYLE CAUSES. The chief predisposing factors involved in yeast overgrowth are listed in Table 11, in the approximate order of importance:

TABLE 11, POSSIBLE CAUSES OF YEAST OVERGROWTH
Use of antibiotics, which kill the normal, healthy bacteria that live in the intestines, where they naturally discourage yeast. Long-term use of tetracycline for adolescent acne in particular can set the stage for yeast overgrowth.
A diet which is high in sugary and starchy foods, including sweet fruits. Sugar feeds yeast organisms.
Use of oral contraceptives (birth control pills), or other hormonal birth control. The synthetic estrogen and progestogens in birth control pills cause changes in the vaginal wall which allow yeast to multiply more rapidly, causing vaginal yeast infections.
Use of cortisone and related drugs (prednisone, for example). Because these drugs by design suppress the immune response for therapeutic purposes, the immune system may be less able to keep yeast under control.
Hormonal fluctuations in women, including those of the menstrual cycles or those of pregnancy.[4]

NUTRITION FOR YEAST OVERGROWTH. Improved nutrition is the first line of defense against yeast overgrowth. Anti-yeast nutrition works on the principles of cutting off the yeast's food supply (sugar and starches), reducing the intake of yeast-containing foods, re-establishing healthy bacteria in the intestines to naturally "crowd out" the yeast, and providing the body with excellent nutrition to decrease inflammation and to bolster the immune system.

There is a good analogy to help understand this. "Friendly" bacteria may be considered to be like grass; they naturally grow in your large intestine like grass does on a healthy lawn. Of course, like grass, they need some maintenance. Yeast organisms may be considered weeds, which are unnecessary but harmless in small numbers. If, though, the grass is burned out or otherwise damaged or destroyed, what grows back first? The weeds, of course, and without the healthy grass to crowd them out, they can take over. Taking in friendly bacteria in supplement form or eating high-quality yogurt is like planting grass seed. This is especially important after taking antibiotics, which kill the good bacteria as well as the bad. Eating sugary foods and taking steroid drugs such as cortisone and oral contraceptives is like feeding the weeds! Eating good foods and taking vitamins, minerals, and essential fatty acids is like fertilizing the lawn; good nutrition tends to promote the friendly bacteria so that they crowd out the yeast organisms and keep them at a harmless level. Seed, weed, and feed![5]

DIET. Sugar, honey, sweet fruits, refined carbohydrates, and sometimes even healthy carbohydrates such as whole grains must be eliminated, at least for a while. Yeast-containing breads, condiments containing vinegar, fruit juices, processed meats, alcohol and mushrooms are eliminated, at least temporarily. Dr. John Trowbridge, author of *The Yeast Syndrome*, calls this restrictive early diet "MEVY," for Meat, Eggs, Vegetables and Yogurt, the foods which are permissible or, in the case of plain yogurt, especially beneficial. He considers this diet almost as helpful as the anti-fungal drug Nystatin in counteracting yeast overgrowth.[6]

FRIENDLY BACTERIA SUPPLEMENTS. "Probiotics" is the term for friendly bacteria that are taken as supplements to "reseed" your intestines. Friendly bacteria crowd out the yeast and are extremely valuable to overcoming yeast overgrowth. Acidophilus, bifidobacterium, and lactococcus are examples of friendly bacteria available in supplement form. Look for a brand containing a mix of live bacteria and take daily as directed on the label.

Supplementing probiotics if you must take an antibiotic is one of the most effective ways of preventing yeast overgrowth related to antibiotic use. Take the probiotic supplements during and for several days after using the antibiotic. Probiotics also promote health in several other ways. They enable the liver to rid the body of toxins more effectively. This includes helping the liver to get rid of excess estrogen, a most beneficial function. Probiotics help prevent bladder infections as well.[7]

VITAMINS, MINERALS, AND ESSENTIAL FATTY ACIDS. Magnesium, vitamin B6, zinc, and essential fatty acids such as those found in cod liver oil and flax oil may prevent candidiasis or promote healing of it. Vitamin A (but not its precursor, beta-carotene) is also useful.[8] Multivitamins and minerals in amounts similar to those in Table 7 (Chapter 3) are also recommended by doctors who treat this disease.[9] A number of herbal remedies are helpful, including grapefruit seed extract, which is safe for pregnant and nursing mothers, babies, and children.[10] Other herbal remedies are available at health food shops.

Diet and supplements alone may control moderate cases of yeast, but severe overgrowth may require management with anti-candida drugs in addition to the nutritional strategies. To use the analogy again, such drugs are like herbicides which specifically target the weeds while sparing the grass.

For completely documented but concise information on this subject, refer to *Chronic Candidiasis* by Michael Murray, N.D. Dr. William Crook's *The Yeast Connection and Women's Health* has a more informal tone, but it is up-to-date and linked to the website *www.yeastconnection.com*. *A Natural Guide to Pregnancy and Postpartum Health*, by Drs. Dean Raffelock and Robert Rountree, also contains an excellent chapter, "Healing Your Digestive Tract," that explains both leaky gut syndrome and yeast overgrowth. It contains practical strategies for quickly overcoming both. (See "Further Reading.")

—— DISCONTINUING BIRTH CONTROL PILLS ——
OR OTHER HORMONAL BIRTH CONTROL

Congratulations on your decision to discontinue birth control pills or other hormonal contraceptives! You have taken a giant step toward better health. As hormone specialist Diana Schwarzbein, M.D., has written, you cannot achieve optimum hormonal balance while you are on the Pill, because hormones interact with each other.[11]

On the other hand, when you discontinue birth control pills, your body may have to go through a period of readjustment to its own natural hormones. Coming off the Pill or other artificial hormones used for contraception may be followed by *delayed ovulation, a pattern of constant less-fertile mucus, and possibly heavy menses*. As an NFP instructor, I have seen many charts from women who have recently discontinued hormonal birth control. My experience has been that about half of them have very regular cycles immediately after coming off the Pill, whereas the other half have one, two, or three irregular cycles of adjustment, especially cycles with poor mucus patterns.

DIET AND SUPPLEMENTS FOR BETTER CYCLES POST-PILL. Many women who are coming off the Pill view it as an opportunity to improve their health generally. Whether or not your cycles are immediately regular, why not read through Part I of this book and consider general dietary improvements? Eating more fresh whole foods, reducing your intake of trans fats, sugary treats, and artificial sweeteners is a good place to start. Use the 80-20 rule (Rule 12 in Chapter 1) so that you do not get discouraged. Aim for improvement, not perfection!

When it comes to vitamins, minerals, and essential fatty acids, research evidence shows that oral contraceptive users have a significant decrease in vitamin B12,[12] vitamin E, and beta-carotene levels in their blood.[13] They have a significant decrease in the essential fatty acids and in the healthy EPA.[14] They have a significant increase in vitamins A and D, which drop once the Pill is discontinued.[15] Use of the Pill is also associated with higher levels of the "bad" LDL cholesterol levels and lower levels of the "good" HDL cholesterol.[16]

Dr. Ellen Grant, a British medical doctor who formerly conducted research on the birth control pill but who now considers them unsafe, recommends zinc, magnesium, essential fatty acids, vitamin E, and B vitamins for those recovering from Pill use.[17] Cod liver oil contains EPA as well as vitamins A and D, which both drop after the Pill is discontinued. You may wish to use flax oil as a source of the essential fatty acids, but either fish oil or flax oil should be taken along with vitamin E, as explained in Chapter 3. Fish oil and vitamin E are well known to have positive effects on blood cholesterol composition.

Any of the multivitamin/multimineral brands suggested in Chapter 3 contain the zinc, magnesium, B vitamins and vitamin E recommended by Dr. Grant. Professional Prenatal Formula, ProCycle, or Optivite all come close to "covering all the bases," but if you choose to use Optivite, you may wish to include extra folic acid, at least 400–800 mcg in addition to the 200 mcg in the full dose. (See "Appendix A" and "Resources.")

OTHER PROBLEMS RELATED TO THE PILL. The Pill is known to worsen PMS in some women. It has also been associated with yeast overgrowth. Chapter 5 covers PMS, and "Yeast Overgrowth" is the topic above. If you were on the Pill to lighten heavy bleeding or to reduce menstrual cramping, you will find natural answers to these problems in Chapter 6. If you were on the Pill to "regulate" your cycle, try referring to the section on low thyroid function, underweight, overweight, or other relevant sections of Chapters 7 and 8. If you have been using the Pill in an attempt to overcome acne, you may be interested to read Chapter 8, which covers polycystic ovary syndrome (PCOS). The high levels of "male" hormones typical of PCOS are a major trigger for acne. See also Chapter 16, "Questions & Answers: Part II" for nutrition to help overcome acne.

—— SENSITIVITY TO NIGHT LIGHTING ——

When I was a first-year graduate student, I worked in a lab dedicated to understanding the pineal gland and its major hormone, melatonin. It was a fascinating topic. The graduate students investigated the link between day length, light-dark cycles, and reproductive readiness in birds, frogs, snakes, and lizards. In these animals, the pineal gland serves as the biological coordinator between the day length and the ability of the animal to reproduce at the most favorable time of year. Most vertebrates, including humans, produce the hormone melatonin from the pineal gland in response to changes in light and darkness. In many animals as well as in human beings, when light hits the eyes, it sends a neural message to the pineal gland, located within the brain, that decreases the production of melatonin. Oppositely, when it is dark, melatonin rises rapidly.

In many mammals, birds, and reptiles, naturally high levels of melatonin inhibit the reproductive hormones. That explains why birds cannot reproduce in the fall and winter when the days are short and the nights are long; their melatonin levels are high, inhibiting reproduction. It explains why, as the day length increases and the nights grow shorter, birds regain their reproductive capability and are able to mate and produce young in the spring. The longer day length reduces the production of melatonin.

WOMEN AND MELATONIN. What about human beings? Since humans are capable of reproducing all year around, it is clear that day length is not the chief factor in human fertility. Yet ongoing research is adding evidence that melatonin levels may affect cycle regularity and fertility, at least in some women.

When human beings are in a very dark environment, melatonin levels rise rapidly. When light, even dim light, hits the eyes, it reduces melatonin output. Bright light does so better than dim light, so that light reduces melatonin output in a "dose-dependent" fashion — more light, less melatonin. The increase in melatonin in the dark seems to be one reason why it is easier to sleep in the dark than in the light, since melatonin promotes sleep.[18]

Is melatonin pro- or anti-fertility in women? Accumulating research suggests that the right amount promotes fertility, whereas either too much or too little can inhibit the fertility cycle. For example, in women who are physically stressed by intense exercise or anorexia nervosa (the disordered eating pattern that results in underweight), cycle irregularities such as delayed ovulation, short luteal phases, anovulatory cycles, and complete absence of cycles occur. In such women, melatonin levels are abnormally high and prolonged during the night. In Finnish women who live relatively close to the North Pole, where winter nights are extremely long, winter melatonin levels are high and LH levels are low.[19]

Conversely, though, since artificial lighting is an integral part of modern life, many women may have too *little* melatonin for optimal reproductive health. For example, a number of studies have shown that women who work night shifts are more prone to breast cancer compared to women who work day shifts. Night shift work tends to reduce melatonin levels, since people work with the lights on. Melatonin is a powerful antioxidant in itself, but there is another link. When melatonin is too low, estrogen rises.[20] Interestingly, nighttime melatonin levels naturally fall during premenopause and remain at their lowest levels in women after menopause.[21]

NIGHT LIGHTING AND NFP. Since 1976, Joy DeFelice, R.N., director of the Natural Family Planning Program at Sacred Heart Medical Center, Spokane, Washington, has studied the effect of eliminating nighttime illumination on the menstrual cycle and on fertility in women who use NFP. She has found that eliminating light from the sleeping area can improve cycle irregularity and infertility. Women who have carefully reduced night lighting in their bedrooms have experienced improvement in their cycle lengths, their bleeding patterns, their mucus patterns, and their temperature patterns, including longer, more normal luteal phases. Such changes generally occur within three menstrual cycles of reduced night lighting. Pregnancy among couples previously experiencing infertility has been achieved following elimination of night lighting, and early miscarriage rates have been reduced by eliminating night lighting while sleeping.[22]

Do you wonder how small amounts of light at night can adversely affect a woman's fertility? Light rays are quite capable of penetrating the eyelids, and in dim light, the retina is exquisitely sensitive even to very low levels of illumination. A special neural route from the eyes sends information about lighting to the pineal gland, reducing melatonin. Getting rid of the light increases melatonin, and sufficient melatonin increases progesterone levels,[23] which may be a major factor in the seemingly amazing results Mrs. DeFelice reports.

PRACTICAL CONSIDERATIONS. For most women, the sources of night illumination in the bedroom are easily identified and controlled. They include hall lights, digital clocks, street lights, headlights, moonlight, and so forth. An irregular bedtime does not seem to be a factor in this phenomenon, provided the woman receives sufficient hours of darkness, and getting up in dim light for short periods to care for a child or to use the bathroom does not disrupt the protocol.[24]

In rare cases, women who do not show improved menstrual cycles after three cycles of night darkness may respond to a temporary regimen of reduced night lighting during all nights except for three nights of low to moderate illumination. These three nights begin two days after more-fertile mucus begins. However, for those who have recently discontinued birth control pills, have experienced a miscarriage, are ending the natural infertility of breastfeeding, or are bottle-feeding a new baby, Mrs. DeFelice does not recommend the regimen of three nights with lighting, but only the constant night darkness. In these situations, the cycles should be allowed to "settle down" on their own for six months before trying the temporary addition of night lighting.[25]

NUTRITION AND MELATONIN. Caffeine reduces melatonin, and caffeine plus night lighting profoundly reduces melatonin.[26] Since melatonin is a natural sleep aid, this may account for what you have probably observed — caffeine late in the afternoon or evening disrupts your sleep. The effect of caffeine on melatonin may also help to explain the effect of caffeine consumption on pregnancy achievement and miscarriage, discussed in the topic that follows.

Supplements of niacin (100 mg), vitamin B6 (75 mg), magnesium (500 mg), and calcium (1,000 mg) are recommended by Julian Whitaker, M.D., author of *Health and Healing* (see "Further Reading") in order to boost the natural production of melatonin.[27]

It is possible to purchase supplements of melatonin at most pharmacies. At least one study suggests that supplements of melatonin of 1 to 3 mg may be beneficial to infertile women.[28] However, in young women in their fertile years (under age 40), the best way to increase melatonin is to do as Mrs. DeFelice's studies have indicated — get rid of night lighting. Besides melatonin, the pineal secretes other factors which might also be a valuable part of the observed effect of reduced night light. For women in perimenopause and afterward who are interested in better sleep only, the same advice holds. However, if three months of careful elimination of night lighting have not improved your sleep, you may wish to try melatonin supplements, as suggested in the question and answer on this subject in Chapter 4. If you do wish to use melatonin supplements, especially if you are trying to achieve a pregnancy or are breastfeeding, seek the counsel of your medical doctor.

OTHER FACTORS THAT AFFECT MELATONIN. Melatonin levels can be affected by some drugs, including nonsteroidal anti-inflammatory agents, steroids, some anti-depressants, beta blockers, calcium channel blockers, and tobacco. Alcohol early in the evening may decrease melatonin, but right before bed may increase it.[29]

Mrs. DeFelice has published a booklet, "The Effects of Light on the Menstrual Cycle: Also Infertility, Clinical Observations," that explains why and how to eliminate night lighting in order have more regular cycles and improved fertility (see "Further Reading"). Will it work for you? People vary considerably; for example, many women have regular cycles and normal fertility despite the presence of night lighting. You will not know whether or not your menstrual cycles will improve in response to reduced night lighting unless you give it a try. If nothing else, though, carefully making your bedroom very dark will probably improve your sleep. Quality sleep is a key to reducing stress.

Please keep in mind that sleep, facilitated as it is by darkness and melatonin, is a basic physical need that cannot be replaced with better nutrition. Likewise, higher melatonin levels and improved sleep cannot make up for poor nutrition. Mrs. DeFelice recommends that diet, exercise, and stress should be considered as well as night lighting when cycle irregularities or infertility occur.[30] I have been disappointed to have NFP clients work hard to eliminate night lighting from their bedroom, without removing junk food from their kitchen!

CAFFEINE CONSUMPTION

Whether or not caffeine consumption affects fertility has been a controversial topic for quite some time. As long ago as 1988, a systematic study concluded that women who used more than the equivalent of one cup of coffee per day took significantly longer to conceive than did those who used less, and high caffeine users experienced longer delays in conceiving than did lower level users.[31] This finding was quickly confirmed by other researchers who studied large numbers of women.[32] However, other studies have found no such relationship.[33]

The issue of caffeine consumption and fertility is again timely due to a large, well-designed recent study that found that more than 200 mg of caffeine daily, the amount in two average cups of coffee, increased the risk of miscarriage.[34] This new information is relevant to any woman who is hoping to become pregnant.

COULD THIS BE YOU? I once counseled a woman who was experiencing secondary infertility of about 18 months. I suggested that she cut out sugar and caffeine, eat nutritiously, and try to drop a few pounds, as she was rather overweight. She conceived two months later and reported that the only change she had made was to reduce her coffee consumption from six or seven mugs per day to one or one and a half cups daily. She also reported that in the year previous to conception, her cycles had become longer and longer, causing her, a non-NFP user, the inconvenience of repeated pregnancy testing.

If you are astounded that anyone could consume so much coffee, you are probably not a caffeine "addict"; if you didn't bat an eye, perhaps you should cut down on your caffeine! This is true even if you are not presently experiencing any direct adverse effects.

I believe that heavy caffeine users are attempting to overcome fatigue related to hypoglycemia (see Rule 7, Chapter 1, and the discussion of hypoglycemia in Chapter 5). Emphasis on the B vitamins, especially folic acid (about 2,000 mcg/day), is helpful. Your meals and snacks should contain a mix of protein, complex carbohydrates, and natural fats. Limiting sweet treats as much as possible is another great help to overcoming low blood glucose.

TEA DRINKING. There is one surprising finding when caffeine consumption has been studied for its effect on fertility: Consumption of tea has been associated with an *increase* in fertility. Tea generally contains considerably less caffeine than coffee or some sodas. In addition, it contains "polyphenols" which are healthy to the chromosomes. It is also possible that tea drinkers have a generally healthier lifestyle than others, according to the researchers who observed this relationship.[35] And some types of tea, such as green tea, are particularly rich in antioxidants, which contribute to fertility.

Anyone experiencing cycle irregularity or any type of infertility should reduce caffeine-containing foods, drugs, and beverages to the equivalent of two cups of coffee per day. More information on caffeine is contained in Rule 8 and Table 6, in Chapter 1. Caffeine consumption also lowers melatonin levels, especially when illumunation levels are high. You may wish to refer to the previous section, "Sensitivity to Night Lighting."

—— CELIAC DISEASE ——————————————

Once thought to be a rare disease that began in childhood, celiac disease is now estimated to affect at least one in 300 people worldwide, and many adults with it go undiagnosed. It has recently been recognized as a cause of cycle irregularity, infertility, recurrent miscarriage, low birth weight babies and pre-term birth.[36] This genetically-determined disease is caused by a specific intolerance to gluten, a protein found in wheat, rye, and barley, and in oats which are processed on equipment that has been used for these grains.[37] In individuals with celiac disease, even tiny amounts of gluten cause a reaction in the small intestinal wall that results in inflammation. Inflammation in this vital organ damages it, leading to the inability to absorb nutrients from food properly, thus causing nutritional deficiencies that impact the entire body.

SYMPTOMS. Untreated celiac disease can cause digestive upsets, including nausea, abdominal pain, diarrhea, and constipation. It may lead to weight loss. Anemia is an important problem that often occurs with it,[38] perhaps because so many vitamins and minerals are needed to make blood cells. It may cause the feeling of being "tired all over," as well as irritability or mood swings. On the other hand, in some people it may produce few symptoms, but it can affect fertility.[39]

Even once it is treated, celiac disease may underlie cycle irregularity and unexplained infertility, which may be related to the multiple nutritional deficiencies that occur as a result of damage to the small intestine. The awareness of celiac disease as a possible cause of infertility has greatly increased recently, but if you have any doubt as to whether or not you may have this disease, you should request medical tests to diagnose it.

DIET FOR CELIAC DISEASE. There is effective treatment for celiac disease. It is the absolute and lifelong avoidance of wheat, rye, and barley, any foods containing them, as well as avoidance of oats, which apparently are often contaminated by wheat dust when processed. When gluten is strictly avoided, over time the inflammation of the intestinal wall subsides.

If tests show that you have celiac disease, you will need a dietitian's assistance to help you become aware of which foods you can eat and which you cannot, as many processed and restaurant foods contain gluten. It will be an adjustment, but your newfound health and vitality will motivate you to continue to avoid gluten as is necessary to control the disease. There are many, many whole natural foods that you can eat: meat, poultry, fish, milk, eggs, fruits, vegetables, beans, nuts, and even grains such as corn and rice.

In fact, because of the growing awareness of this disease, it has become far easier to obtain gluten-free foods. Health food shops and even grocery stores carry a variety of products labeled gluten-free. For example, the private health food shop that I frequently visit has recently posted signs throughout the store pointing out gluten-free products, especially gluten-free flours made from various grains.

As your health improves on the gluten-free diet, gaining weight if you have been underweight will help improve your cycle regularity. However, weight gain alone may not be sufficient to restore optimal health, ideal cycles, and fertility. Overcoming vitamin and mineral deficiencies related to damage to the intestinal wall is a key step in improving cycle regularity and fertility in women with celiac disease.

VITAMINS, MINERALS, AND OTHER SUPPLEMENTS. Harvard School of Public Health researchers Drs. Chavarro and Willett, in *The Fertility Diet*, hypothesize that even when gluten is strictly avoided, past damage to the intestinal wall results in deficiencies of folic acid, iron, vitamin D, vitamin K, and other micronutrients that are involved with fertility. They offer evidence that the infertility that may occur with celiac disease is somehow related to low levels of the B vitamins folic acid and vitamin B_{12}. They summarize published anecdotes of women with untreated celiac disease and infertility who became pregnant soon after taking large doses of folic acid daily.[40]

Vitamin, mineral, and essential fatty acid supplements are especially valuable if you are trying to overcome cycle irregularity and infertility. It is quite easy to find supplements labeled "gluten free." However, it is important to start to take supplements slowly, so that they help to heal, not to irritate, the small intestinal wall. The assistance of a nutritionally-oriented physician is a must as you begin supplements.

Ideally, you would take all supplements as listed in Chapter 3. Whether or not you are actually able to do so depends on the health of your intestines and on your doctor's recommendations. If you are dealing with infertility, folic acid in the amount of 4,000–5,000 mcg per day may be especially helpful, and is safe during pregnancy. Vitamin B_{12} (1,000 –2,000 mcg/day) and zinc (25–50 mg/day) also assist folic acid in its beneficial effects on fertility, and are helpful in achieving pregnancy.

OTHER CONSIDERATIONS. As you consider your chart, look for specific signs of cycle irregularity that are discussed elsewhere in this book. For example, the anemia which is so common in women with celiac disease may contribute to heavy bleeding, which in turn contributes to painful periods. Chapter 6, "Shorter, Lighter and Pain-free Periods," has information on nutrition for overcoming anemia. Underweight related to poor absorption of food molecules can cause long cycles. Or, if your basal temperatures are low (average pre-ovulatory temperatures of 97.2° F or below), see "Low Thyroid Function" in Chapter 7. If you continue to have cycle irregularities, make sure that your physician helps you to identify other problems that may occur unrelated to the celiac disease. In summary, if your cycles and fertility do not respond to diet and supplements aimed at treating celiac disease, do not overlook other factors that might also be involved.

A FINAL CAUTION. Some people are sensitive to gluten, and feel much better when they avoid wheat products and the other sources of gluten. However, sensitivity to gluten and celiac disease are not the same thing. It is not wise to attempt to undertake a gluten-free diet on the outside chance that celiac disease might be the cause of your cycle irregularity, infertility, or other symptoms. If you think celiac disease might be your problem, an accurate medical diagnosis is the first step, and it will ultimately save you much time and frustration, whether or not you have this disorder.

If you would like practical information on implementing a gluten-free diet, see *www.gicare.com*, which has a concise discussion of the disease as well as charts of permitted and forbidden foods. The Celiac Disease Foundation at *www.celiac.org* and the Celiac Sprue Association at *www.csaceliacs.org* are also very useful, but neither can substitute for personal care from a doctor and dietitian, at least as you get started on the road to recovery.

—— AGE-RELATED INFERTILITY ——

Based on my experience in counseling NFP and nutrition, I now recommend a specific nutritional strategy for women who are over 40 and are having difficulty conceiving or maintaining a pregnancy. Such over-40 problems occur because of the age-related decline in the quality of the ova (eggs). I also recommend the same strategy for women of any age with stubborn infertility of unknown cause. However, if you are also dealing with overweight, underweight, endometriosis, short luteal phase, or any of the many other possibilities discussed previously, be sure to address those issues at the same time — your problem may not be completely age-related.

Please refer back to the Introduction to Part II, which explains that, amazingly, the unfertilized ovum must complete its cell division, called "meiosis I," during the two days prior to ovulation. As the ova age, their ability to do this properly declines, contributing to infertility, early miscarriage without proper development of the newly conceived child, and even Down syndrome. In addition, the reproductive hormones FSH and LH decline in the early years of premenopause, so that their hormonal "push" of the ovum to complete meiosis I may be insufficient.

The vitamins, minerals, and essential fatty acids listed below are intended to accomplish two ends: first, to provide the body with the nutrients needed to produce adequate progesterone. If progesterone levels during the second half of the cycle are normal, it is likely that FSH and LH in the first half of the cycle are also normal. Studies cited in Chapters 5 and 7 show that vitamin B6 and vitamin C can raise progesterone levels. Other B vitamins and the mineral magnesium support the activities of vitamin B6.

The second goal is to provide the ovum itself with nutrients known to be involved in meiosis and cell division. These nutrients include folic acid, vitamin B12, zinc, and the essential fatty acids, particularly the omega-3 alpha linolenic acid. Vitamin E is an antioxidant that reduces the oxidation of the essential fatty acids.

DIET. Improve your overall diet, as outlined in Chapter 1, with special attention to avoiding trans fats, aspartame (NutraSweet) and other artificial sweeteners, caffeine, and sugary treats. If you are overweight, whether extremely overweight or just moderately so, try to lose some weight — perhaps 10 pounds. If you are underweight, you will need to gain weight.

SUPPLEMENTS. Consider vitamins, minerals, and essential fatty acids as in Chapter 3, including these higher amounts of the following daily:

TABLE 12, DAILY NUTRIENTS FOR AGE-RELATED INFERTILITY			
Vitamin B6	300 mg[41]	Zinc	25-50 mg
Folic acid	4,000 mcg[42]	Flax oil	5-10 g (5-10 capsules)
Vitamin B12	1,000 mcg[43]	or Fish oil	1 teaspoon
Vitamin C	1,000-1,500 mg	Probiotics, such as acidophilus	
Vitamin E	400-800 IU		

You can start with any of the vitamin brands recommended in Chapter 3. Just add these additional nutrients so that the daily overall total is at the level listed here. Vitamin B12 is easily available in small, flavored tablets that can dissolve under your tongue. Folic acid is available in 800 mcg tablets.

NIGHT LIGHTING. If you can reduce the night lighting in your bedroom, as described in "Sensitivity to Night Lighting" above, you may be able to increase your melatonin levels, which in turn, may help to normalize your progesterone levels.

IMPORTANT NOTE: If you get pregnant using these guidelines, do not discontinue them during the pregnancy! It is not wise to "pull the rug out" from yourself nutritionally once you achieve pregnancy. All of these are safe for use during pregnancy, but of course you should work together with a doctor who is knowledgeable about the benefits of good nutrition.

FOURTEEN YEARS OF INFERTILITY AND COUNTING: 1, 2, 3, 4! Charlene A. of Fort Wayne, Indiana, conceived with ease three times in her twenties (miscarrying between the births of two daughters). Thereafter, however, she was unable to become pregnant. When she was 38, a doctor told her and her husband that there was "nothing wrong" but that she was too old to pursue treatment. At age 41, after 14 years of infertility, she and I met when she enrolled in my university class in human anatomy and physiology. I was pregnant at the time, and more than once she commented to me about her yearning for another child and her long-standing infertility despite regular cycles.

Meanwhile, she constantly complained about the difficulty of my university class, and to talk her out of dropping it, I suggested she drop caffeine and sugar instead. (I have suggested this to many overstressed students over the years, with pretty fair success.) She took this advice to heart, and each week thereafter, when the class met, she raved to me about the difference nutrition made: "I feel so much better...I've lost ten pounds without even trying... I'd never go back to sugar...I've even talked my husband into good nutrition." The two of them soon enrolled in an excellent fitness course emphasizing sound nutrition and moderate exercise. Two months later, to her absolute astonishment and joy, she realized that she was pregnant. I will never forget her incredible joy — the morning of the final exam — as she exclaimed again and again, "It's a miracle!"

You probably expect that this anecdote ends with the birth of a baby, but the story continues. Charlene had a healthy daughter the following August, and shortly afterward enrolled in our NFP course. When the baby was 13 months old, she weaned in order to conceive again. Doubting her ability to do so naturally, she sought the services of her obstetrician. After four months of inducing her to ovulate with the oral fertility drug Clomid, he dismissed her somewhat rudely: "You're never going to get pregnant."

Six months later, using a combination of charting, timing, maintenance of the weight at which she had previously conceived, ideal diet and supplements similar to those in Table 7 (Chapter 3), she did conceive! She had a wonderfully healthy pregnancy and birth; her lovely daughter, her fourth, was born when she was 43.

Charlene's remarkable story has yet another chapter. While her fourth child was still quite young, she again turned to fertility treatment, because she still doubted her own fertility. Five cycles of treatment with Clomid and four with the more powerful drug Perganol combined with progesterone only made her feel sick. The doctor, a fertility specialist, blamed her age and discouraged her from further therapy.

Charlene had continued vitamins and was maintaining her optimum weight, but early in the first cycle without treatment she binged on sugar and contracted a vaginal yeast infection. She immediately eliminated all sugar and took generous supplements of "friendly" acidophilus bacteria to combat the infection. During this cycle she conceived again. Her fifth child, a boy, was born after another healthy pregnancy when Charlene was 45.

Are you ready for the final chapter of this story? Using good nutrition and one cycle of medical treatment (Perganol injections) once more, Charlene had another healthy boy, her sixth child, when she was 47!

This, my favorite anecdote, illustrates several factors that may have been involved — diet, supplements, and body weight. Other points are also important to mention: the simultaneous improvement of both spouses' diets; a positive attitude despite the clear ticking of the "biological clock" and the discouragement of doctors who would not or could not help; and the willingness to continue self-help techniques during and after unsuccessful medical intervention. Last but not least was bringing the infertility in prayer before the Lord.

I am sure that Charlene would not recommend that you experience 14 years of infertility before you try nutrition, and it is useful to realize that the large majority of normally fertile couples who have non-contraceptive intercourse regularly (say twice a week) will conceive within six months. If conception has not occurred by then, timing of intercourse, excellent nutrition, sleeping room light reduction, and the other fertility strategies listed in Appendix B, "Focus on Infertility," should all be implemented by both husband and wife. If in six or nine months conception has still not occurred, seek the assistance of an infertility specialist. A specialist who works with infertility on a daily basis can bring a systematic, comprehensive approach to diagnosing and treating infertility that contrasts sharply with the more limited approach of the obstetrician-gynecologist who deals with this problem only sporadically.

Once you proceed with fertility treatments, excellent nutrition is more necessary than ever if your body is to respond well to the added stress of synthetic or natural fertility drugs or surgery. Also consider the possibility that prolonged or inappropriate treatment may actually delay conception, as may have been the case with Charlene's fourth and fifth pregnancies.

A TRUE SURPRISE PREGNANCY. Here is an article that I wrote for *Family Foundations* in 2000.

> As members of CCL, we tend to think of surprise pregnancies as breaking the rules, ignoring the rules, or rarely, a method failure — any of which could result in an unintended pregnancy. There is another "true surprise" pregnancy, though — the one that follows infertility. Ron and I have experienced our very first surprise pregnancy this way. At age 47, I am now five months pregnant! Our youngest biological child, Ellen, was born when I was 41. My cycles returned during breastfeeding about the time I turned 43, but even though I have ovulated more or less regularly, it certainly appeared that my fertile years were over. Of course I took my own advice, but to no avail. In 1997 we applied for adoption, and we brought Vahn home in June of 1998. My interest in achieving pregnancy dropped once Vahn was in my arms, and I stopped charting. I could honestly say that after the adoption, my recurring periods had no more meaning to me than they did when I was single. We did nothing to avoid a pregnancy, but were completely convinced that it would not happen. In fact, we were confidently discussing the possibility of initiating a second adoption in 2000.
>
> Meanwhile, my cycles became quite irregular last winter — my first sign of approaching menopause. They straightened out again for several cycles until last August, when another long cycle began. Since I wasn't charting, I didn't know for sure what was happening, but I thought to myself, "Here comes menopause again." I started charting, but even before I had 21 high temperatures charted, I was convinced that the rapid physical changes were indicative of a healthy pregnancy. By God's grace all is well so far, my health is excellent, and we are anticipating the birth in early May. Ron and I are beside ourselves with surprise and happiness.
>
> Did nutrition make any difference? One can never say for sure. I take vitamins daily similar to what I recommend for infertility, mostly because it makes such a difference in my energy level to do so. In May or June, however, I started taking 1,000 mcg of vitamin B_{12} daily, again for the energy. In August, when I conceived, I was taking all my vitamins especially carefully, including flax oil, folic acid [2,000–3,000

mcg], and the whole laundry list. I have done some reading and in fact have been able to verify that B12 is important for fertility. Who knows? When my doctor, who was truly astounded, asked me what I thought might have made the difference, I answered sincerely, "The Lord."[44]

This article preceded the birth of our healthy baby daughter, Monica Grace Shannon, two months before I turned 48. I never requested an ultrasound during the pregnancy, yet I felt confident that the baby would be healthy. If you are interested in the research that helped give me that confidence, please refer to Chapter 11, "Repeated Miscarriage & Birth Defects."

By the way, I think Monica, who is now 8, is a budding scientist. A naturalist at heart, she loves plants and animals, including insects. She gardens avidly (and organically), hand-picking the caterpillars off her prize broccoli. She asks many, many questions! Like, "Do bees sleep?" "What's a pig's tail for?" "Can toads see in the dark?" "How big is an ant's stomach?" and, "Do chickens have knees?"[45]

➤ A number of subtle health problems or situations may interfere with cycle regularity, or they may contribute to infertility without obvious changes in the cycle at all. They include:

1) yeast overgrowth, in which the usually harmless intestinal fungus, Candida albicans, causes infection, allergic reactions, or reactions to toxins;

2) discontinuing birth control pills or other hormonal birth control;

3) sensitivity to night lighting, which apparently can affect fertility by decreasing the hormone melatonin;

4) excess caffeine consumption;

5) celiac disease, in which an abnormal reaction to the protein gluten in certain grains damages the small intestine, resulting in multiple nutritional abnormalities; and

6) age-related infertility, the natural life progression that results in hormonal changes and poor ovum quality.

➤ Each of these may respond to specific nutritional or other strategies aimed at overcoming them.

10

Pregnancy &
Postpartum Nutrition

And so Joseph went up from Galilee from the town of Nazareth in Galilee to Judea, to David's town of Bethlehem — because he was of the house and lineage of David — to register with Mary, his betrothed wife, who was with child. — Luke 2:4-5

Ideally, pregnancy is a time of great joy, anticipation, and wonder. It is a miracle — a child, the fruit of your love, developing within you! There is sweet anticipation on sharing the secret with others, donning your maternity clothes for the first time, and feeling the first fluttery kicks. You are already a mother, and your protective instincts are already powerfully engaged. What you eat, what medicines you take, and what type of exercise you engage in are all done with your growing baby constantly on your mind and in your heart.

No one needs to convince you what good nutrition means to your unborn baby. But more than at any other time in your life, what you eat, how much you eat, and what supplements you take will also make an immense difference in how much you enjoy your pregnancy. However, even if excellent nutrition does not give you the energy you would like, or does not prevent morning sickness, stretch marks, or some of the other annoyances of pregnancy, it will enable your baby to develop the healthiest nervous system and immune system that he or she can. Good nutrition is the best insurance that your baby will be born at term and at a healthy weight. Good nutrition will help you feel your best during the postpartum period so that you can delight fully in that all-too-fleeting time when your newborn is so tiny and helpless.

—— *PREGNANCY* ——————————————

HOW LONG SHOULD YOU PREPARE BEFORE PREGNANCY? There is no absolute answer to the question of how long you should work to improve your nutrition before trying to become pregnant. It depends on your health at the time. Many women's health advocates recommend about three months of preparation, including taking prenatal vitamins. If you have cycle problems such as short luteal phase or polycystic ovary syndrome, implementing the self-help strategies in the earlier chapters of this book for two or three months gives you time to reap the benefits of improved nutrition. If you are coming off birth control pills or other hormonal birth control, it is prudent to let your own hormones readjust for three months as you improve your nutrition and start taking good supplements. If you have been sick with an illness that has caused you to lose weight, such as pneumonia, two or three months gives you time to recover your health and regain your weight.

On the other hand, if you are in good health and are already eating nutritious foods, starting your prenatal vitamins and other supplements at the beginning of the cycle before the one in which you hope to conceive is certainly adequate. I also believe that waiting just one cycle is adequate for women who have unfortunately experienced an early miscarriage, as long as it has not been complicated by heavy blood loss or surgical intervention.

But what if you decide, on short notice, that you would like to conceive this month? Or what if you discover you are pregnant, quite by surprise? Right then is the best time for you to fully implement a diet and supplements aimed confidently at the healthiest pregnancy possible.

NUTRITIONAL PREPARATION FOR PREGNANCY. As you prepare for pregnancy, cut down on sugary treats and soda pop (including diet pop), and limit caffeine to the equivalent of two average cups of coffee daily.[1] Replace junk food with good food, as recommended in Part I of this book. As much as possible, eliminate trans fats, and make sure you have sources of the beneficial monounsaturated fats and the essential fatty acids, as explained in Rule 3, Chapter 1. Pay special attention to nutritional choices aimed at stabilizing your blood glucose levels, as explained in Rule 7, Chapter 1. A holistic diet will make you confident that you will give your baby the best start possible. Beginning your pregnancy with good blood sugar control as a result of good diet will also go a long way toward decreasing morning sickness.

No doubt you are aware that the B vitamin folic acid has been shown to reduce the incidence of several types of serious birth defects called neural tube defects. Research on the effectiveness of folic acid in preventing such problems has indicated that supplementing this vitamin for several weeks before conception and for twelve weeks after conception is most effective. That is why the beginning of the cycle *before* the one in which you hope to conceive is a good time for you to start your vitamins, unless you have already been taking at least 400 mcg of folic acid (and preferably more, especially if you are an older mother).

But do not supplement just folic acid. Take a comprehensive multivitamin/ multimineral and essential fatty acids supplement, as recommended below. As one British researcher wrote in a review article on supplements for pregnant women: "Since the Medical Research Council study in 1991 on folic acid and the prevention of neural tube defects, it has become evident that there are nutrients in supplement form that can have a significant impact on the outcome of pregnancy. Folic acid is only one of the B vitamins, but what about all the nutrients that are contained in food?"[2]

MORNING SICKNESS

The nausea and vomiting of morning sickness can take enjoyment out of even the most long-awaited pregnancy. More importantly, though, it can be severe enough to cause you to lose weight early in pregnancy. Fortunately, it usually subsides by the second trimester, when you really need to increase your intake of good food to meet the growing needs of your baby and yourself.

I am a proponent of the theory that the nausea and vomiting of early pregnancy are related to low blood glucose, which in some women stimulates the vomiting center in the brain. A diet rich in protein foods, vegetables, fruits, and grains, without sugary junk food, will naturally tend to stabilize blood sugar. Ideally, such a diet would be started well before you get pregnant. However, even if you have morning sickness already, you may find that you actually do feel better after you eat small meals of protein, carbohydrate, and natural fat. This is often true despite the fact that your appetite may be poor and you just do not feel like eating.

Adrenal exhaustion, described in Chapter 14, may also be a factor in morning sickness, because healthy adrenal glands support normal blood glucose levels and normal blood pressure. (I have noticed that many women with morning sickness have low blood pressure, which may explain why some women say that frequently eating salty foods early in pregnancy helps them.) Reading Chapter 14 and implementing its nutritional recommendations to the extent that you are able may help you. All of the recommendations within that chapter are safe for pregnant women.

SUPPLEMENTS FOR MORNING SICKNESS. Studies show that vitamin B6 is effective in reducing morning sickness.[3] Taking 50–300 mg daily is helpful in pregnancy, but make sure to get your doctor's approval first, especially if you take more than 200 mg daily.[4] Complete vitamin/mineral supplements are useful to keep blood glucose levels steady, but often they contribute to nausea by irritating the stomach. If this is true for you, take only the supplements that you can with a meal at the time of day you feel best. Folic acid and vitamin B6 are the most important supplements in early pregnancy. Folic acid prevents birth defects, but it also supports fasting blood glucose levels and therefore may help with morning sickness.

For example, my friend Ann had her ninth baby at age 43. We took our kids swimming at a beautiful wooded lake on a sunny summer day when her new baby boy was just two weeks old. Ann looked and felt wonderful, and the baby was a really content little guy. She mentioned that during this pregnancy, she took a prescription vitamin pill for morning sickness that reduced her morning sickness from a "7 or 8" on a scale of 1 to 10 during her previous pregnancies, to a "2 or 3" this time. This product, called PremesisRx, contains 75 mg of vitamin B6, 1,000 mcg of folic acid, and 200 mg of calcium carbonate as a buffer against stomach upset. (She also took additional folic acid.)

Ginger, in the amount of 1 g daily, helps some women to overcome morning sickness and is safe to use during pregnancy.[5] Capsules of ground ginger root are available at health food shops and can be taken with meals or made into a tea. Digestive enzymes, also available at health food shops, may also reduce nausea in some women by promoting digestion of food by the stomach.

MYTHS ABOUT MORNING SICKNESS. Morning sickness is not in the least psychological in origin — you already know that if you have had it! — but sometimes others who have never experienced it may imply that it is. If you have had it, you probably agree that the name itself is a myth, because it can happen at any time of the day or even all day long. I believe, though, that the traditional name, morning sickness, is based on the fact that most people's blood sugar levels are lowest when they wake up in the morning, and low blood glucose stimulates nausea in some people.

Morning sickness is certainly not a "healthy sign," as some doctors tell women. Yes, it does indicate that the hormonal changes of pregnancy are happening, but many women, myself included, have had several healthy pregnancies without even an hour of this distressing, demoralizing condition. Nor is it inevitable, even if you have had it during past pregnancies — consider my friend Ann's improvement. Even if you are prone to it, the nutritional strategies discussed here can make it far less severe.

My booklet, *Managing Morning Sickness*, has more information on this topic. (See "Further Reading.") However, if you cannot keep your food down and gain weight with self-care as you begin the second trimester, your doctor's treatment is essential for your health and for that of your baby.

DIET DURING PREGNANCY

There is simply no substitute for nutritious food during pregnancy to ensure both your health and your baby's. As an expectant mother, your need for protein increases progressively, especially as you enter the second half of your pregnancy. Your need for calories increases as well, so that your body can use the protein for the baby's rapid growth and for your own increased blood volume, uterine size, and so forth. Not enough overall calories causes protein to be "burned" as fuel, rather than used as an essential building material for mother and child. On the other hand, enough calories but not enough protein foods cannot do the job either. You absolutely need both — adequate protein, and enough overall calories from carbohydrates and natural fats.

PREECLAMPSIA (TOXEMIA OF PREGNANCY). You may have wondered why prenatal care includes blood pressure monitoring and urine checks more and more frequently as you approach your due date. These are done in order to detect early signs of a potentially serious problem, preeclampsia, or metabolic toxemia of late pregnancy. "Toxemia," as it is still often called, can be recognized clinically by high blood pressure and protein in the urine. Severe edema (fluid retention) often occurs with it.

If early signs of toxemia occur, the expectant mother is usually advised to rest in order to help keep her blood pressure down, and to limit salt in order to reduce the edema. If the situation worsens, the doctor frequently induces labor or performs an emergency caesarian section to prevent the dangerous stage that follows, called eclampsia. If it is left untreated, eclampsia can progress from seizures to coma, and even to death of the mother and unborn child.

Perhaps you know a woman who has had her labor induced early due to her elevated blood pressure and other abnormalities, even though it meant that the baby was born several weeks prematurely. The induction of labor was not undertaken lightly. The attending physicians had to weigh the risk of eclampsia against the long-term problems that often occur when a baby is born early. That is how serious toxemia of pregnancy is. Inducing labor can prevent a disaster.

As with so many other things in life, prevention is infinitely preferable to dealing with the problem once it has occurred. Avoiding toxemia is by far the best strategy, yet toxemia along with premature birth to avoid the effects of this disease is distressingly common.

THE BREWER DIET TO PREVENT TOXEMIA. Tom Brewer, M.D., spent a long career advocating the use of a healthy daily diet aimed at preventing toxemia in pregnant women. The diet he developed is high in protein and rich in plant foods, and he implemented it successfully with thousands of women in various parts of the United States. As part of his dietary plan, he specifically advised pregnant women against restriction of weight gain.[6]

The Brewer diet is simple to learn and is made up of ordinary foods. It recommends the following daily: One quart of milk, two eggs, one or two servings of meat or fish; two servings each of dark green vegetables and a vitamin C source; five servings of grains or starches, three servings of fats and oils, and one source of vitamin A.[7] These recommendations, with minor modifications, serve as the basis of Table 13, "Suggested Daily Food Goals for Pregnant and Nursing Women" (see pages 146–147).

Dr. Brewer additionally recommended that pregnant women salt their food to taste, drink plenty of water, and eat at least one snack daily. His website, The Blue Ribbon Baby Pages (*www.blueribbonbaby.org*), contains further information on this topic and includes a checklist that you can use to make certain you have eaten all the recommended foods daily. It also contains food substitutions for a vegetarian diet.

As you begin your pregnancy, the hearty intake of food recommended by the Brewer diet is neither necessary nor possible, but as you get into the second and especially the third trimester, your appetite picks up and eating healthy food becomes almost a craving!

ALLERGIES TO MILK OR EGGS. If you are allergic to milk, it is important to realize that it is a major source of protein and you need to compensate for avoiding it. You can substitute two 3-ounce servings of lean meat or fish for one quart (four glasses) of milk. It is best to supplement calcium, along with magnesium and vitamin D, if you do not use dairy products.

TABLE 13
SUGGESTED DAILY FOOD GOALS FOR PREGNANT AND NURSING WOMEN

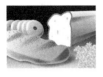 ## Whole Grains

5 servings daily
(1 serving = 1 slice bread or 1/2 cup cooked cereal)

Whole grain bread	Whole grain pasta	Millet
Oatmeal	Whole grain pancakes	Tortillas
Whole grain breakfast cereal	Rice	Bagels

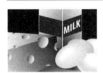 ## Dairy/Eggs

6 servings daily
(1 serving = 8 oz. milk, 2 oz. cheese, 1 egg)

| Whole milk | Yogurt | Cheese | Kefir | Ice cream | Eggs |

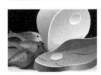 ## Complete Protein

1-2 servings daily
(1 serving = 4 oz. meat)

Poultry	Grain + Legume
Fish (preferably twice weekly)	(Peas, beans, peanut butter, nuts, lentils)
Beef	Dairy + Grain
Pork	Dairy + Legume
Lamb	

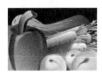 ## Yellow Fruits and Vegetables

1 serving daily
(1 serving = 1/2 cup cooked or 1 cup raw)

| Carrots | Sweet potatoes | Mangos | Peaches |
| Squash | Pumpkin | Apricots | Cantaloupe |

This table may be photocopied, covered with adhesive backed clear plastic and taped to

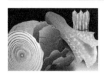

Leafy Green Vegetables

3 servings daily
(1 serving = 1/2 cup cooked or 1 cup raw)

Lettuce
(leaf, Romaine,
Bibb, iceberg)
Spinach
Escarole
Endive

Beet greens
Alfalfa sprouts
Cole crops
(cabbage, broccoli,
Brussels sprouts,
cauliflower, kohlrabi)

Asparagus
Chard
Kale

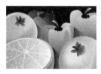

Vitamin C Source

2 servings daily
(1 serving = 1 medium fruit or 1/2 cup berries)

Citrus fruits
(oranges, grapefruits,
tangerines)

Tomatoes
Melons
Berries

Peppers
Potatoes

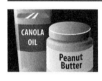

Unsaturated Oils

3 servings daily
(1 serving = 1 tablespoon)

Monounsaturated
Olive oil
Peanut oil
Unprocessed peanut butter
Avocado oil

Polyunsaturated
Soy oil *
Walnut oil *
Safflower oil
Sunflower Oil
Corn oil

Both
Canola oil *
Sesame oil

* Source of the essential omega-3 alpha-linolenic acid.

your refrigerator. Check off the boxes daily with a dry erase marker.

Eggs have a number of wonderful nutrients in them, so much so that my midwife used to refer to them as "big vitamin pills." However, one 3-ounce serving of meat can replace the protein of two eggs.

OVERWEIGHT WOMEN. I am always troubled when I hear a woman recount a story that goes like this: "I was overweight when I got pregnant. My doctor told me to gain no more than 30 pounds. I really tried to keep my weight down. But by seven months, I already had gained the full 30. The doctor told me in no uncertain terms that I had gained my quota. So I really cut down, just as much as I could. I started swelling, and my blood pressure went sky high. They did an emergency C-section at seven and a half months. My baby was in neonatal intensive care, and I had to pump milk and bring it to the hospital. It was really a stress all the way through."

Dr. Brewer made a distinction between gaining weight on junk food and carbohydrates versus weight gain based on his protein-rich diet. He pointed out that women who are obese or overweight when they get pregnant still need to eat healthy food daily and that pregnancy is not the time to diet. On the other hand, women who begin their pregnancies while overweight or obese may find that with his diet plan, they in fact do not gain much weight, or may even lose a little, which in such a case is not a problem.[8]

Unfortunately, studies of how weight gain, or lack of weight gain, affects pregnancy in women who are obese still fail to include consideration of what type of diet these women were eating.[9] How much of the diet is carbohydrate or fat versus protein? During pregnancy, it makes an immense difference.

UNDERWEIGHT WOMEN. If you are overly thin, part of your preparation before pregnancy should be an earnest attempt to bring your weight up. Once you become pregnant, working up to the Brewer ideal should be your goal. While some health experts state that 25–35 pounds of weight gain is adequate, an additional 10 or 15 pounds (35–50 pounds total) may be completely normal and healthy for a thin or slender woman.

MAINTAINING YOUR FIGURE. If you are troubled by the idea of "losing your figure" or by the time it takes to lose weight after childbirth, remind yourself that you are feeding your baby's developing brain every day. You are forming your baby's immune system with what you eat. A woman's body is designed to store several pounds of fat during pregnancy. This is necessary for the health of both mother and baby, and the fat reserves are gradually nursed away over a period of a few weeks or months. Failure to gain enough weight on good food is the leading cause of low birth weight and prematurity, both of which may have lifelong physical and mental consequences for the baby.

IF YOU HAVE ALREADY GAINED "TOO MUCH." What about the woman in the anecdote above? What should you do if you have already gained "too much" weight, yet still have two or three months to go? The answer is straightforward: whether you were of normal weight or obese when you got pregnant, you need to continue nourishing your baby and eat especially the protein and other nutrients that both you and your baby must have. There is no substitute for daily nutritious food, and the need for overall calories and protein is highest during the last trimester.

RECENT RESEARCH ON NUTRITION FOR TOXEMIA. I am dismayed to see that the role of actual food type — protein versus fat or carbohydrates — is ignored in major research studies concerned with preventing toxemia. A number of different vitamins, minerals, and fatty acid supplements have been studied for their effect on toxemia, but except for the B vitamins, most have ended with disappointing results.[10]

One study assessed the effect of a high-fiber diet on the risk of developing toxemia. While fruits, vegetables, low-fat and high-fat dairy products were evaluated, overall protein intake was not. Nevertheless, the authors did observe that foods rich in fiber, such as cereal, whole-grain bread, low-fat dairy, and fruits and vegetables were generally associated with a reduced risk of toxemia.[11]

Another recent study indirectly confirms Dr. Brewer's work. This study found that women with a low intake of milk had a higher risk of developing toxemia (preeclampsia), and those with the lowest milk intake were most likely to suffer from the dangerous eclampsia. The researchers observed that two and one-half glasses of milk daily was average for women who had preeclampsia, and noted "an evident protective effect" against preeclampsia of five glasses of milk daily; that much milk consumption lowered the risk of toxemia almost *five times.* Yet the discussion centered on the role of calcium, and the authors stated, "The mechanisms by which calcium may prevent preeclampsia are still unknown."[12] They then noted that other large studies in which calcium was supplemented did not reduce the risk of toxemia.[13] Two and one-half glasses of milk daily average about 20 grams of protein; five glasses, about 40 grams. How is it that the role of protein in preventing toxemia can be overlooked even when it is staring you in the face!

"The Blue Ribbon Baby Pages" (***www.blueribbonbaby.org***) have all of the information you need to know about what and how much to eat when you are pregnant, even if you have had problems with previous pregnancies. It will help you whether or not you are milk intolerant or eat a vegetarian diet. You may also wish to read Dr. Brewer's classic book, *What Every Pregnant Woman Should Know: The Truth About Diet and Drugs in Pregnancy.* (See "Further Reading.")

VITAMIN AND MINERAL SUPPLEMENTS DURING PREGNANCY

Both over-the-counter prenatal vitamins as well as prescription prenatal vitamins vary widely in their potencies, so you need to read labels whether or not your prenatal supplement is under prescription. In fact, prescription prenatal vitamins are often surprisingly low in potency. I recommend supplements in amounts similar to those listed in Table 7, Chapter 3. Professional Prenatal Formula comes the closest of any supplement I know to meeting all the needs for pregnant women. It is labeled for six tablets per day, allowing you to adjust your intake downward if you wish, or if you cannot tolerate a full dose.

ProCycle PMS is also safe and healthy for pregnancy, though it contains no iron.[14] You may need to supplement iron separately if tests show that you need more. Optivite PMT is also safe for pregnancy, and may even reduce nausea and vomiting. [15] It contains only 200 mcg of folic acid per full dose, so additional folic acid must be added. (See "Appendix A" and "Resources.")

If you have taken other vitamins, minerals, or a product such as Fertility Blend to achieve pregnancy, do not stop taking them now! You need the nutritional support for your hormones more than ever. With your doctor's approval, you can continue Fertility Blend.[16] You could combine it with a two-thirds or three-fourths dose of Professional Prenatal Formula, Optivite, or ProCycle.

One of the principles of this book is that vitamins, minerals, and essential fatty acids work together to maintain health. Nowhere is this principle more evident than during pregnancy, as more and more new studies illustrate. I would like to offer some important examples of this.

THE BIG Bs: FOLIC ACID, VITAMIN B12, AND VITAMIN B6. Supplements of folic acid decrease the risk of neural tube birth defects, including spina bifida and anencephaly. But folic acid plays other important roles in pregnancy. It is involved in cell division and has a vital role in the implantation, development, and health of the placenta, which develops from a single cell into an organ weighing over a pound. Low levels of folate have been found in women who have had abruption of the placenta, the dangerous situation in which the placenta separates from the uterus, threatening mother and fetus.[17] Supplements of multivitamins containing folic acid in the second trimester also lower the risk of preeclampsia.[18]

However, folic acid works together with two other B vitamins — vitamin B12 and vitamin B6 — to support certain biochemical processes necessary to protein metabolism. These three B vitamins decrease the overproduction of a potentially harmful amino acid, homocysteine. Homocysteine is under intense study to understand its role in several different diseases, including heart disease. With reference to pregnancy, there is a growing acceptance of the possibility that homocysteine is the actual chemical that causes neural tube defects.[19] Homocysteine is elevated in women who have preeclampsia.[20] In addition, it has been implicated in early miscarriages, intrauterine growth retardation (failure of the fetus to grow normally), and low birth weight babies.[21] These topics are explored more fully in Chapter 11.

What does that mean to you? Multivitamin supplements which contain folic acid, vitamin B12, and vitamin B6 are preferable to folic acid supplements alone. Taking such supplements before pregnancy helps if you cannot tolerate vitamins during the first trimester, and taking complete supplements throughout your pregnancy, along with good diet, should give you confidence in your own health and that of your baby.

FOLIC ACID AND IRON. Supplementing folic acid together with iron is more effective than iron alone in enabling pregnant women to overcome iron-deficiency anemia.[22] Folic acid and iron may also help to reduce an annoying problem, restless legs syndrome, which some women develop during pregnancy.[23] See Table 7, Chapter 3, for recommended amounts of both.

FOLIC ACID AND VITAMIN B12 FOR ENERGY. Some women feel much better when they take larger amounts of folic acid than the usual 400 mcg. Some international organizations and researchers recommend ten times that amount (4,000 mcg) or more (5,000 mcg) beginning before pregnancy for women who have had a child with a neural tube defect[24] or for all women's prenatal vitamins.[25] I recommend that you try up to 4,000 mcg daily if you are an older mother, or if you struggle with fatigue during your pregnancy. In addition, Dean Raffelock, D.C., and Robert Rountree, M.D., authors of *A Natural Guide to Pregnancy and Postpartum Health*, recommend for "severe fatigue during or after your pregnancy, try taking up to 5,000 mcg of vitamin B12. This is a safe way to energize your body, and it will not harm your baby."[26] You will very likely find that small tablets of 1,000 mcg of vitamin B12, dissolved under your tongue, contain enough vitamin B12 to enable you to overcome pregnancy fatigue.

VITAMIN B6 AND MAGNESIUM FOR EDEMA. Texas physician John Ellis, M.D., spent years studying the relationship between vitamin B6 deficiency and various disorders, including pregnancy edema, toxemia, and eclampsia. The following excerpts from his book, *Vitamin B6: The Doctor's Report*, summarize the results of his clinical experience:

> Numerous signs and symptoms appear during pregnancy that are responsive to B6. These include painful neuropathies in the fingers and hands, swelling (edema) in the hands and feet, leg cramps, hand and arms "that go to sleep," and, most of all, B6 is a factor in the prevention and treatment of toxemia of pregnancy and the convulsions of eclampsia...Edema of pregnancy, long discussed in both medical and lay circles, has become so common that many doctors have come to accept it as being normal during pregnancy, and patients have grown resigned to suffering through it. It is not normal at all. It is not normal at any time. The patient feels bad. There is nothing healthy about being swollen with fluids. Based on my investigations with 225 pregnant women on B6 therapy, in most cases vitamin B6 will completely relieve and prevent edema of pregnancy as it has been known to the scientific community. This is a large statement, but it has been proved over and over. Because of the skepticism that some readers may entertain, it would be wise to repeat that in these 225 cases no diuretics were given to any patient, and there was no restriction on either salt or fluids.[27]

Dr. Ellis presented a series of conclusions based on his research, including emphasis that salt restriction is not necessary when vitamin B6 is adequate, and that the babies born to mothers who have taken large doses of B6 do not show increased need for this vitamin. He also noted the role of magnesium, which works synergistically with vitamin B6:

> ...All pregnant women should have at least 50 milligrams of B6 [daily] as a supplement throughout their pregnancies, and many of them will require considerably more than that. All pregnant women should also receive at least 500 milligrams of magnesium daily, and with the appearance of the signs of toxemia the magnesium should be increased to 1,000 milligrams daily.[28]

While I consider this older research valuable enough to recommend here, please note that there is no substitute for adequate protein to prevent toxemia of pregnancy. However, vitamin B6, like folic acid and vitamin B12, does improve the use of protein in the body through its effect on reducing homocysteine. During my own pregnancies, I found that Dr. Ellis's findings were true for me — for example, I can confirm that the numbness of the hands that some women complain of is much improved by vitamin B6. In addition, I think that vitamin B6, along with other B vitamins, is helpful to preventing "brain fog."

PUTTING IT ALL TOGETHER: The following anecdote, contributed by a young medical student, illustrates the beneficial effects of adequate supplements during pregnancy:

> My wife and I were expecting our third child. Both of our older children had been born at home, and our plans were to deliver this child at home as well. However, a potentially serious problem presented an obstacle to a safe delivery at home. Despite care in maintaining good nutrition, in each of the other two pregnancies my wife had retained water and experienced nausea far beyond the normal length of "morning sickness." In addition, she had other related problems, such as tingling and numbness in her fingers and hands, joint aches and pains, elevated blood pressure, and a general feeling of not being well. These symptoms had occurred earlier in the second pregnancy than the first, and now, in the third, were occurring earlier still; she was only in the fourth month of pregnancy and had already gained 35 pounds. We both felt strongly that she had been only slightly better than a marginal candidate for home delivery with the last baby, and that if she wasn't in substantially better health with this pregnancy (largely because 6-1/2 years had passed, and she was now 30 years old with a family history of diabetes), it would not be safe to have this baby at home. However, we were even less enthusiastic about a hospital birth.

> As we were in the middle of this quandary, I had the opportunity to discuss the subject with the author, with whom I taught a class weekly. She shared with me information on the importance of good multivitamin supplements, and recommended a balanced nonprescription prenatal multivitamin. [The full dose of this supplement contained 75 mg/mcg of most B vitamins, 100 mg of B6, 450 mg of magnesium, and

other vitamins and minerals in amounts similar to those in Table 7, Chapter 3. Professional Prenatal Formula is very similar.]

As soon as my wife began taking these vitamins (and I mean within one day), she began shedding excess water, and experienced a visible improvement of the edema in her hands and feet. She lost nearly six pounds in the first week, and continued to improve until we could see the veins on the tops of her feet. Her blood pressure remained normal, there was no numbness, and she only occasionally felt nauseous. The improvement was so pronounced that we no longer felt reservations about continuing with plans for a home birth.

The effectiveness of this improvement in nutrition was demonstrated very pointedly some weeks later, when we ran out of the vitamin supplement, and found that the health food store where we had purchased them was also out of stock. In the week that my wife was not taking this supplement, she quickly became fatigued, nauseous, and edematous [swollen with fluid]. As soon as we had obtained a new supply and she had begun to take them regularly again, the problems disappeared.

My wife enjoyed excellent health throughout the remainder of the pregnancy, and delivered a healthy baby boy at home.[29]

OTHER STRATEGIES TO REDUCE EDEMA. Good multivitamin/multiminerals, combined with good diet, really help to reduce water retention and swelling. But here are some more tips to prevent edema: eat more protein and reduce extra carbohydrates if you are retaining fluid. Drink plenty of water, which in itself is a natural diuretic. Do not sit for too long, and elevate your feet when you rest. Keep cool! Try going wading in deep, cool water. The cool water causes vasoconstriction of the blood vessels in the skin, a change that generally stimulates the kidneys to produce more urine. The actual pressure of the water on the body also signals the kidneys to excrete extra fluid. If you cannot go wading, try soaking your feet in a tall bucket of cool water.

FISH OIL AND FLAX OIL SUPPLEMENTS

FISH AS BRAIN FOOD. A recent research article noted that the advice for pregnant women to limit their seafood consumption due to the possibility of toxins, especially mercury, may be counterproductive. Why? The less seafood pregnant women consume, the higher the risk that their children will have developmental problems, including those involving fine motor skills, communication, and social skills. The researchers concluded that based on their large study, "risks from the loss of nutrients were greater than the risks of harm from exposure to trace contaminants in 340 g [12 oz., or three 4-oz. servings] seafood eaten weekly."[30] That is, mothers who ate more than the government-recommended amounts of seafood had children with better developmental outcomes from six months of age until eight years of age, which is the age limit of the study.

Why should seafood matter when there are many other sources of protein? In this case, it is not the protein. It is the DHA (docosahexaenoic acid) found in fish that is critical to the brain development of the fetus in the womb. If DHA is insufficient, neuron-to-neuron connections in the developing brain are not made properly.

Seafood is a good source of many nutrients, but instead of worrying about mercury, use the Internet to access recommendations as to the least contaminated species of fish. (See the question and answer on this topic in Chapter 4.) However, supplementing with certified contaminant-free, good-tasting cod liver oil is another option that is supported by new research. Supplements of fish oil enhance the development of the brain of the baby before birth; in fact, the need for DHA is highest during the last trimester of pregnancy, when the baby's brain is growing the fastest. Such supplements may even reduce the risk of premature birth, especially in women who have had premature babies previously.[31]

Udo Erasmus, Ph.D., in his book, *Fats That Heal, Fats That Kill*, noted that the "Catholic custom of fish on Fridays may have had health benefits, at least before it degenerated into fish-n-chips — low-fat fish and potatoes, both deep-fried in damaged and damaging oils."[32]

FISH OIL AND FLAX OIL SUPPLEMENTS. Drs. Raffelock and Rountree, in *A Natural Guide to Pregnancy and Postpartum Health*, recommend an amount of purified fish body oil that supplies 150–300 mg of DHA and 180–300 mg EPA daily.[33] They do not recommend fish liver oil because of the vitamin A content, but I disagree with them on this point. The amount of fish liver oil with these amounts of DHA and EPA is in the range of only one-half teaspoon daily (3 1-g capsules), and the vitamin A in fish liver oil of this amount is only 350–600 IU, far below the limit of safety for a pregnant woman, which is 8,000–10,000 IU of true vitamin A.[34]

These doctors also recommend a tablespoon of ground flax seed daily.[35] This is equivalent to about 1 teaspoon or five 1 g capsules of flax oil, which is a source of the essential omega-3 fatty acid, alpha-linolenic acid. They recommend the same for postpartum women, especially those who are breastfeeding. In any case, be sure to take about 400 IU of vitamin E as an antioxidant to protect these valuable oils.

—— THE POSTPARTUM TIME

Life changes profoundly when the new baby arrives! The entire family dynamic is reshuffled. If it is the first child, the husband and wife become parents. A single child becomes a big brother or sister. The current baby becomes an older sibling. Schedules change; sleep patterns are disrupted; visitors come and go. The mother is entirely focused on her new baby, ideally with help from caring relatives and friends. It is easy for everyone to forget that profound hormonal changes are occurring in the new mother. There is simply no other situation in healthy human physiology that comes remotely close to the speed and magnitude of the hormonal readjustments that happen to a new mother.

Mom's first meal after labor and birth is the best meal many women have ever had! I still savor the memories of the biggest and tastiest pizza I ever ate, which our best neighbors brought to our home after a very long labor ending with the birth of our third child, Stephen. These neighbors had kept our two older children at their house during the labor and birth, but they arrived soon afterwards with the kids (and the pizza). Here is the story they told us: When Ron finally called them with the news, they told John, who was six, and Rosemary, who was four, that Mom and Dad had had a baby boy, and so now they had a new baby brother. "But I wanted a girl brother!" Rosemary wailed.

EMOTIONAL NURTURING. When it comes to "postpartum nutrition," the emotional nurturing of the mother comes first. Birth is an intense physical stress; the adjustment to the new baby is an intense emotional stress; and the excitement of it all is an intense overall stress, albeit a positive one. Having trusted helpers around who know how to reduce that stress will provide the mother with joyful memories for the rest of her life. Conversely, thoughtless remarks that she might construe as a criticism during this hormonally and emotionally unsettled time will easily upset her. The new mother needs complete support, as much rest as she can get, and the positive assurance that everything around her is being taken care of. One of the nicest things that you can do for a new mother is to drop off a meal, spending a few minutes to congratulate the family and admire the baby.

BREASTFEEDING NUTRITION

The physical stress of late pregnancy far exceeds the physical stress of breastfeeding. Before the baby is born, you are not only eating for him (or her), but you are also breathing oxygen for him and excreting his wastes. You are carrying him around in an internal bathtub "24/7," as they say. As a breastfeeding mother of a young baby, you are now only eating for him, and carrying him some of the time. But that is a job, too! Ideally, as you get started, you should have the assistance of at least one experienced, compassionate woman who has nursed her own babies successfully.

FLUIDS. Water is the first nutrient that you need as a breastfeeding mother, and you need to make sure you are drinking enough, whether or not your sense of thirst is a reliable guide. Just as you can judge your baby's fluid intake by his or her output, you can get a sense of the adequacy of your own input by your output. When you are fully breastfeeding, you are producing about a quart or more of milk daily. Nevertheless, you should be producing as much urine as before you were pregnant. That means you need to drink considerably more than when you were pregnant. Many women experience a distinct sensation of thirst when the baby first latches on — it relates to the hormonal response of milk "letdown." It is a good idea to keep a large water bottle handy so that you can drink plenty of water before that sensation fades.

DIET. You will likely find that your appetite drops after the birth compared to when you were pregnant. It is usual to lose some weight immediately, and then to gradually lose the "baby weight." A modified version of the Brewer diet will serve you well as you breastfeed. High-quality protein and natural fat in the diet are the most important of the major nutrients for milk production. If you are tolerant of milk, you will probably agree that "milk makes milk." On the other hand, if you do not drink milk or use dairy products, substituting two servings of meat or fish for a quart of milk enables you to keep up your protein.

About 50 percent of the calories that breast milk provides comes from fats. The fat composition of breast milk reflects the mother's diet. Eating trans fats is to be avoided, as they end up in the breast milk. Using olive oil and expeller-pressed canola oil helps to provide the fatty acids that the baby requires.

Plenty of nursing mothers find that certain foods make their babies fussy, but that does not mean that a food that seemed to bother your older child will necessarily bother the newest one. Lists of foods that bother some babies often include caffeine-containing drinks and foods, spicy foods, and gas-producing vegetables. As a baby gets older, foods that you may have had to avoid earlier may be fine for you to eat.

SUPPLEMENTS. Fish oil especially (or flax oil or both) will continue to nourish your baby's growing brain now that he or she is born. Your breast milk will contain the valuable DHA that enables proper development of your baby's brain tissue, as long as DHA is available through your diet. Use about the same amounts of fish and flax oil as recommended in the preceding section on pregnancy. You need at least as much of the essential fatty acids when you are breastfeeding as when you are pregnant.

Good vitamins, minerals, and essential fatty acids will nourish both you and your baby. Supplements, such as those in Table 7, Chapter 3, or as recommended in the preceding section on supplements for pregnancy, will help you meet your own increased nutritional needs as well as those of your baby.

POSTPARTUM THYROIDITIS

At some point after giving birth, often before the baby is six months old, a small percentage of women experience thyroid problems. About one to four months after the birth, some new mothers (approximately 4 percent) develop an overactive thyroid gland. They may feel heart palpitations and fatigue, both of which develop rather rapidly. They may develop a small, painless goiter. About two-thirds of such women will return to normal on their own, or they may actually go on to develop low thyroid function.[36]

Approximately 2–5 percent of women develop low thyroid function (hypothyroidism) about four to eight months postpartum, but sometimes even earlier. Often it corrects itself on its own by the time the baby is a year old, but replacement of thyroid hormone may be necessary, at least temporarily. Of the women who develop either overactive thyroid or hypothyroidism after giving birth, about one-third develop permanent hypothyroidism, which must be treated medically.[37]

THE NFP CHART. I have observed very low temperatures, often in the range of 96.8° F and below, on the charts of some women with young babies, reflecting the low thyroid function that may occur postpartum. I have also seen the temperatures rise over a period of two weeks to a month after such women have supplemented vitamins, minerals, and essential fatty acids as recommended in Chapter 7 under the topic "Low Thyroid Function." If you see very low temperatures on your chart, whether or not you are breastfeeding and whether or not you have had your periods return, give the supplements recommended in Chapter 7 a try for a month or two. However, you should be in touch with a medical doctor as well.

Mary Shomon, author of *The Thyroid Hormone Breakthrough*, explains postpartum thyroid problems thoroughly in an excellent chapter dedicated to this topic. (See "Further Reading.") For example, she explains how women with previous thyroid problems may have to be tested regularly after they have a baby because their needs for thyroid medication may change. She explains how either hyper- or hypothyroidism can reduce milk production in a nursing mother, and offers strategies to increase milk output.

HAIR LOSS. Mary Shomon also makes the distinction between the hair loss that is common after a woman has a baby versus hair loss that is a symptom of low thyroid function. In addition to comprehensive multivitamin/multimineral supplements, she recommends 500 mg of evening primrose oil daily to overcome hair loss.[38] However, if you are nursing your baby, instead of evening primrose oil, I recommend flax oil (five to ten 1 g capsules or 1–2 teaspoons daily), along with vitamin E (400 IU).

OVERCOMING POSTPARTUM BLUES

ADRENAL FUNCTION. If you are dealing with the "three-day baby blues," or other minor anxiety or depression related to birth, please read Chapter 14, "Increasing Your Energy & Decreasing Your Stress." During pregnancy, the placenta produces large amounts of hormones which stimulate your adrenal glands to produce their hormones. In the right amounts, adrenal hormones help you to feel good if you are otherwise healthy. However, once the placenta is lost after birth, your adrenal glands lose that stimulation and need to readjust to this change. If the adrenal hormone cortisol is too low, it can contribute to depression. Nutrition aimed at improving the ability of the adrenal glands to produce their hormones is discussed in Chapter 14. The B vitamins, vitamin C, and the minerals zinc, selenium, manganese, and magnesium are all involved in supporting the adrenal glands, as are the omega-3 fatty acids from flax oil and fish oil.

SLEEP. Do not overlook the role of sleep in dealing with the baby blues. Sleep directly helps the adrenal glands to recover. Your spouse, a trusted relative, or a friend can help you rest by caring for other children, and perhaps for the baby, so that you can get the sleep you need. Enough sleep is a key issue in preventing or overcoming postpartum mood problems. However, if you are breastfeeding, do not use melatonin supplements as a sleep aid.[39]

THYROID FUNCTION. It is possible that your thyroid gland is the source of the postpartum fatigue, depression, anxiety, or "brain fog" that may develop while your baby is young. Postpartum thyroiditis, described above, could be the underlying cause, especially if you see very low temperatures on your NFP chart. If you have had previous thyroid problems, you will need to have your thyroid function re-evaluated. *The Thyroid Hormone Breakthrough* addresses the link between hypothyroidism and postpartum depression.

NATURAL PROGESTERONE. Supplements of natural progesterone are helpful to many women who experience postpartum mood problems. Dr. John R. Lee recommended small amounts of over-the-counter progesterone cream for nursing mothers with the baby blues, in the range of 10 to 15 mg daily.[40] Drs. Raffelock and Rountree recommend the same, but in addition they caution against artificial progestins, and especially against the artificial hormones in birth control medications.[41] In any case, discuss natural progesterone supplements with your doctor, and be aware that supplements of oral "micronized" natural progesterone are available by prescription. (See Women's Health America in "Resources.")

A PRACTICAL HANDBOOK. Dr. Raffelock and Dr. Rountree's book, *A Natural Guide to Pregnancy and Postpartum Recovery*, is a unique resource if you have struggled with postpartum depression or anxiety and are looking for effective self-care options. (See "Further Reading.") Very readable, it has many practical recommendations for preventing or overcoming postpartum mood problems. It explains in laymen's terms several topics of nutrition that you may have heard about but have not had explained. In particular, the information on leaky gut syndrome and on the role of the liver in detoxifying wastes and ingested toxins is excellent. While its focus is on nutrition, it also covers the topic of using natural hormones to recover health.

➤ Diet and supplements aimed at stabilizing the blood sugar are the best strategies to prevent or lessen morning sickness. Vitamins B6 and folic acid are both helpful to blood sugar control.

➤ During pregnancy, there is no substitute for a protein-rich diet that supplies enough calories. Eating such a diet reduces the risk of preeclampsia, as well as other complications of pregnancy such as prematurity.

➤ Comprehensive vitamin, mineral and fatty acid supplements are the next priority. Folic acid is well known to prevent certain birth defects, but it also helps prevent other problems, such as abruption of the placenta. In various health functions it works together with iron, vitamin B12, and vitamin B6. Vitamin B6, along with magnesium and other B vitamins, is helpful for preventing swelling (edema) that occurs so commonly in pregnant women. The nutrients found in fish and fish oil are vital to the healthy development of the unborn baby's brain.

➤ Once the baby is born, "emotional nurturing" of the mother is as important as her physical nutrition.

➤ Extra fluids are essential to the breastfeeding mother, and her supplements should be similar to that of a pregnant woman. Plenty of protein in the diet is necessary to promote the production of breast milk, but the amount of overall calories needed is usually less while breastfeeding than while pregnant.

➤ Postpartum thyroiditis occurs in some women after childbirth, and is usually temporary. Postpartum blues may respond to nutrition aimed at restoring adrenal gland function. Postpartum health also depends on enough sleep.

11

Repeated Miscarriage & Birth Defects

Truly you have formed my inmost being; you knit me in my mother's womb. I give you thanks that I am fearfully, wonderfully made; wonderful are your works. My soul also you knew full well; nor was my frame unknown to you, when I was made in secret, when I was fashioned in the depths of the earth. — Psalms 139:13-15

If you have had personal experience with either of these topics, I am sorry for the sadness it has brought you. May you find courage and especially hope in the face of your disappointment and heartache. Let me emphasize also that the purpose of this chapter is not to stir up "what if's" or "if only's," those self-doubts that parents so often experience after the loss of an unborn child or the birth of a child with a major birth defect. Even experts seldom know with certainty the underlying cause of a particular miscarriage or a particular birth defect, and even the most optimistic agree that not all prenatal loss or developmental errors will ever be prevented.

But knowledge is power, and knowing the risk factors and ways to reduce them enables you to "change the things you can, and accept the things you cannot change." My goal is to point out known risk factors and to offer nutritional or other lifestyle strategies so that you can look forward to another pregnancy with confidence and joy.

— MISCARRIAGE

Miscarriage refers to the loss of a child after conception but before twenty weeks of gestation. (Such a loss after that time is termed stillbirth.) "Early" miscarriage refers to a loss that occurs in the first trimester of pregnancy, about the first twelve weeks. For a number of reasons, the first trimester is the most common time of pregnancy loss. About 12 to 15 percent of confirmed pregnancies end in miscarriage.[1] Very early miscarriage, occurring before a woman is aware that she is pregnant, is another possibility, but it is difficult to estimate accurately how frequently it occurs.

Having two consecutive miscarriages occurs in about 3 percent of women,[2] and having three consecutive miscarriages occurs in about 1 percent of women.[3] Experiencing three consecutive miscarriages is recognized as a clinical problem and is called recurrent miscarriage, but two miscarriages in a row may be considered recurrent as well. The statistics on the frequency of recurrent miscarriage are reassuring in one sense — even though the heartbreak of miscarriage is all too common, it is the exception to have even two in a row. That is, women who have experienced a miscarriage can usually have good hope that their next pregnancy will result in a full term baby.

CAN THE RISK OF MISCARRIAGE BE REDUCED? The answer is yes; research literature confirms this. Nutrition has an important role to play in reducing the incidence of miscarriage. Other lifestyle factors such as smoking affect the chance of having a miscarriage. Some risk factors, such as older age of the mother, cannot be changed. Nevertheless, there are definite self-care steps you can take, even if you are in a situation of higher risk. Both the nutrition for overall health in Part I of this book and the information aimed at overcoming specific reproductive problems covered in Part II apply importantly to reducing the risk of miscarriage. The discussion of pregnancy nutrition in Chapter 10 is especially applicable to preventing pregnancy loss.

CAUSES OF MISCARRIAGE

There are a number of known causes of miscarriage, though in many cases what triggered a particular miscarriage is never discovered.

EVENTS BEFORE OVULATION. Many miscarriages actually result from events that occur before the unfertilized ovum is ovulated. This is so because the unfertilized ovum must complete a critical cell division, called meiosis I, during the 24 hours before ovulation. Meiosis I is the cell division that converts the ovum from a "diploid" cell containing 46 chromosomes to a "haploid" cell containing 23 chromosomes. Meiosis I serves the vital role of preparing the ovum for fertilization with a sperm, which is also a haploid cell containing 23 chromosomes. The newly conceived child, then, has 46 chromosomes, half from each parent.

If meiosis I occurs properly, the ovum can be fertilized and is likely to develop normally. However, if this cell division does not occur as it should, the unfertilized ovum will contain too many or too few chromosomes. In most cases, fertilization cannot take place because the chromosomal abnormality is too great. Sometimes, though, conception does occur, but the genetically abnormal child, tiny as it is, cannot develop properly and within a few days or weeks, it passes away. In such a case an early miscarriage will ensue, usually without evidence of a fully formed embryo.

Proper completion of meiosis I in the few hours before ovulation depends on the hormonal "push" and timing of FSH and LH, as well as on nutrients that are known to promote efficient cell division. The Introduction to Part II discusses this topic in more detail, and "Age-Related Infertility" in Chapter 9 lists the nutrients that are most helpful to the cell division of meiosis.

IMPLANTATION. About a week after conception, the tiny embryo must implant into the lining of the uterus, the endometrium, in order to tap into the mother's nutrient provisions. Successful implantation depends on a thick, healthy endometrium, which in addition to adequate nutrition, depends on hormones, especially progesterone. If the endometrium is not well-developed, or if the embryo cannot attach properly, an early miscarriage may occur within a few days or weeks.

HORMONAL SUPPORT. Progesterone levels are affected by other hormones, including thyroxine (thyroid hormone), estrogen, and cortisol. Hormonal imbalances contribute to miscarriage. Some of these may respond, at least in part, to improved nutrition or body weight; in other cases medical intervention is needed.

OLDER AGE OF THE MOTHER. As you are probably aware, the risk of miscarriage rises as a woman ages. The quality of her ova declines with age, and her reproductive hormones change.

OTHER FACTORS. Physical problems with the uterus, such as fibroid tumors, can interfere with proper implantation and formation of the placenta, leading to miscarriage. Problems with blood clotting are yet another factor. Infections such as sexually transmitted disease or damage from them can be contributing factors. Rarely, there are genetic factors involving both parents that affect the embryo. If a woman has been infertile, she is unfortunately at a higher risk for miscarriage if she becomes pregnant. Yet infertility treatment itself raises the incidence of miscarriage,[4] making self-help for overcoming infertility an important first step.

GENERAL GUIDELINES TO PREVENT MISCARRIAGE

If you have particular reasons to be concerned about pregnancy loss, the ideal time to attempt to prevent it is during the two to three months before and immediately following conception. If possible, use the three preconception months to improve your diet and begin multivitamin/multimineral supplements, as outlined in Part I and Chapter 10 of this book.

DIET. How important is a healthy diet? In a large population study of British women, pregnant women who ate fresh fruits and vegetables daily had a rate of miscarriage only half as high as women who did not do so. Eating dairy products frequently also related to a reduced risk of miscarriage. The authors did not consider these foods as specific "anti-miscarriage foods," but rather interpreted eating such nutritious foods often as evidence of an overall well-balanced diet.[5]

VITAMIN AND MINERAL SUPPLEMENTS. In the study just mentioned, taking vitamins, especially multivitamins containing folic acid or iron, reduced the miscarriage rate by half compared to women who did not do so.[6] In another study, vitamin B12 deficiency was found to relate to fetal loss, and supplementing it in deficient women restored fertility and reduced the number of miscarriages, even among women who had suffered many recurrent miscarriages. In fact, one woman with undiagnosed vitamin B12 deficiency had had seven miscarriages without a single term birth. After taking vitamin B12, she quickly became pregnant and went on to have a total of three full term births in a row.[7]

Virtually every vitamin and mineral is involved in some aspect of pregnancy, literally from "A to zinc." Comprehensive supplementation, as suggested in Chapters 3 and 10, is far preferable to taking just one or two vitamins or minerals as you prepare for pregnancy.

BODY WEIGHT, MEDICATIONS, AND LIFESTYLE FACTORS. If you are underweight or overweight or if you are coming off the Pill, use the appropriate parts of this book to help yourself attain a better body weight or a better hormonal balance. Before you become pregnant is also the best time to eliminate unhealthy habits such as smoking or excess alcohol consumption.

Cut your caffeine intake to the equivalent of two cups of coffee per day, as more than 200 mg of caffeine daily has been associated with an increased risk of miscarriage. More caffeine increases this risk.[8] Be careful that any medications you take are acceptable for use during early pregnancy. If necessary, make arrangements to minimize exposure to workplace toxins. Exposure to heavy metals, organic solvents, pesticides, and many other chemicals may increase the risk of miscarriage.[9]

If you have a history of miscarriage, you may wish to try eliminating night lighting, as explained in Chapter 9 under the topic of "Sensitivity to Night Lighting." Exposure to light affects the hormone melatonin, which in turn may affect progesterone levels.

STRESS AND MISCARRIAGE. The role of stress in miscarriage is not well established, but one study has shown that women who had very early miscarriages did have higher levels of the adrenal stress hormone cortisol.[10] With or without such research, pregnancy is itself a stress, though a healthy and natural one. Reducing other stresses if you are able is prudent.

There is no doubt that many women in their childbearing years are under a great deal of stress. How do you decrease it? First, eat the best diet you can, and take your vitamins and minerals. Get enough sleep, or at least lie down and rest in a very dark room if you have trouble sleeping. If you get very little exercise, try to find a way to incorporate some moderate exercise into your routine. Conversely, if you are exercising excessively, cut down on it. It is a stress to your body, even if you enjoy it. Instead, exercise moderately, and find a slower, more relaxing physical activity that you can enjoy to take the place of overly demanding workouts.

Most important of all, if you are planning to become pregnant and are under great stress, do your best to eat as much good food as you know you need, even if your appetite is very low. When under stress, many women just don't feel like eating, and the stress of low blood glucose creates a "vicious cycle" that adds more stress. You can stop that cycle by eating small, healthy meals, even if you just don't feel like it. Use your bathroom scales to check your progress.

Finally, see Chapter 14, "Increasing Your Energy & Decreasing Your Stress" for nutrition to support adrenal health. Supporting your adrenal health decreases your body's response to stress even when you can't remove the actual stressors in your life. And try not to stress out over your daily stress! Work to reduce physical stresses, such as poor nutrition, inadequate sleep, and inadequate (or excess) exercise, and you will find that the daily stresses of life feel much more manageable. Your cortisol levels will also drop.

SPECIFIC RISK FACTORS FOR MISCARRIAGE

If your charts show problems such as very short luteal phase, low thyroid function, or other irregularities discussed in the previous chapters of this book, you may wish to wait up to three months to conceive as you work to improve them.

LUTEAL PHASE DEFICIENCY. Abnormal levels of FSH or LH before ovulation may ultimately result in the formation of a corpus luteum which releases insufficient progesterone for an insufficient number of days. This is called luteal phase deficiency, and it appears on the NFP chart as fewer than the normal number of post-ovulatory elevated temperatures. In addition, the abnormal FSH and LH may cause ovulation of an immature egg, as described previously. In such a situation pregnancy may be difficult to achieve, but even if it does occur, the newly conceived life may not be capable of normal development, or the corpus luteum may not produce enough of the progesterone necessary to sustain the pregnancy. Repeated early miscarriage is a known consequence of luteal phase deficiency.[11]

In Chapter 7, the topic "Luteal Phase Deficiency" explains the relationship between luteal function, the charted signs of fertility, and certain nutrients. This information is pertinent to you if you have observed short luteal phase cycles with less than ten to twelve days of elevated temperatures in non-conception cycles. It may also help you if you have experienced an unexplained early miscarriage, especially if fetal development did not occur. In such a case you may have been told that you had a "blighted ovum," or an "empty sac" pregnancy, or that the miscarriage was the result of a "random genetic error." Improved diet as well as vitamin B6, vitamin C, other nutrients, and even certain herbs, as explained in Chapter 7, have helped women to overcome luteal phase deficiency and to achieve term pregnancies.

LOW THYROID FUNCTION. The thyroid gland, which sits at the base of the neck, produces hormones that stimulate the function of most of the body's cells. When the thyroid hormones are too low, they can cause a number of female reproductive problems. Infertility and miscarriage are among these problems. Thyroid hormones produced by the mother affect the embryo and fetus from a very early stage of development, including implantation and formation of the placenta. Early miscarriage, stillbirth, prematurity, and developmental problems with the baby's nervous system are other consequences of low thyroid function in a pregnant mother.[12]

Nutrition can improve thyroid function, as explained in Chapter 7, under the topic "Low Thyroid Function." If your charts shows signs of low thyroid function, especially basal temperatures in the range of 97.2° F or below in the pre-ovulatory phase, implement nutrition aimed at improving thyroid function, but also look for medical assistance. Even if you need to take thyroid hormone replacement, improved nutrition can enable your own thyroid gland to function better.

If you already take thyroid medication because of low thyroid function, before you become pregnant you should make sure that your prescription is up to date for your current needs. Thyroid hormone replacement greatly reduces the incidence of miscarriage in women who need it, but not if the level of replacement is too low.[13] You will also need your thyroid levels monitored as your pregnancy progresses. *The Thyroid Hormone Breakthrough* devotes an excellent chapter called "Pregnancy Challenges" to women with thyroid dysfunction. (See "Further Reading.")

POLYCYSTIC OVARY SYNDROME. Polycystic ovary syndrome (PCOS), discussed in Chapter 8, may cause an increased risk of miscarriage. Apparently it is the "insulin resistance" that is the culprit, and increasing insulin sensitivity may provide effective treatment.[14] However, women who have elevated levels of androgen ("male" hormones) are at an increased risk for miscarriage, even if they do not have full-blown PCOS.[15] In either case, please refer to Chapter 8 for an explanation of insulin resistance as well as the nutritional strategies to overcome it. Overcoming insulin resistance also helps to decrease the production of androgens. Moderate weight loss, regular exercise, a low-sugar diet, and vitamin and mineral supplements are the self-care means of dealing with the problems of insulin resistance and high androgen levels.

OBESITY. Obesity increases the risk of miscarriage and stillbirth, according to a recent review.[16] It is very easy for researchers who report such data simply to suggest that obese women who are contemplating pregnancy lose weight, but if it were so simple, such women already would have done so! Yes, try your best to manage your weight problem, but above all eat the healthy foods you need and take high quality supplements before and during your pregnancy. Once you become pregnant, do not begin dieting in an attempt to lose weight. On the other hand, eating healthy foods, especially adequate protein and natural fat, may make it so that if you are obese, you can have a healthy pregnancy without much weight gain.

UNDERWEIGHT. Low body weight or low body fat can result in infertility and complete absence of cycles, but they can also cause or be related to short luteal phase and low thyroid function, especially if a woman is excessively athletic. If an underweight woman or a woman with low body fat becomes pregnant, she has a higher risk of miscarriage compared to women of normal weight. A large study of women in the United Kingdom who had early miscarriage showed that having a body mass index of less than 18.5 increased the risk of miscarriage.[17] This is equivalent to a weight around 110 pounds in a woman whose height is 5 ft., 5 in.

However, body mass index is an inexact measure of appropriate body fat, and your chart gives you better information about possibly being underweight.

For example, if you are small-boned but have regular cycles, you may have adequate body fat for your frame, even though your body mass index number seems rather low. Or, you may be slender, and your ovulations may be a few days later than average, but if your luteal phase is at least twelve days in length and your temperature levels are normal (pre-ovulatory temperatures averaging around 97.3° to 98.2° F), it is my opinion that your body weight is adequate for healthy hormones and a healthy pregnancy. On the other hand, if you perform vigorous muscle-building exercise and have replaced body fat with muscle, you could lack sufficient body fat despite a normal weight. Often delayed ovulation, a short luteal phase or low basal temperatures will reveal the stress to your body. As discussed in Chapter 7 under the topic "Underweight or Inadequate Body Fat," bringing your body fat up to normal will restore normal charts.

CELIAC DISEASE. Celiac disease is a disorder in which the body makes antibodies to gluten, a protein found in wheat, rye, and barley. It causes inflammation of the small intestine, and consequently decreases the absorption of nutrients. Apparently, because of the nutrient deficiencies, including iron-deficiency anemia, untreated celiac disease is responsible for a high risk of repeated miscarriage. Treatment with a strict gluten-free diet has been shown to reduce the incidence of miscarriage to as low as that of the general population.[18] The prevalence of celiac disease is higher than was once thought, and the disease may be "silent" in terms of obvious gastrointestinal problems. If you have had recurrent miscarriages without explanation, you should have your doctor arrange for a test for this disorder. See Chapter 9 for more information about celiac disease and the supplements that are helpful in overcoming nutritional deficiencies that may occur because of it.

CLOTTING DISORDERS. In some women, abnormal "antiphospholipid antibodies" increase blood clotting abnormally. This disorder, called antiphospholipid syndrome, decreases blood flow to the placenta during pregnancy, and the result may be recurrent miscarriage in such women. Low-dose aspirin during pregnancy is often recommended to decrease the clotting and therefore the risk of miscarriage. Omega-3 fatty acid derivatives from fish oil (4 or 5 g of mixed EPA and DHA) have been used in two studies to achieve the same effect, and the omega-3 treatment was as effective as aspirin in enabling women with antiphospholipid antibodies to carry their pregnancies to term.[19] While the anti-inflammatory properties of fish oil are becoming better known, you should discuss this new alternative with your doctor if you have reason to believe that you may have a clotting disorder. Fish oil, though, is an excellent supplement for most women before and during pregnancy.

UTERINE PROBLEMS. Anatomical problems within the uterus can interfere with implantation of the embryo or growth of the fetus. One such problem is fibroid tumors,[20] which are benign growths within the muscle layer of the uterus. Endometrial growths called polyps are another possibility. Occasionally a woman is born with a uterus that is abnormally separated into two halves. If necessary, surgery to correct the uterine anatomy can help prevent future problems in a woman who has had miscarriages due to this abnormality.[21] However, it is wise also to consider your overall health and your chart so that other problems such as the ones just discussed are not overlooked.

AGE-RELATED MISCARRIAGE. Increasing age of the mother, especially past age 35, is a well-established risk factor for miscarriage. Nevertheless, estimates on the risk of miscarriage as related to age vary. One researcher estimated the risk of miscarriage at age 37 to be 20 percent, at age 44 to be 30 percent, and at age 48 to be 40 percent of all pregnancies.[22] A large British study found that women had no age-related risk before age 35, but between age 35 and 39, their risk was 75 percent higher compared to the low-risk years of 25 to 29. Once over age 40, these women's risk of miscarriage progressed to five times greater than at age 25 to 29.[23]

Much of the problem that occurs as women age has to do with the quality of their remaining ova and delays in becoming pregnant often occur as well. Chapter 9's final topic, "Age-Related Infertility," contains specific nutritional and other lifestyle recommendations for achieving pregnancy when age is a factor. These are exactly the guidelines that I recommend to reduce the risk of age-related miscarriage, because they are intended to provide the ova with the nutrients they need and to support healthy progesterone levels as well.

In counseling women in their 40s who would like to have more children despite having had a recent miscarriage, I encourage more than just nutrition. There is a kind of internal courage, an emotional resolve, that is required. That is, if you are hoping to have more children, you need to hold the hope for another child firmly against the pain and fear of another loss.

I counseled a lady who consulted me after having two miscarriages in a row in her early forties. She had given birth to five children without difficulty when she was younger, and she told me that she could not bear the grief of another miscarriage. What could I say? If she avoided a pregnancy, she would never experience such a loss again. But she would never have the chance for the joy of giving birth to another child again, either. Yes, we discussed nutrition, and she closely followed the guidelines that I recommend for older mothers (see Chapter 9). After she gave birth to her sixth child, she contacted me to share the wonderful news. She said that what made the greatest difference to her was the counsel that she would need courage to try again. She went on to have a second "over-40" baby as well.

PREVIOUS MISCARRIAGES. A history of miscarriages in itself is considered a risk factor for miscarriage, though many women who have experienced it, even with their first pregnancy, go on to give birth to several full-term babies without any other losses. Keep in mind that studies that report such data involve women who have not specifically implemented strategies aimed at reducing their particular risks for miscarriage, as discussed above.

INFERTILITY. It is apparent that there is a relationship between infertility and miscarriage; it is known that women who take longer to conceive are more prone to miscarriage. What does that mean to you? First, if you are having a problem with infertility, do all the self-help steps listed in Appendix B, "Focus on Infertility." You will be healthier for it, and better health will reduce your chance of miscarrying, as you can see from the research above.

Equally as important, if you seek medical care for your infertility, keep up the good nutrition! You will respond best to medical care if you are as healthy as you can be. Finally, if you become pregnant while using the nutritional or other self-help suggestions in this book, do not discontinue them. All recommendations in this book are safe and healthy for pregnancy, unless your doctor has counseled you otherwise. To discontinue good nutrition or whatever else has seemed to help — weight gain, weight loss, reduction of night lighting — could interfere with your hormones during the vulnerable first trimester.

—— BIRTH DEFECTS

Are you ready to be encouraged? The amazing research that follows should help you put aside the unfounded fears that so many women have about giving birth to a baby with a major birth defect. In short, when it comes to reducing the risk of *many* different birth defects, the B vitamin folic acid has a leading role, but as you will see, not the only role.

NEURAL TUBE DEFECTS
It has been well established in the last twenty years that supplements of folic acid sharply reduce the incidence of birth defects that are collectively referred to as "neural tube defects," even in mothers who have had a previous child with such a developmental error. Neural tube defects are a major cause of death among newborns, second only to congenital heart defects.[24]

There are several types of neural tube defects, including spina bifida. When spina bifida occurs, the child may require several surgeries in order to prevent fluid accumulation around the brain and to promote the ability to walk. Anencephaly, or failure of the brain to develop completely, is an even more severe neural tube defect than spina bifida. Sadly, anencephaly usually results in stillbirth or death soon after birth.

FOLIC ACID, MULTIVITAMINS, AND OTHER BIRTH DEFECTS
Folic acid and multivitamin supplements around the time of conception not only reduce the incidence of neural tube defects, but a number of studies show that they also significantly reduce the risk of congenital heart defects, which are the leading cause of death of newborns. In addition, folic acid and multivitamins taken before and during pregnancy have substantially reduced the occurrence of oral clefts (such as cleft lip or cleft palate), urinary tract defects, limb formation defects, omphalocoele (a defect of the intestines and umbilical cord), and even childhood brain cancers and leukemia.[25] It is worth noting that in many cases, the studies do not make it clear whether it is the

folic acid or another nutrient in the multivitamins that has provided these very, very encouraging results.

FOLIC ACID, VITAMIN B12, AND VITAMIN B6. Ongoing research is shedding light on the nutrients in multivitamins that might be involved in the reduction of birth defects in the babies of women who take folic acid along with a multivitamin. It is known that folic acid works together with two other B vitamins — vitamin B12 and vitamin B6 — to reduce the production of the amino acid homocysteine. It is beyond the scope of this book to explain the biochemical details, but in low concentrations homocysteine is normal to the cells. If folic acid, especially, or the other two B vitamins are deficient, homocysteine builds up and creates havoc within cells. For example, it causes problems within the linings of the blood vessels, making it a risk factor for cardiovascular disease. This also explains why it is harmful to the placenta, which is a vascular organ. When it comes to pregnancy, homocysteine may be the actual culprit involved with the birth defects listed above, as well as with problems such as abruption of the placenta.[26]

In addition to vitamin B12 and vitamin B6, the mineral zinc works along with folic acid. Vitamin C is necessary for the absorption of folic acid. It may be that several nutrients found in multivitamins together make a difference in preventing birth defects.

FOLIC ACID AND OTHER SUPPLEMENTS: WHEN SHOULD YOU START TAKING THEM? Since the neural tube closes by 22–28 days after conception (one to two weeks after a woman misses her period), it is clear that folic acid should be started *before* conception in order for it to prevent neural tube defects. How long before conception? Some researchers have suggested three weeks, others eight weeks, and still others three months before conception. Such early preparation is ideal, but many pregnancies are unplanned — or planned on very short notice!

The best insurance is for every woman who might become pregnant to supplement folic acid and a multivitamin/multimineral as part of her daily good health habits. However, beginning supplementation just as soon as you realize that you may be pregnant is the next best strategy. Supplemental folic acid is quickly absorbed and is immediately biologically active, even more so than the natural "folate form," which is found in food.[27] So if you discover you are pregnant by surprise, don't delay. Start the folic acid immediately.

FOLIC ACID AND OTHER SUPPLEMENTS: WHEN CAN YOU DISCONTINUE THEM? Many researchers suggest that folic acid be supplemented until twelve weeks of pregnancy, but because this vitamin decreases the risk of intrauterine growth retardation, pre-eclampsia, abruption of the placenta and fetal death, "it seems highly advisable to administer folic acid during the second and third trimester of pregnancy in order to prevent hyperhomocysteinuria [elevated homocysteine levels] which in many cases could be partially or totally responsible for the vascular damage [to the placental]."[28] As noted, multivitamins have been shown to reduce the occurrence of childhood cancers, but in at least one large study of childhood brain cancers, the effect occurred only if the vitamins were taken in both the first and second trimester of pregnancy, and a greater effect (a stunning 50 percent reduction) occurred if the multivitamins were taken during the third trimester as well.[29]

FOLIC ACID: HOW MUCH? Since 1992, the U.S. Public Health Service has recommended that all women who may become pregnant take 400 mcg of folic acid daily. In addition, the U.S. Centers for Disease Control in 1991 recommended that women who have had a previous child with a neural tube defect or who are otherwise at high risk should take 4,000 mcg of folic acid when they are trying to become pregnant, and for the first twelve weeks of pregnancy.[30] These guidelines are similar to those in some other countries.

However, some prominent Canadian researchers interested in folic acid and its effect on birth defects believe that all women, regardless of whether or not they have risk factors for birth defects, should take 5,000 mcg (5 mg) of folic acid daily.

The Joint Society of Obstetricians and Gynaecologists of Canada (SOGC) and The Motherisk Program Clinical Practice Guideline (2007) recommends 5,000 mcg of folic acid daily for all women who have had a previous child with one of the birth defects discussed above (neural tube defects, heart defects, and the others), beginning three months before conception and continuing through twelve weeks of pregnancy, after which they recommend 400–1,000 mcg until breastfeeding is complete. They additionally recommend a multivitamin of unspecified potency, noting only that true vitamin A (retinol) should not exceed 10,000 IU per daily dose, as it has been associated with birth defects.[31] For women with obesity, diabetes, or epilepsy, or women with a family history of neural tube defects, they recommend the same. For low-risk women who plan their pregnancies and eat a good diet, and who are conscientious in taking supplements, they recommend 400–1,000 mcg daily beginning three months before conception and continuing as long as breastfeeding continues. For women who are not health conscious and have risk factors such as smoking, alcohol use, and so forth, they recommend 5,000 mcg of folic acid along with a multivitamin, exactly as for the known high-risk groups.[32]

A review article by Canadian researchers of The Hospital for Sick Children in Toronto, Canada echoes these recommendations. They also address the issue of folic acid possibly masking vitamin B_{12} deficiency by suggesting that supplementation of vitamin B_{12} may allay such concerns. They point out that even though controlled studies show that 800–1,100 mcg daily of folic acid is adequate to protect women from having a child with a folic acid-related birth defect, in practice women do not unfailingly take their vitamins. For example, even women who describe themselves as motivated to take vitamins averaged less than 60 percent compliance in taking their vitamins in a controlled study. These authors believe that larger amounts of folic acid, together with "impaired compliance" (hit-or-miss taking of vitamins), will enable many more women to avoid having a child with a birth defect. Finally, in addressing the safety of large amounts of folic acid, they state that "case-control and some prospective studies have repeatedly shown a 20–30 percent decline in cancer associated with folic acid."[33]

FOLIC ACID AND TWINNING. A large Hungarian study that was done to add evidence that folic acid reduces the risk of having a child with a neural tube defect was re-evaluated in 1994, and the original researchers reported a 40 percent increase in the incidence of twinning among women who had taken folic acid around the time of conception.[34] However, scrutiny of these results by other investigators revealed that women in the study who conceived while using fertility drugs accounted for 40 percent of the multiple births.[35]

Several other studies followed to address this issue. A very large Chinese study showed no effect on twinning when women took 400 mcg of folic acid daily around the time of conception,[36] but a Swedish study showed a doubling of the rate of fraternal twinning among women who used folic acid, mostly in the same amount.[37] Another large Hungarian study evaluated women who had taken on average large doses of folic acid (6,000 mcg daily) along with multivitamins, and only a very small increase in the incidence of twinning was seen.[38]

FOLIC ACID AND MISCARRIAGE. Studies have shown that low folate status in women increases the risk of miscarriage, which apparently relates to elevated levels of homocysteine.[39] It came as a surprise in 1997 that the same Hungarian researchers who re-evaluated their studies on the effect of folic acid on twinning also reported a 16 percent increased occurrence of miscarriage. These researchers speculated that folic acid might actually decrease the occurrence of neural tube defects by the improbable route of causing unborn children with such developmental errors to be "selectively" miscarried.[40]

This disturbing hypothesis stirred up the interest of other researchers, some of whom suggested that if such data were accurate, another hypothesis is that folic acid and multivitamins may enable what would have been a very early, undetected miscarriage to continue long enough to be recognized as such.[41] In light of the research on the beneficial effect of folic acid and multivitamins on the health of the placenta, that hypothesis seems much more likely, and in fact the original Hungarian researchers did offer this possibility to explain the increase in miscarriages that they observed. They also noted a pro-fertility effect of folic acid; there were more pregnancies and more births to the women who supplemented folic acid compared to those who did not.[42] When more pregnancies occur, the chance of miscarriage also increases.

A 2005 review of several studies which investigated the relationship between miscarriage and folic acid, as well as the studies on twinning, ends with the following: "It is reassuring that data do not support the reports that folic acid supplements increase the occurrence of miscarriage or multiple births because women of childbearing age in many countries are advised to take folic acid supplements daily to prevent NTDs [neural tube defects]. Women of reproductive age and their health care providers can support the periconceptional folic acid supplementation without concern that this practice will increase the occurrence of multiple births or miscarriage."[43] As noted previously, a large study of early miscarriage in British women showed that taking multivitamins before pregnancy reduced the incidence of miscarriage by half.[44]

DOWN SYNDROME

Down syndrome is a genetic disorder that occurs at the time the child is conceived. Instead of having 23 pairs of chromosomes, 23 from each parent, the child has three number 21 chromosomes; thus, "trisomy 21," the genetic name for Down syndrome. Children with this disorder have developmental disabilities, including mental retardation, and they may have physical health problems such as poor immune function, low muscle tone, hypothyroidism, and sometimes heart defects.

Compared to many genetic diseases, though, Down syndrome may be considered a mild disorder. With the care of a loving family and the support of health professionals and educators, many children born with Down syndrome can expect to have good health, go to school, and grow to adulthood. The Human Genome Project has led to increased understanding of the various manifestations of the syndrome, and in turn, treatment for individuals with Down syndrome has improved.

NUTRITION FOR INDIVIDUALS WITH DOWN SYNDROME. Before considering prevention of Down syndrome, I would like you to be aware that there is nutritional therapy available to treat children and adults with this genetic disorder. A nutritional supplement called Nutrivene-D has been designed for newborns, children, and adults with Down syndrome.

Nutrivene-D is intended to compensate for specific metabolic defects that occur because of the trisomy 21 error, which affects all cells. A major problem is excessive oxidative stress on the body's cells, including the brain cells. High oxidative stress occurs because the extra chromosome 21 causes cells to overproduce oxidized cellular wastes faster than they can get rid of them. To compensate, Nutrivene-D contains large quantities of antioxidants: vitamins A, C, E, beta-carotene, selenium, coenzyme Q_{10}, and alpha-lipoic acid. Another challenge occurs because children with Down syndrome do not produce enough of the structural protein collagen to promote proper muscle tone and joint stability. Certain amino acids have been included in Nutrivene-D to enable connective tissue cells to produce more collagen. Folic acid and B vitamins are also part of the formula, again compensating for particular metabolic deficiencies.[45]

While I have not had personal experience with a child with Down syndrome, I wholeheartedly encourage parents of children with Down syndrome to consider the targeted nutritional therapy discussed above as an adjunct to the medical, educational, and social assistance you no doubt already have in place. To gain a fuller understanding of the biochemical challenges that people with Down syndrome face, as well as the possibilities for solving some of these through nutrition, see the website of pediatrician and geneticist

Lawrence Leichtman, M.D., of Virginia Beach, Virginia, who treats children with Down syndrome using targeted nutritional therapy as well as other approaches. If you are interested in more information, see ***www.lleichtman. org*** and ***www.nutrivene.com***.[46] (Both are listed in "Resources.")

CAN THE RISK OF DOWN SYNDROME BE REDUCED? The greatest risk factor for conceiving a child with Down syndrome is older age of the mother. Even so, having a baby with Down syndrome is much more common in younger mothers since they have many more babies overall. Research has not answered this question definitely, but there are several very hopeful studies that, in fact, point to the same nutrients that decrease the risk of neural tube defects — folic acid and others which work together with it.[47]

The genetic error that results in Down syndrome occurs in the hours shortly before ovulation, when the unfertilized ovum completes meiosis I, as explained in the Introduction to Part II. At that time the ovum normally divides so that instead of 23 pairs of chromosomes, it contains only 23 single chromosomes. In what is called a "nondisjunction" error, the two 21 chromosomes stick together. When the ovum is fertilized, then, trisomy 21 occurs. About 95 percent of Down syndrome conceptions occur because of improper cell division in the unfertilized ovum as opposed to the sperm.[48] Among other functions, folic acid is necessary for the events of meiosis to proceed normally.

A number of investigations have found that many women who have given birth to children with Down syndrome have a genetic abnormality in the way they metabolize folic acid; in effect, these mothers have an increased need for folic acid to maintain normal cellular processes.[49] Some studies have found that homocysteine is elevated and/or folic acid levels are depressed in mothers of children with Down syndrome.[50]

It is clear from these studies that these genetic errors are not necessary for a woman to have a child with Down syndrome, and that other factors besides these errors must be involved. One possibility is a deficiency of folate. Inadequate folic acid in a woman prior to conception may result in problems similar to those caused by the metabolic inability to use folic acid properly.

The jury is still out on whether or not folic acid supplements reduce the incidence of Down syndrome. Simply fortifying food with folic acid has not changed the incidence of Down syndrome, according to one study.[51]

What does this mean, practically speaking, given the evidence that Down syndrome occurs more frequently in the children of mothers who cannot use folic acid properly? My strong recommendation is to take folic acid in the amounts suggested previously *before conception* to reduce the incidence of neural tube defects, and be aware that it may possibly reduce the incidence of Down syndrome. Your childbearing years may be over before all the studies are in.

Folic acid works together with zinc and vitamin B12, and it requires vitamin C to be properly absorbed. Vitamins do not function in isolation, and taking a good multivitamin/multimineral supplement is an excellent preparation for pregnancy, as suggested in Chapter 10. If you are a woman over 40 or if you have other reasons to be concerned about Down syndrome, I recommend the amounts of vitamins in Chapter 9 under the heading "Age-Related Infertility."

A PERSONAL NOTE. When I got pregnant with my daughter Monica at age 47, it was quite a joyful surprise, since my last baby had been born when I was 41. I had given up hope quite a while before. I had been aware at that time (1999), that research on the link between folic acid and prevention of Down syndrome was in progress, because in 1996 I had attended a national conference on the nutritional treatment of Down syndrome.

There I had the opportunity to meet nutritionally-oriented physician Dr. Julian Whitaker, who in response to my question about preventing Down syndrome said, without hesitation, "Folic acid. You are going to see research forthcoming on the link between folic acid and prevention of Down syndrome. Right now the evidence is circumstantial. But the biochemical evidence is coming."[52] Almost three years later, when I realized I was pregnant, I was glad that, for general good health, I had been taking 3,000 mcg of folic acid (along with 1,000 mcg of B12 and comprehensive vitamins) for three or four months. I did not request an ultrasound, but I felt very positive that the baby would be normal. Nevertheless, the encouraging information on treatment for Down syndrome children made me very relaxed throughout the pregnancy.

It was in October of 1999, when I was only three months pregnant, that the original article on the topic of folic acid for prevention of Down syndrome was published. I must admit that I went through that pregnancy much more confident about having a healthy baby then, at age 47, than I did at age 41, when I was six years younger, but not aware of any information linking nutrition to the prevention of Down syndrome.

A DEBT OF GRATITUDE. All of us want the best for our children, and it is a normal maternal instinct to want your children to be as healthy as they can be. For me, the initial research on folic acid and Down syndrome was a huge encouragement when I was pregnant so late in my fertile years, because it gave me great hope and confidence that the baby would be genetically normal. I also felt that if Down syndrome did occur, I would have plenty of nutritional information aimed at helping the baby be as healthy as he or she could possibly be. I also had a firm trust that God knew what we could handle.

As it turned out, Monica was a completely healthy baby and continues to be a healthy, happy little girl. Nevertheless, I still consider my attendance at the national conference on treatment of Down syndrome children with nutrition in 1996 as one of the high points of my life. The passion of the health professionals there on behalf of those children was electrifying. The hope that they offered to the many parents of Down syndrome children in attendance was real, as several of them were parents of children with Down syndrome themselves. One presenter had adopted three children with Down syndrome!

I count it a great honor to have met Dr. Lawrence Leichtman there, with his passion for the health of these precious children. Most of all, I loved their recommendation as to when to start the nutritional intervention: "Theoretically, they should begin as soon as it is diagnosed, and if not, certainly as soon as they are born."[53]

* * *

THE FATHER'S ROLE

The role of the father in miscarriage and birth defects is a factor which is infrequently considered. Damage to a man's sperm may cause infertility, but it is apparently rare for a damaged sperm to survive in the female reproductive tract long enough to fertilize the ovum, especially when millions of healthy sperm are more able to do so.

Older age of the father may be a contributing factor to miscarriage,[54] and researchers estimate that about 5 percent of Down syndrome is related to an extra number 21 chromosome in the sperm involved in conception.[55]

Sperm have a very high need for oxygen because of their high energy use as they swim. Because they are very small cells, they carry few protective antioxidant enzymes with them. "Oxidative stress" is what damages sperm. Exposure to toxins, whether from workplace materials, cigarette smoking, alcohol, or house and garden chemicals, ultimately results in oxidative stress. The effect of aging on sperm is also explained as oxidative stress. The damage that prolonged heat exposure causes to sperm is summarized as oxidative stress. The all-important DNA, the genetic contribution of the father, is damaged by oxidative stress.[56]

Avoiding exposure to toxins and excessive heat reduces oxidative stress and sperm damage. Improved nutrition provides antioxidants that counteract oxidative stress.[57] These nutrients — vitamins A, C, and E, folic acid, zinc, and others — are detailed as part of the discussion of male fertility in Chapter 15.

In any type of infertility, including repeated miscarriage, both parents should strive for the best nutrition possible, as outlined in Part I. Keep in mind that it takes perhaps two months for improved nutrition practices to affect complete sperm development (see Chapter 15). Once conception has occurred, the father's physical contribution to his child is complete, but his continued emphasis on good nutrition will not only enhance his own health; it will also be the best encouragement to excellent nutrition that he can offer to his expectant wife.

Summary – Chapter 11

➤ While miscarriage is unfortunately common, recurrent (repeating) miscarriage is not. Many of the same factors that cause cycle irregularities or infertility increase the risk of miscarriage, but good diet and taking multivitamins before and during pregnancy can reduce the risk of miscarriage.

➤ Supplements of folic acid and/or multivitamins significantly reduce the risk of several types of birth defects, including congenital heart defects and neural tube defects. In addition, supplements of folic acid and multivitamins reduce the occurrence of umbilical defects, limb defects, and urinary tract defects. They decrease the risk of childhood brain cancers and leukemia; taking folic acid throughout pregnancy reduces the risk of childhood brain cancer by 50 percent.

➤ Folic acid and other B vitamins decrease the production of the damaging amino acid homocysteine, which may be the actual culprit in many birth defects.

➤ New evidence suggests that supplements of folic acid and/or multivitamins may decrease the incidence of Down syndrome, as research shows that women who have a genetic inability to use folic acid properly have increased levels of homocysteine, and an increased incidence of having children with Down syndrome.

➤ Targeted nutritional support is now available to help children with Down syndrome to compensate for the biochemical problems caused by this genetic disorder.

➤ The father's role in miscarriage and birth defects may be smaller than that of the mother, but good nutrition for overall male fertility is the most prudent course to take when a couple is concerned about pregnancy loss or birth defects.

12

Premenopause,
Perimenopause, & Menopause

May you see your children's children, peace be upon Israel! — Psalms 128:6

This ancient blessing succinctly reveals the biological purpose of menopause. The normal, natural, and predictable loss of fertility that has been part of womanhood throughout the ages ensures that women have a life span potential well beyond their childbearing years. Menopause makes it possible for women to nurture the children to whom they have given birth. Menopause allows women to live long enough to help their grown children as they become parents, and to enjoy the age-old delight of seeing their "children's children."

Menopause actually refers only to the woman's last period, which typically occurs around age fifty. Two other terms are much more useful when dealing with the longer process traditionally called "the change of life." **Premenopause** is the beginning phase of a woman's gradual decline in fertility. Premenopause generally begins in the late thirties or early forties, and on average lasts through the forties. During this time, the ovaries slowly decrease their output of the reproductive hormone progesterone. You may be surprised to learn that the hormone estrogen may increase during premenopause, leading to a hormonal imbalance often called "estrogen dominance." Estrogen, however, eventually drops to approximately half of what it was during the fertile years.

Women generally experience about two years of cycle irregularity before the actual menopause — the last period — occurs. This time of transition before the menopause is called the **perimenopause**. During the perimenopause, progesterone drops to very low levels. However, even after menopause, both the ovaries and the adrenal glands continue to secrete sex hormones, and the body fat plays a major role in producing estrogen. Many of the changes of the perimenopause are completed during the five years that follow menopause.

Good nutrition and other good health habits continue to be the keys to vibrant good health during premenopause, perimenopause, and afterward. You will notice that many of the topics addressed below refer you to previous chapters of this book. The years of declining fertility are part of a continuum, and the strategies for optimal reproductive health are not essentially different from what they were in earlier years.

SEEKING OR AVOIDING PREGNANCY

If you are attempting to become pregnant in your forties, you should know that fertility declines significantly during the early forties and sharply after age 45. Yet many women can become pregnant and have children in their early forties. Some women can become pregnant when they are 45 or 46. A few women will be able to conceive during the year that they are 47. Once you have your 48th birthday, there is little basis to hope to become pregnant or to fear that you might.[1] This is true even if you are charting normal-looking cycles indicating ovulation, because it is the eggs that have degenerated, along with the ability of the tubes to transport the ova and the endometrium to nourish a fertilized ovum.

SEEKING PREGNANCY. If you are hoping to have a baby but are having difficulty conceiving in your forties, see the section in Chapter 9 titled "Age-Related Infertility" for specific nutritional recommendations which may be helpful to achieve pregnancy at this age. See also Chapter 11, "Repeated Miscarriage & Birth Defects," because the incidence of miscarriage unfortunately climbs as women approach the end of their childbearing years. Please note that the above information relating to age and fertility refers to seeking pregnancy *naturally*, but even medical treatment for infertility may not overcome the age-related decline of the forties.

AVOIDING PREGNANCY. If you are avoiding a pregnancy, continue to chart and to follow the Couple to Couple League's guidelines for the premenopause time, no matter what your age. It is worth reminding you that nutrition to improve your cycle regularity makes NFP easier to use at every stage of life, including premenopause and perimenopause. Your goal should be for a smooth, healthy, and happy transition from the fertile years to menopause and beyond. NFP will literally help you to "chart the course," giving you insight into what is happening as your hormones change — another wonderful benefit of NFP.

CYCLE IRREGULARITIES

Cycle irregularities are to be expected during the final two years or so before menopause. Your cycles may gradually shorten during *pre*menopause, only to become much longer in the transition of *peri*menopause. Your menstrual periods may become lighter and shorter than before, but you also might experience a few heavier and longer periods. It is common in perimenopause for the real period to be preceded by one, two, or three days of light spotting, called "irregular shedding." It is also common for the period to end with a brownish color to the menstrual flow, instead of the ordinary pinkish color. Both irregular shedding before the actual period and brownish bleeding at the end of the period are signs of low progesterone.

Your charts might also reveal a pattern of short luteal phases (less than 10 or 11 elevated temperatures after ovulation), which are another indication of lower levels of progesterone. Occasional anovulatory cycles ("cycles" without the temperature shift indicating ovulation) may occur, and your last few periods may follow anovulatory cycles. Sometimes spotting will occur between episodes of more typical menstrual bleeding.

However, you should also not be too quick to accept any cycle irregularity as an inevitable part of pre- or perimenopause, especially if you are only in your early or mid-forties! Instead, try to uncover other possible causes of the irregularity. For example, PMS is well known to worsen with age, but it can also be improved at any age, so taking a look at Chapter 5, "Premenstrual Syndrome (PMS)," may be helpful to you. Here are several other possible causes of cycle irregularities:

LUTEAL PHASE DEFICIENCY. Luteal phase deficiency, discussed under that title in Chapter 7, refers to inadequate progesterone in the second half of an ovulatory cycle. It may be detected with charting, as described in Chapter 7, because ovulation followed by less than ten or eleven post-ovulatory elevated temperatures is typical of this hormonal imbalance. The pattern may repeat, month after month. Luteal phase inadequacy is common in the forties, and may underlie the bothersome mood swings of PMS at any age. Reread Chapter 5, "Premenstrual Syndrome (PMS)," because the nutritional strategies to overcome PMS are very helpful in improving an inadequate luteal phase. In fact, even if you have tried the PMS nutritional plan in the past but have discontinued it, you may be pleasantly surprised at the difference it makes during this stage of life.

THYROID DYSFUNCTION. You may have had a lab test for suspected thyroid problems, but it is still all too common for the diagnosis of hypothyroidism to be missed. Undetected low thyroid function can cause cycle problems at any stage of a woman's life, but it can also begin for the first time during premenopause and later. Long cycles or anovulatory cycles, if they occur along with very low temperatures on the NFP chart (pre-ovulatory temperatures below 97.2° F), are signs that you may have low thyroid function. Or you may experience short luteal phase occurring with low pre-ovulatory temperatures. Often the mucus pattern is that of ongoing less-fertile mucus.

One cause of low thyroid function is the rise in estrogen during the premenopause years, since excess estrogen (estrogen dominance) interferes with the action of the thyroid hormone.[2] There are other causes, including unmet nutritional needs of the thyroid gland. See "Low Thyroid Function" in Chapter 7 for information on detecting and correcting thyroid problems.

If after menopause the common menopausal complaints such as hot flashes, mood disturbances, and cognitive disturbances (memory problems) do not resolve, you should be checked for thyroid dysfunction. Either hypothyroidism or hyperthyroidism can cause such problems, and addressing the cause with medical intervention can improve the symptoms.[3]

LOW BODY FAT. Being underweight or lacking sufficient body fat (see "Underweight or Inadequate Body Fat" in Chapter 7) can cause long cycles or a total lack of ovulation and periods at any age, but if you lose too much body fat during your forties, you may believe you are in perimenopause when you are not! If you are in serious doubt as to whether you are truly in perimenopause or if there is another explanation for your long cycles or lack of periods, you can have your FSH and LH tested. These two hormones become and remain irreversibly elevated after menopause, making true menopause easy to ascertain via testing. Conversely, inadequate body fat is one common cause of *low* FSH and LH, which also causes irregular or absent periods.

I have counseled several women in their mid-forties who believed that they were going through menopause, yet the answer to their cycle irregularity or lack of periods was a strenuous exercise program and dieting for weight loss, not menopause. If you have begun dieting or vigorous exercise and have developed irregular cycles, anovulatory cycles, or have lost your periods completely, consider this possibility carefully. It is worth regaining some body weight or cutting down on the exercise to restore your normal hormone levels and cycles, as bone loss may accompany amenorrhea (loss of menstrual cycles) caused by loss of body fat.

EXCESS BODY WEIGHT OR WEIGHT GAIN. Just as low body fat affects the reproductive hormones, so does excess body fat. If you have had fairly regular cycles during your most fertile years, and do not have polycystic ovary syndrome (PCOS), gaining weight during the premenopause can be both the cause and the effect of estrogen dominance. Excess body fat is a source of estrogen, and estrogen affects several other hormones in such a way as to favor fat storage. High estrogen levels during premenopause may underlie such problems as fibroid tumors, tender breasts, mood swings, gallbladder disease, anxious depression, weepiness, and foggy thinking.[4] I believe that the best approach to dealing with weight gain in premenopause is with a diet relatively low in starchy and sugary carbohydrates, along with regular exercise, as is described in "Overweight without PCOS" in Chapter 8. Dropping even a modest amount of weight can help some women have more regular cycles.[5]

HEAVY OR PROLONGED BLEEDING
Heavy or prolonged bleeding may be caused by uterine fibroid tumors, which are benign growths within the wall of the uterus. Many women have them without symptoms, but if you begin having heavy, painful, or prolonged periods, suspect fibroids and seek a diagnosis by a medical doctor. Estrogen dominance during the premenopause time stimulates the growth of fibroids, sometimes causing them to grow as large as a grapefruit. (In such cases you may be able to notice the increase in the size of your abdomen.) Once estrogen declines significantly during perimenopause and beyond, fibroids usually shrink. See Dr. Kristine Severyn's article in Appendix C, "Uterine Fibroids: How I Kept my Uterus," for excellent information about how and why to try and save your uterus, even if you are past childbearing.

If a doctor has confirmed that you do not have fibroids or any other significant medical condition, please refer to Chapter 6, "Shorter, Lighter, & Pain-free Periods." The nutritional suggestions there apply to women of every age. My experience as an NFP counselor is that heavy bleeding not caused by fibroid tumors or other medical conditions is one of the easiest problems to overcome with improved nutrition, no matter what the age of the woman.

HOT FLASHES AND NIGHT SWEATS

Hot flashes and night sweats are caused by low estrogen levels. They usually occur in the perimenopause time of transition, and they are a sign that the change of life is really in progress. On the other hand, sometimes much younger women experience hot flashes or night sweats in the weeks after childbirth, when their estrogen levels are low. Significant weight loss or loss of body fat due to strenuous exercise may occasionally cause them at younger ages also.

How do you know if you are having a hot flash? If you need to ask, you probably have never had one! They are named well — you suddenly feel quite overheated, and you may break out in a sweat. You may or may not appear to blush. Hot flashes usually last for just a minute or two. They may occur many times a day or only every few days. They are not usually accompanied by anxiety, as you might suppose, but anxiety, stress, or embarrassment can bring them on. Being too warm is a major cause, but often there is no obvious trigger — they just happen.

While hot flashes do relate to low estrogen, there are a number of small changes you can make to reduce their frequency and intensity. Taking care not to dress too heavily is very helpful. Avoid hot drinks, which can provoke them. Thick blankets at night can cause the sleep-disturbing nighttime variety, accurately named night sweats. Carrying ice-cold bottled water with you and drinking it as needed can put a stop to an unwelcome hot flash. Here is another trick that may help you if you want to avoid blushing during a hot flash: exhale and hold your breath as the hot flash comes on. This initiates a reflex that causes the blood vessels in your skin to constrict, counteracting the blood vessel dilation of the hot flash.

Body weight may affect hot flashes. If you are somewhat overweight, the extra insulation of the body fat may make you prone to them. Conversely, if you tend to be underweight, you may be prone to them because a lack of body fat results in reduced estrogen levels.

If your hot flashes are mild and not too frequent, you may experience them as almost amusing, as a minor episode not even significant enough to be called an annoyance. That's how I experienced them during my change of life. I always considered myself to have been "born cold and never warmed up." It was funny for me to find that even using a hair dryer could trigger a mild hot flash!

Vitamin E (400–800 IU), together with flax oil (about five to ten 1 g capsules per day, or 1–2 teaspoons of the liquid), is especially helpful for reducing the incidence and severity of hot flashes. Even more flax oil, up to 6 teaspoons or 30 grams, is safe and healthy for hot flashes.[6] Take vitamin E when you use flax oil, as vitamin E protects the essential fatty acids in the flax oil from oxidative damage.

Here is a special note about vitamin B6, which is so central to decreasing the symptoms of PMS (See Chapter 5, "Premenstrual Syndrome"): Dr. Guy Abraham, who performed double-blind studies relating vitamin B6 to a reduction in PMS symptoms, has pointed out that vitamin B6 makes hot flashes worse because it reduces estrogen.[7] Because I was aware of this, I avoided B6 for three years during my perimenopause, even though the hot flashes I experienced were mild. I have recently increased it again to about 200–300 mg per day, and now I am wondering why I ever avoided it! Yes, it did bring on a few mild hot flashes, especially as I began taking it again, but the energy, mood improvement, and especially the mental sharpness I've experienced since resuming vitamin B6 have been well worth it. Along with the other supplements discussed in Chapter 3, try to get at least 50–100 mg of vitamin B6 daily,[8] unless you find that it is responsible for increasing hot flashes to an annoying level.

VAGINAL DRYNESS AND SEXUAL DESIRE

Estrogen is responsible for stimulating vaginal secretions, and a decline in estrogen underlies vaginal dryness, a common symptom of perimenopause and beyond. Dryness in the vagina can cause an uncomfortable sensation of irritation; it can make intercourse difficult, and it increases the risk of vaginal and urinary tract infections. Vitamin A, vitamin D, vitamin E, zinc, flax oil, and cod liver oil in amounts as listed in Table 7, Chapter 3 are all helpful to this condition. Vaginal lubricants can be used during intercourse if necessary. According to the late Dr. John Lee, author of *What Your Doctor May Not Tell You about Menopause*, a small amount of prescription cream containing the natural estrogen estriol, without other forms of estrogen, is safe to apply to the vagina twice a week to relieve vaginal dryness. Vaginal suppositories of estriol may also help overcome bladder incontinence and prevent bladder infections.[9]

Interestingly, vaginal dryness at this time of life is not necessarily related to low sexual desire. Why not? As estrogen declines, a woman's natural androgens ("male" hormones) from her ovaries and adrenal glands are less hidden by estrogen, unmasking the effects of the androgens. Sometimes this leads to a minor increase in unwanted body hair, but androgens also stimulate female desire. Because androgens come from the adrenal glands as well as from the ovaries, supporting the adrenal glands through improved nutrition, as discussed below, may increase sexual desire.

However, if a drop in sexual desire does occur during pre- or perimenopause, there are several possible explanations. It should not be considered normal or inevitable. One possibility is low thyroid function. Refer to "Low Thyroid Function" in Chapter 7 for more information on this topic and ways to correct it. Another is being very thin or lacking enough body fat. The stress of low body fat causes hormonal changes that reduce the output of the sex hormones. Gaining a modest amount of weight may improve desire. Oppositely, overweight or obesity can also cause low sex drive. It is not necessarily due to poor body image, as you might guess. Rather, excess body fat converts the natural androgens from the ovaries and adrenal glands into estrogen. A moderate amount of weight loss — perhaps 10 percent of the total body weight — may help to restore sexual desire.

If, nevertheless, decreased desire is still a problem, natural progesterone cream applied to the skin during the second half of the cycle, *after ovulation is confirmed by the NFP chart*, may be helpful. Once you stop having periods, the progesterone cream can be used during the second half of each calendar month. While Dr. Lee recommended over-the-counter natural progesterone cream for women with low desire,[10] in some cases, very small amounts of prescription testosterone cream may be helpful instead.[11] Read *Dr. John Lee's Hormone Balance Made Simple: The Essential How-to Guide to Symptoms, Dosage, Timing, and More* in order to acquaint yourself with the uses of natural progesterone, estrogen, and testosterone (See "Further Reading"). One note of caution: I believe it is prudent to have your doctor's counsel before you use progesterone cream for any reason, even though it is not under prescriptive control. See "Low Sexual Desire" in Chapter 13 for more information.

MOOD SWINGS, ANXIETY, AND DEPRESSION

Premenopause and perimenopause have the reputation of being times of unstable moods, poor mental focus, and decreased energy levels. There are many ways to avoid or lessen such problems. First is better nutrition. If you are troubled by mood swings, meaning short-term changes between normal moods and anxiety, irritability, or "the blues," look first at stabilizing your blood sugar levels. Proper function of your adrenal glands, which sit atop each kidney toward the back of the waist, is key to accomplishing this task.

Drops in blood glucose force the inner part of the adrenal glands, the adrenal medullae, to secrete the stress hormones norepinephrine and epinephrine, formerly called "adrenaline." These hormones do raise the blood glucose levels, but they also produce nervousness, irritability, and anxiety. A sugary treat that suddenly elevates blood glucose levels may seem to help out for a while, but other hormones, especially insulin, will soon produce a reactive drop in blood glucose levels. Along with the blood sugar drop come fatigue, brain fog, and another spurt of stress hormones! Regular meals and snacks, each a combination of protein, unrefined carbohydrates, and healthy fats, are the best way to get off the blood glucose roller coaster. See Rule 7 in Chapter 1 for more information on the effects of refined sugar on blood glucose levels.

Mood swings, anxiety, and low energy can also be improved by nutrition aimed at bolstering the function of the adrenal cortex (plural is "cortices"), which is the separate, outer part of each adrenal gland. Most people are hardly aware of the adrenal cortices, unless they have heard that they produce the stress hormone cortisol. Yet the adrenal cortices do an amazing amount of "behind the scenes" work. They coordinate the physical response to all types of stress, whether the stress is from illness, infection, sleeplessness, pain, low blood glucose, overwork, or emotional causes. They are essential in managing the stress of the changes of perimenopause. Moreover, they produce androgens, the "male" hormones. These hormones promote sexual desire in women; equally as important, some androgens are converted to estrogen by the body fat.

Nourishing the adrenal glands pays off well with calmer nerves, improved sexual desire, and normal levels of estrogen in the body. The adrenal cortices actually produce about fifty different hormones, and they can become exhausted, favoring production of some of their hormones at the expense of the others. Reducing stress in your life is helpful to them, but nutrition aimed at meeting their needs is at least as beneficial as stress reduction.

The adrenal glands need a variety of nutrients: vitamin A, the B vitamins, especially pantothenic acid, plenty of vitamin C, vitamins D and E, and the minerals magnesium, zinc, and manganese. They must have an adequate supply of the essential fatty acids to produce their hormones. Fresh, unheated salad oils such as canola oil and supplements of flax oil (five to ten 1 g capsules or 1–2 teaspoons daily) supply these fatty acids. Cod liver oil, which supplies the ready-made EPA and DHA as well as vitamins A and D, may be used instead. Adequate salt is another nutrient that the adrenal glands require.

Reducing caffeine intake is also very helpful to the adrenals. Caffeine acts on them like a whip on a tired horse — short-term stimulation, for sure, but long-term consequences as the adrenal glands become exhausted by the overstimulation. No doubt one of the unhealthy ways that caffeine affects the adrenals' stress response is by causing sleep disruption. You need more sleep at this time of life, and so do your adrenal glands! Sleeping and waking at regular times actually entrains a healthy pattern of secretion of the adrenal hormones. Try not to let caffeine interfere with your sleep, and do not let lack of sleep interfere with your adrenal glands. One of the best ways to reduce stress is to get more sleep.

Among the many tasks they perform, adrenal cortical hormones also keep blood glucose levels up between meals. Because low blood glucose can make it difficult to concentrate, attention to the nutritional needs of the adrenals will help prevent the common complaint of "brain fog" during the change of life.

For a comprehensive, easy-to-understand book that emphasizes nutrition for pre- and perimenopause moods, focus, and energy, read nutritionist Ann Louise Gittleman's *Before the Change: Taking Charge of Your Perimenopause*. (See "Further Reading.") In addition to better diet and supplements, it explains the role of exercise, stress reduction, adrenal support, and natural hormone replacement during this period of life. It recommends supplements such as black currant oil and borage oil, which may be valuable to some women. This book, I believe, is the best currently available to help you make an emotionally smooth, healthy, and happy transition from the fertile years to menopause and beyond. It is also excellent for those past menopause.

MAINTAINING HEALTHY BONES

With the medical and media spotlight on osteoporosis for the last two decades, many women rank concerns about this disease as their greatest fear of menopause. They are concerned about breaking a hip and becoming disabled. They are concerned about vertebral fractures and becoming stooped. They are equally concerned about the side effects of medications to prevent bone loss. Yet there are four effective self-care strategies for maintaining healthy bones for life: weight-bearing exercise, bone-building nutrition, healthy body weight, and safety habits aimed at preventing fractures.

WEIGHT-BEARING EXERCISE. Bone is living tissue, and the microscopic bone-laying cells, called osteoblasts, don't like to be squashed! When they "feel the squeeze" — that is, when pressure is put on them by your walking, jogging, running, jumping, or lifting, they respond by laying solid bone material around themselves until they have fortified a microscopic pocket with bone and are left safe and still alive within it. Weight-bearing exercise "puts the pressure on" the osteoblasts, and the result is strong bone. This bone will eventually deteriorate, but bone-dissolving cells called osteoclasts periodically invade worn bone, and like a crew of miniature miners, they clear out a tiny stretch of old bone. That sets the stage for new osteoblasts to come in, get "squashed," and respond by laying new solid bone material around themselves. Pressure on bones is an essential ingredient for new bone formation. By contrast, did you know that astronauts in weightless space suffer rapid and substantial bone loss? Their osteo*clasts* keep removing old bone, but their bone-building osteo*blasts* have no motivation to do their job!

Regular weight-bearing exercise — putting the pressure on your osteoblasts — is not optional if you wish to have strong bones for life. If you are not currently exercising regularly, find some activity that you enjoy, whether it is walking the dog, working out at a gym, or jogging around your neighborhood. That exercise will additionally help to regulate your insulin levels and burn calories, contributing to weight control. It will elevate your mood, especially if you do it in the great outdoors and try not to do too much.

BONE-BUILDING NUTRITION. Exercise alone cannot do the job of building up bone, because bone requires a large number of raw materials to renew itself. Many people name calcium first when they think of providing the body with the raw materials to make bone, but this is only one aspect of nutrition for healthy bones.

I am intrigued with the dietary suggestions that Susan Lark, M.D., offers for bone health, and I would like to share them with you. She points out that calcium and other minerals from the bones are naturally released to neutralize acid in the blood. A diet that chronically produces excess acid requires the bones to give up extra calcium to buffer that acid. As people age, the constant loss of minerals used to buffer the acid begins to take its toll, and thinning bones results. Oppositely, a diet that is more alkaline (basic) allows the bones to hold on to their calcium, reducing bone loss.[12]

About one-third of bone is the thread-like protein collagen, which decreases the brittleness of bone. Adequate protein is therefore important to bone health, but *excess* animal protein, especially from red meat, poultry, and dairy, causes acidity as it is metabolized within the body. Dr. Lark instead recommends moderate use of protein foods, as well as emphasis on protein sources which produce less acid: whole grains (except wheat), beans, nuts, fish, and eggs. Many fruits are quite acidic, so she believes they should be limited. But most vegetables are somewhat alkaline, and are good sources of magnesium and potassium, both of which she calls "bone-sparing" nutrients. Sugar, caffeine, alcohol, and "fizzy" soft drinks, even those without sugar, produce excess acid in the body. Plenty of water tends to dilute acid within the body, and she recommends drinking more water. Her recommendations are generally consistent with the "Twelve Rules for Better Nutrition" in Chapter 1.[13]

What about the micronutrients? Calcium is key, but it cannot be absorbed out of the intestines and into the blood unless vitamin D is present. Vitamin D can be made by the action of sunshine on the skin, but for people who work indoors and live in a climate with a cold winter, supplements of vitamin D are very beneficial. There are good "side effects" to vitamin D intake: A recent scholarly review of the research has revealed that this wonderful vitamin also decreases the risk of cancer.[14]

While calcium and vitamin D are important in preventing osteoporosis in later years, calcium should be balanced with magnesium, which is plentiful in the bone and enables the body to use calcium. If you have reason to be concerned about your bone health, I recommend supplements that include "MCHC" (microcrystalline hydroxyapatite concentrate), a mix of naturally-occurring bone minerals, including calcium and phosphorus, along with magnesium and vitamin D. I personally am very pleased with a supplement called Bone Builder, manufactured by Ethical Nutrients, which includes all of these nutrients as well as the bone-healthy mineral boron.

You may wish to subtract 250 mg of calcium from your supplemental intake of calcium for each cup of milk or serving of other dairy products in the diet, and you may wish to adjust the ratio of total calcium (dairy plus supplements) to supplemental magnesium to equal 1:1, or approximately 1,000 mg calcium (dairy plus supplements) to 1,000 mg of supplemental magnesium. As noted in Chapter 3, "Supplements to Consider," magnesium in the form of magnesium oxide may be too laxative for many people. A mix of magnesium oxide and "chelated" magnesium in the form of magnesium aspartate, magnesium citrate, or magnesium gluconate is less likely to cause loose bowels.

In addition to the "big three" for bone health — calcium, vitamin D, and magnesium — there are a number of other nutrients that enable the bone cells to lay down new bone: zinc, silica, boron, vitamin K, vitamin C, and the essential fatty acids.[15]

HEALTHY BODY WEIGHT. Good nutrition also includes maintaining an adequate body weight. The reproductive hormones estrogen, progesterone, and testosterone stimulate bone health. During perimenopause, progesterone falls essentially to zero, and the body fat becomes the major source of estrogen. In the fertile years, including premenopause, if enough body fat is lost, the reproductive hormones will decrease. Lack of ovulation and loss of periods result. Thin women have a well-established increase in risk of osteoporosis compared to women of normal weight.

The modest increase in weight that many women experience during pre- and perimenopause is a natural and healthy readjustment of the body to the change in its hormonal status. This is not to advocate obesity, but rather, a comfortable weight for your age. It may be 10 or 20 pounds higher than when you were 25, even a bit more if you were quite slender back then. In fact, a body weight of 132 pounds or more offers protection against bone fractures.[16] Did you know that one reason thin women are more prone to bone fractures than heavy women is because thin women have less padding than their heavier sisters?

FRACTURE-PREVENTING SAFETY HABITS. The final key to bone health is preventing fractures through proper safety habits. Gillian Sanson, author of *The Myth of Osteoporosis*, advocates strongly for behavioral changes to decrease the chance for fractures. She rightly points out that it is bone *fractures*, not bone density in itself, that will impact your quality of life as you age. (See "Further Reading.")

Hip fracture is one of the most debilitating bone injuries that can occur, and preventing such a fracture should be a high priority for everyone, including men. Only a small percentage of hip fractures occur spontaneously — that is, the neck of the femur (thigh bone) breaks under the weight of the body without a fall or other accident causing it. The vast majority of hip fractures, about 95 percent, occur in response to falls.[17]

One of the most effective things you can do to prevent bone fractures as you age is to implement safety measures to prevent falls. Now is the time to form the habits of using hand railings on steps, taking extra precautions on wet or icy outdoor decks, and keeping small items and pets from underfoot. Do you walk up and down your household steps with large clothes baskets held in both hands? Do you dash down your stairs in slippery socks? Are you ready to change unsafe habits such as these? It may be a humble concession to age to start safety habits while you feel youthful and vigorous, but good, well-ingrained safety habits may prevent disaster when you are much older.

Compressive fractures of the vertebrae (backbone) may not cause intense pain, but they can cause deformities of the spine and poor posture, limiting ease of movement. On the other hand, poor posture may just be a bad habit. This is an excellent time to evaluate your posture. How much poor posture is the habitual but reversible failure to "stand tall"?

If osteoporosis is a concern of yours, read *The Myth of Osteoporosis*, with its careful referencing of the medical literature. (Despite the title, the author does not consider the serious bone disorder osteoporosis a "myth.") While the author downplays the value of the Dexa Scan test of bone density, I disagree, and I believe that it should be routinely done in women well before the premenopause years. I urge you to have such a test soon, if you have never had one. If your test lets you know that your bones are dense and strong, keep up the good work!

If your test should come back showing low bone density, *The Myth of Osteoporosis* will be an excellent resource. It will alert you to the possible inaccuracies in your test or in its interpretation. It will reassure small-boned women that in fact their petite body build may contribute to poor test results despite healthy bones. Most of all, it will inform you of the marginal usefulness but major side effects of drugs intended to increase your bone density. Instead, the book recommends the keys to bone health reviewed above: weight-bearing exercise, bone-building nutrition, adequate body weight, and fracture-preventing safety habits.

PROGESTERONE CREAM. Dr. John Lee advocated natural ("bio-identical") progesterone cream for prevention of osteoporosis.[18] Even though it is available over the counter, if it is of interest to you, you should look for a medical doctor familiar with its use to assist you. Natural progesterone is certainly no substitute for the combination of exercise, improved nutrition, body weight awareness, and fracture prevention, but it may be a useful addition to your bone health approach. Women's Health America (*www.womenshealth.com*) is a wonderful resource that can assist you in finding a medical doctor who can help you to take a natural approach to maintaining bone health through natural hormone therapy.

BEAUTIFUL SKIN

The aging process most noticeably affects the skin, of course, but there are several approaches to maintaining beautiful skin. The first, I think, is to recognize the beauty of age. For example, my husband's Aunt Lorraine lived to be almost 101, and spent the first 100 years of her life in vigorous good health. She was an elementary schoolteacher (back in the one-room schoolhouse days), the adoptive mother of a fine son, a grandmother and great-grandmother, an avid gardener, a hard-working farm wife, and the loving caretaker of her husband, whom she outlived by fifteen years. Deeply involved in her small town community and church, she wrote letters regularly to a host of correspondents, was interested in everybody, and was loved by everybody. Her 100th birthday party was hugely crowded with family, friends, and well wishers. She was a beautiful woman, inside and out, for all the 30 years that I knew her. She had beautiful skin, too. Aged skin? Wrinkled skin? Well, yes, I suppose she did. It wasn't relevant. That's what I mean by recognizing the beauty of age, and accepting it in yourself is the first step to beautiful skin.

However, nutrition also helps the skin, as it does every other organ of the body. The outer layer, the epidermis, is particularly helped by the fat soluble nutrients vitamins A, D, E, and K, and the essential fatty acids. Flax oil in particular (about 10 grams or 2 teaspoons daily) or fish oil and other healthy oils such as olive oil condition and moisturize the epidermis from the inside out.

The deeper layer, the dermis, is the connective tissue layer and it has somewhat different needs. It requires vitamin C for the synthesis of its structural proteins collagen and elastin. It requires sulfur-containing amino acids. These are most plentiful in eggs and the "cruciferous" vegetables — broccoli, cabbage, Brussels sprouts, and other members of the cabbage family. Both the epidermis and dermis require protein.

Almost everyone knows that prolonged exposure to the sun damages the skin, but moderate summer sunshine exposure for just 10 or 15 minutes daily to a person in shorts and a T-shirt is very effective in enabling the skin to make vitamin D, with its powerful anti-cancer potential. Exercise is healthy for the skin because it increases the blood flow through it. Conversely, smoking is extremely damaging because it causes the blood vessels of the skin to vasoconstrict, decreasing its blood flow. Using only natural cosmetics with absorbable oils helps to keep the surface of the skin conditioned and healthy.

Finally, if you need one more reason to motivate yourself to cut down on your sugar consumption, here it is: According to cosmetic dermatologist Frederic Brandt, M.D., reducing your sugar intake can make your skin look ten years younger, because sugar accelerates the breakdown of the collagen and elastic proteins in the dermis. Elevated blood glucose levels cause glucose to bond with body proteins, resulting in a damaging process called glycation that affects virtually all tissues, including these two skin proteins. Dr. Brandt's thirty-day "detox" diet for beautiful skin is much like the recommendations in this book, particularly the recommendations for those attempting to overcome yeast overgrowth (Chapter 9). That is, he recommends a sugar- and starch-free diet for thirty days, but non-starchy vegetables, non-dairy animal protein, and a few fruits are allowed. As a side effect, he mentions how much more energetic and clearer-thinking eliminating sugar makes you! You will no doubt be hearing more about the damaging molecules caused by glycation, which are called "advanced glycation end products" — AGEs for short. They are serious factors in blood vessel disease, age-related brain dysfunctions, as well as skin aging.[19]

May I end with just one more anecdote about Aunt Lorraine? She gardened avidly until she was 100, and she ate what she grew. She always had a row of vitamin bottles on her neat kitchen counter. But perhaps as significant, she was well known for how she dealt with dessert. If there was party or a potluck, someone would usually bring an angel food cake, without icing. Aunt Lorraine would have just one thin slice. Everyone knew that that was the way she liked it, and one piece was all she would eat!

➤ Menopause is a natural life transition designed to enable women to live long enough to rear their children.

➤ While the term menopause refers to the last menses, the transition from the fertile years to infertility begins with **premenopause** in the late 30's or early 40's, and is completed during **perimenopause**, the last two to three years before menopause, around age 50.

➤ A number of changes take place, mostly relating to the decline in progesterone and the rise and then decline of estrogen.

➤ As the body readjusts, NFP charts are a great aid to understanding what is happening and when.

➤ Improved nutrition, the same as during the fertile years, is still the best way to maintain vibrant good health. Nutrition can help with some cycle irregularities, heavy bleeding, hot flashes, vaginal dryness, sexual desire, and mood changes.

➤ Long-term bone health is promoted by weight-bearing exercise, bone-building nutrition, healthy body weight, and fracture-reducing safety habits.

➤ Beautiful skin is promoted by a variety of vitamins and minerals, adequate protein, and avoidance of sugary foods.

13

Miscellaneous Problems that Affect Women

My lover belongs to me and I to him. — Song of Songs 2:16

Natural family planning users are truly the most health-conscious women I know. They are interested in all aspects of reproductive health, and are diligent in using self-help options if they exist. Using NFP in itself reduces a number of reproductive health risks, which is one reason that draws women to natural means of family planning. But there are a few miscellaneous problems that may occur anyway. Self-care strategies for preventing or overcoming them are offered below. (This chapter excludes sexually transmitted diseases, which must be dealt with medically and are not covered in this book.)

— VAGINAL INFECTIONS

There are two major types of vaginal infections — yeast infections and the less common bacterial infections. NFP is a great help in avoiding them since it does not decrease the protective mucus, as hormonal birth control often does, and it does not irritate the vagina, as barriers and spermicides do. In addition, by practicing NFP, you become aware of the ordinary, healthy cervical mucus discharge and therefore have the benefit of early recognition should infection occur.

YEAST INFECTIONS

Vaginal yeast infections occur all too frequently in women. The common yeast *Candida albicans* is normally found in the healthy vagina, but several factors can cause it to get out of balance and cause infection. The decreased acidity and increased production of glycogen, a natural carbohydrate, that occur during pregnancy or use of hormonal birth control can trigger yeast infections. Since yeast thrives on sugar, overconsumption of sugars and refined starches is a major risk factor. Antibiotics are an important contributor to yeast infections because they destroy the "friendly" bacteria that inhabit the vagina and naturally inhibit yeast organisms. Irritations in or around the vagina can also trigger outbreaks of yeast. Tight clothing, synthetic underwear, douches, and feminine hygiene sprays are sources of such irritation.

How do you know if you have a yeast infection? Yeast causes a discharge that tends to be whitish, thick, and caked. The discharge does not have a bad odor;

it may smell a little bit like baking bread. There is often itching of the vulva or vagina, and there may be reddening of the labia and even the upper thighs.

As usual, an ounce of prevention is worth a pound of cure. With reference to the role of sugar, one hundred women with chronic vaginal yeast infections were found to have "…excessive oral ingestion of dairy products, artificial sweeteners and sucrose. Eliminating excessive use of these foods brought about a dramatic reduction in the incidence and severity of Candida vulvovaginitis."[1] Translation: Cutting out sweet junk foods, including artificial sweetners, is the first step to avoiding yeast infections. One of my NFP clients ended twenty years of treatment for yeast infections by limiting sugar and caffeine and taking supplements similar to those in Chapter 3. She has not had a recurrence in three years.

If antibiotics are truly necessary, eating yogurt daily during and following treatment will help restore normal intestinal bacteria. Probiotics (capsules of "friendly" bacteria such as acidophilus) may also help prevent vaginal yeast infections.[2] Probiotics differ, so try to obtain a high quality brand with a variety of different friendly bacteria. Vitamins A and E and the essential fatty acids in flax oil (five to ten 1 g capsules or 1–2 teaspoons daily) are generally healing to the mucus membranes. Zinc works along with vitamin A to support the immune system, as does vitamin C.

Cotton underwear and loose-fitting, natural-fiber clothing that "breathes" are helpful to preventing yeast infections. Frequently-changed sanitary napkins are preferable to tampons. If you swim regularly, change into dry clothing immediately afterward, as yeast organisms prefer a damp environment.

Intercourse should be avoided during yeast infections in order not to spread the yeast cells. The penis may also become infected with yeast, so that yeast infections may be passed between the spouses. In one study, semen of the spouses of some women with recurrent yeast infections was found to contain yeast organisms thought to infect the seminal vesicles of the man. Yeast was also found to colonize the mouths of husbands of some women with recurrent yeast vaginitis, suggesting that oral-genital contact might be a source of reinfection in such women. Treating the husbands systemically for yeast in these cases greatly reduced the incidence of vaginal infections in the wives.[3]

Anti-yeast medications that are available over the counter have made annoying infections easier to deal with than in the past, but recurrent yeast infections are a prime symptom of general candidiasis, or yeast overgrowth. This topic is discussed in Chapter 9, under "Yeast Overgrowth." *The Yeast Connection and Women's Health*, by William Crook, M.D., contains a wealth of information on yeast-related problems, including vaginal infections and a related condition, vulvodynia, or genital pain in women. (See "Further Reading.")

BACTERIAL VAGINOSIS
Bacterial infection of the vagina is less common than yeast infection. Bacterial vaginosis, as it is called, typically causes a gray or yellowish discharge that has

a foul or fishy-smelling odor. It may cause itching, general pelvic pain, pain on intercourse, cramps, pain on urination, or low back pain. Intrauterine devices (IUDs) and diaphragms may contribute to these infections, again illustrating the value of NFP.

Prevention of such infections is of course the primary goal. Wiping from front to back is a usual recommendation for preventing bacterial contamination from the feces. The same irritating substances mentioned relative to yeast infections (feminine hygiene sprays, tight clothing, and so forth) should be avoided in order to prevent bacterial infections. Sanitary napkins are preferable to tampons when bacterial infections are a problem.

Since cervical mucus helps protect against infection, you should be especially careful during the "dry" times of the month if you are prone to bacterial infection. Consider nutritional aids, particularly flax oil and vitamin A, if scant mucus is a problem. For postmenopausal women who experience vaginal irritation due to dryness, flax oil is very helpful (5–10 g/day), as are vitamins A, D, and E, and zinc. (See Table 7, Chapter 3, for amounts.) All of these are very healing to the vaginal membranes. There is some evidence that probiotics ("friendly" bacteria taken by capsule) may help prevent bacterial vaginosis, since friendly bacteria tend to crowd out the wrong kind of bacteria in the colon, where the infective bacteria originate.[4]

As with yeast infections, abstinence is advisable when bacterial infections are present. If antibiotic treatment is necessary, be careful to avoid getting a yeast infection. Husbands of women who are troubled by frequent bacterial infections of the vagina should be examined also and treated if infection of the penis or prostate is present, though most prostate infections are not communicated to the woman.

Accurate diagnosis is essential for vaginal infections that do not quickly respond to home remedies. For those with reason to believe that their infection could be sexually transmitted, medical diagnosis and treatment of both spouses by a physician is a must.

—— BLADDER INFECTIONS ————————————

Differences in anatomy explain why women are far more prone to bladder infections than are men. Since the urethra of the female is shorter and infective bacteria come from the outside, it is a shorter trip to the bladder for such bacteria in women than in men. The female urethra is also closer to the anus, where the infective bacteria usually originate. Sexual activity is the most important risk factor for urinary tract infections,[5] as the urethral opening lies close to the vagina.

Urinating within about thirty minutes after intercourse is a useful practice for women who are prone to bladder infections, as is emptying the bladder every two hours or so during the day. This flushes away bacteria and prevents overstretch of the bladder wall, which reduces its blood supply. If you are prone to urinary tract infections, be sure that you empty your bladder as completely as possible each time you urinate, leaning forward a bit and not rushing. Making sure that you do not sit in one place for long periods of time is another helpful habit, especially if you have had past urinary tract infections after long hours of travel. Drink plenty of pure water to dilute the urine and encourage emptying.

Certain foods may cause inflammation of the bladder in some people. Consider whether or not any of the foods listed under the topic below might contribute to your tendency to bladder infections.

INTERSTITIAL CYSTITIS/PAINFUL BLADDER SYNDROME
Some women are bothered by chronic or recurrent episodes of bladder pain and inflammation, termed interstitial cystitis and painful bladder syndrome. Certain foods may increase these symptoms, according to a study based on the experience of people who have such interstitial cystitis. The most commonly reported foods that resulted in bladder pain were as follows: caffeinated foods and beverages, with coffee being the worst, followed by cola drinks, tea, decaffeinated coffee, dark chocolate candy, and milk chocolate candy; carbonated drinks and alcoholic beverages; foods containing hot peppers, such as burritos; other spicy foods; artificial sweeteners, including aspartame and saccharin; juices, including cranberry juice and pineapple juice; tomato products; horseradish and vinegar. Conversely, using baking soda to produce less acidic urine has been reported to be the most helpful self-care.[6]

Note that the commonly-recommended cranberry juice is on the list of bladder irritants! Yes, it somewhat inhibits bacteria, but most cranberry drinks are loaded with sugar, and any acid or spicy food can irritate the urinary tract in women who are prone to bladder infections, allowing the bacteria to take over.

Bladder infections are more easily prevented than cured through self-help strategies, and you may need an antibiotic if you develop one. Here is a final tip if you ever find yourself with a urinary tract infection which makes it painful to empty your bladder: Pour a large glass of warm water slowly over the vulva as you urinate. Those who have had such infections report that this is a tremendous help.

— LOW SEXUAL DESIRE

A young woman once wrote a letter to The Couple to Couple League's *Family Foundations* magazine, asking for help because her sexual desire was high only at mid-cycle, the fertile time. Since the couple was avoiding a pregnancy, this led to a frustrating situation — by the time infertile days were available after ovulation, the wife's desire had faded. The letters from the readers who responded to the writer were insightful, sensitive, and mature. One writer dealt with communication between the spouses regarding the problem, its possible causes, and its resolution. All the respondents charitably encouraged the woman to face this difficulty with graciousness and prayer, and some shared their own similar struggles.

I would like to discuss this issue from the physical aspect, because there is a very good chance that women like the original letter writer experience low libido (low sexual desire) because of physical factors involving overall health and, in particular, hormonal balance. This is not to dismiss other possibilities — the interpersonal, emotional, or spiritual. Nor do I intend to equate the level of desire of a woman to the overall happiness of her marriage. I think everyone agrees, though, that it is easier for a husband to please his wife, and for a wife to please her husband, when her libido naturally makes her appreciative of and responsive to his attention.

LOW DESIRE IN THE POST-OVULATORY INFERTILE TIME

When a woman experiences desire only during the fertile time and loses all desire during the rest of the month, she is experiencing a form of low sexual desire that should be recognized as such. Even if she were seeking a pregnancy and not abstaining during the fertile time, this would be a frustrating problem. Women are sexually receptive at all times of the month, and it is the norm for women to be able to respond sexually whether or not they are in the fertile time. Some studies have shown that women have two peaks of desire: one during the fertile time, and one during the premenstrual days. Some have even written that many women find the infertile premenstrual days a time of higher libido than the actual fertile time.

John Lee, M.D., author of *What Your Doctor May Not Tell You about Menopause*, stated that libido depends more on levels of progesterone than on estrogen or androgens ("male hormones") in women. His experience is that women who use nonprescription natural progesterone cream during the second half of their cycle (the luteal phase, or post-ovulatory phase) report a noticeable increase in desire.[7] This makes sense, because progesterone stimulates thyroid function and also serves as the precursor for some adrenal hormones. Both glands are involved in libido.

If you are in your fertile years, however, you should first attempt to improve your own progesterone levels naturally with diet and nutritional supplements, rather than with hormone supplements. (See "Luteal Phase Deficiency" in Chapter 7). If you do choose to use progesterone cream, always wait until the third day of elevated temperatures that confirm ovulation before doing so. Once you are past menopause, if you wish to use over-the-counter natural progesterone cream, you can do so for two or three weeks of each calendar month. In any case, even though it is nonprescription, you should consult with a supportive doctor first.

Guy Abraham, M.D., developed and tested a diet and supplement plan for overcoming premenstrual syndrome (PMS), which is often caused by low progesterone levels in the luteal phase. He created Optivite, a complete multivitamin/multimineral supplement which, under double-blind conditions has relieved the symptoms of PMS. Vitamin B6 and vitamin C, major nutrients in

Optivite, have been shown to raise the levels of progesterone, at least in some women. (See Chapter 5 for details.)

I spoke by telephone with Dr. Abraham about the effect of Optivite on womanly desire. "Yes, that has been unexpected, but we have received many reports of increased desire in women using Optivite. Husbands will say, 'This is the woman I married again,' after she takes Optivite. Not all women, but some women report that they are more receptive, even more interested in initiating relations during the premenstrual days."[8]

If you are experiencing low desire during the luteal phase, first try to improve your nutritional (and indirectly, hormonal) status with Optivite or the similar ProCycle and improved diet, as outlined in Chapter 5. Equally as important, five to ten 1 g capsules of flax oil a day may make a noticeable difference in desire. When the ovaries have the nutritional building blocks they need, they are more likely to produce optimal amounts of their hormones. This is also true of the thyroid gland and adrenal glands, whose hormones also affect libido.

OVERALL LOW DESIRE

LOW THYROID FUNCTION. For many years it has been known that low thyroid function (hypothyroidism) is a major contributor to low sexual desire. Low thyroid function is common, and many women have been tested for it. But Mary Shomon, author of *The Thyroid Hormone Breakthrough*, points out that thyroid tests are notoriously unreliable, and the understanding that "subclinical hypothyroidism" exists has gained acceptance. Thyroid function affects basal body temperature, and if your pre-ovulatory basal temperatures are in the range of 97.2° F or below, you have good reason to suspect that low thyroid function might be your problem, even if you have been tested and the tests have been normal. See "Low Thyroid Function" in Chapter 7 for information on nutrition and other help for low thyroid function. Mary Shomon's book is an excellent resource as well. (See "Further Reading.")

POOR ADRENAL FUNCTION. The adrenal glands, which sit atop each kidney, have a major role in the physical response to stress. Poor adrenal function should be considered a possibility if sexual desire is low, especially if you have been under prolonged stress. Why? Among the many roles they play, the adrenals produce androgens that increase libido in women. Besides coordinating the response to stress and producing these "male" hormones, they regulate the immune response, they are vital for salt balance in the body, and they keep the blood glucose levels up between meals. Stress of any type, whether physical or emotional, increases the workload of the adrenals. In addition to emotional stress, low blood glucose, underweight, excess exercise, pain, allergy, illness, and sleeplessness can all affect the adrenal glands, increasing their need for nutrients. In order to make their hormones, the adrenals need many nutrients, including vitamin C, the essential fatty acids (five to ten 1 g capsules of flax oil daily) zinc, manganese, and B vitamins, especially pantothenic acid. Attention to the nutrients the adrenal glands need can improve libido. See

Chapter 14 for more information on the adrenal glands.

MENOPAUSE. As fertility declines in the 40s, the adrenals' production of androgens contributes importantly to women's sexual desire. Desire may in fact increase in the 40s and afterward because as estrogen declines, the androgens produced by the adrenals are "unmasked." That is, their effects are more obvious because they are not overshadowed by estrogen. Let me state it clearly: Do not accept the common belief that desire inevitably drops as menopause approaches. If your desire does drop at that time, look to low thyroid function or poor adrenal function, and work to correct the problem.

In some cases, small amounts of testosterone can restore desire in women, especially during the perimenopause and beyond. Dr. John Lee recommends that women try natural progesterone cream for six months, and if desire is still not restored, that they talk with their doctor about natural testosterone, which is available only by prescription.[9]

The amino acid L-arginine increases the blood flow to the genitals, increasing sexual sensitivity in some women. A proprietary blend of L-arginine, Panax ginseng, Ginkgo biloba and damiana leaf, along with several vitamins and minerals, was formulated and tested under double-blind conditions for its effect on sexual desire, sexual satisfaction, and satisfaction with the overall relationship. Taken daily for four weeks, this supplement, called ArginMax for Women, was shown to be most helpful to women in the perimenopausal transition, but was also moderately helpful to overall sexual satisfaction in postmenopausal women.[10] ArginMax is available at *www.arginmax.com*, and is recommended by women's health writer Susan Lark, M.D. Alternatively, Dr. Lark recommends 500 mg of arginine one to three times daily.[11] Be aware, however, that arginine can cause flare-ups of genital herpes, as well as the herpes virus that causes cold sores in the mouth.

OVERWEIGHT. Obesity or substantial overweight may be related to low desire in some women. This is not necessarily due to the "body image" that an overweight woman in our weight-obsessed society may be burdened with, but simply due to the hormonal situation. Overweight results in elevated estrogen levels and lowered androgens, because body fat converts androgens from the adrenals and ovaries into estrogens. High levels of estrogen lower progesterone, and both androgens and progesterone are involved in female libido. A modest, gradual weight loss, coupled with moderate exercise and good nutrition, is helpful to regaining a better balance of hormones and improving desire. (See Chapter 8 for more information on overweight.)

UNDERWEIGHT OR INSUFFICIENT BODY FAT. Dropping too much weight can cause a drop in desire because estrogen and progesterone levels drop. A woman who lacks adequate body fat will ultimately experience delayed ovulation, and even complete amenorrhea if the weight loss is great enough. How much weight is enough? If you are ovulating more or less regularly — by day 18 or so — probably the underweight is just on the border. Even if you are not ovulating at all, usually a gain of just a few pounds, or a decrease in vigorous exercise, will bring back the cycles. The decrease in stress and the increase in sex hormones will very likely improve desire. (See Chapter 7, "Underweight or Inadequate Body Fat.")

YEAST OVERGROWTH. Dr. William Crook, author of *The Yeast Connection and Women's Health,* was a proponent of the theory that some people have abnormal amounts of yeast organisms in their bodies. These organisms, according to this viewpoint, disrupt many systems of the body, including the immune system and the hormone glands. When the hormones are disrupted, loss of sexual desire is one of many possible effects.

Yeast may get out of hand when sugar intake is excessive, when antibiotics are taken for long periods, or when cortisone drugs or birth control pills are used. Avoiding yeast-containing foods, eating good quality yogurt, and maintaining a healthy, low-sugar diet with supplements as listed in Table 7 (Chapter 3) generally enables the body to keep yeast in balance. When yeast organisms are under control, the function of the thyroid gland, adrenal gland, and ovaries improves, and so will sexual desire, according to Dr. Crook. If you are bothered by yeast infections or overall poor health, refer to "Yeast Overgrowth" in Chapter 9 of this book and to Dr. Crook's book also. (See "Further Reading.")

LOW DESIRE POSTPARTUM
The high hormone levels of pregnancy contribute to the increased desire that many women experience if they stay rested and healthy throughout the pregnancy. But the steep drop in hormones after the birth may produce the opposite effect, especially during the first few months of breastfeeding. All of this is quite natural, and recognizing it as a temporary situation gives perspective. Nevertheless, desire can pick up long before fertility returns after childbirth, even as a woman continues breastfeeding.

I have frequently noticed very low temperatures when counseling women who are infertile while breastfeeding. These reflect low thyroid function, called "postpartum thyroiditis." (See Chapter 10 for a discussion of this topic.)

Poor adrenal function is another possibility; the stress of pregnancy, childbirth, and a new baby can increase the needs of the adrenal glands, and their hormones are also involved in milk production. I suggest that you practice nutrition aimed at meeting the needs of both the thyroid and adrenal glands, starting with flax oil (five to ten 1 g capsules/day) and including the other vitamins and minerals listed in Table 7, Chapter 3. The book *A Natural Guide to Pregnancy and Postpartum Health,* by Dean Raffelock, D.C., and Robert Rountree, M.D., is an excellent source of information that you may wish to review. (See "Further Reading.") Some of the information that follows may also apply to postpartum mothers.

OTHER FACTORS IN LOW DESIRE
HORMONAL BIRTH CONTROL. I've heard this line a number of times: "I got on

the Pill so I could have sex any time I wanted it, but it made me so I didn't want it." If this sounds like you, getting off the Pill or other forms of hormonal birth control is the first step to improved desire, as well as improved overall health. But work hard to improve your nutrition so that your body "bounces back" and produces its own hormones in the right amounts. See Chapter 9, "Discontinuing Birth Control Pills or Other Hormonal Birth Control" for nutritional strategies to help out. Should the problem of low desire continue, refer to the other subtopics in this chapter. More than one cause could be involved.

OTHER MEDICATIONS. A number of medications may adversely affect desire in women: statins for cholesterol, antidepressants, blood pressure medicines, stimulants, and antihistamines.[12] In some cases you may be able to decrease or discontinue such medications by improving your diet, your body weight, or your exercise level. Working with a nutritionally-oriented doctor in such a situation is the best way to discontinue such medications.

INADEQUATE SLEEP. Cheating the need for sleep is a sure way to lower sexual desire. I've never seen any research that substantiates it, but I believe that most women need more sleep than most men. It is been written many times before, but it is worth repeating: How can a husband and wife have satisfying times of intimacy if both are exhausted from the day's activities? When a couple is abstaining periodically, they usually have a fairly good idea of when the time of abstinence will end. Planning ahead for time together, taking a nap in the afternoon, or spending time together in the morning are all possibilities. How do we get more rest? When are we both most rested? Can we make time in the morning or early evening? These are questions that spouses should discuss with one another if fatigue is involved with low desire. (See the question and answer on sleep in Chapter 4.)

WEAK PELVIC FLOOR MUSCLES. Having poor tone in the skeletal muscles that support the uterus, bladder, and rectum does not cause low desire, but it can interfere with sexual climax. The Kegel exercise, routinely taught during childbirth classes, is intended to strengthen these muscles, which are stretched somewhat by the enlarged uterus, and greatly by childbirth.

To learn the exercise, you first practice stopping a stream of urine by strongly contracting the pelvic floor muscles. Then, you practice contracting them any time at all. Contracting and holding the contraction strongly for several seconds about twenty-five to fifty times a day increases the tone of these muscles.

The benefits are several: better support for the bladder and uterus; better control of the bladder, especially during pregnancy and later in life after menopause, and better ability to achieve sexual climax, as these muscles are the ones that are consciously contracted during intercourse to produce the female orgasm. I believe that women who find that they are unable to experience orgasm should not first seek psychological counseling, but rather counseling explaining the *physical* components of the sexual response.

PAIN DURING INTERCOURSE. If you are experiencing pain during sexual relations, you should certainly discuss it with a compassionate physician. Sometimes a woman may be injured during childbirth; for example, an episiotomy may be poorly repaired. Sometimes estrogen levels are low — from postpartum changes, from menopause, or from underweight — and in response the vaginal tissues become thin and vulnerable to injury. If this seems to be the case for you, see "Vaginal Dryness and Sexual Desire" in Chapter 12. If the problem is endometriosis, please refer to that topic in Chapter 6 for nutritional strategies that can reduce endometriosis pain. Whatever the cause, it is surely worth serious effort to find the source of the trouble and to follow through with appropriate treatment.

TOO FREQUENT INTERCOURSE. Yes, too much of a good thing can dull desire. Part of the heightened libido typically experienced by women who abstain during the fertile time results from the abstinence itself. By contrast, when relations are had more frequently than your natural level of desire, you may find yourself believing the problem is lack of desire, when it is at least partly caused by sexual satiety. This is a topic best discussed by the two of you, so that both understand that the out-of-sync desire is not a lack of love on your part, nor a lack of consideration on his part. For couples with no reason to abstain, sexual satiety might also contribute to seeming low desire, and a decrease in "quantity" may make for an increase in "quality."

➤ Vaginal infections, whether from yeast organisms or from bacteria, are unpleasant in themselves, but they also can interfere with the mucus sign of fertility.

➤ A sugary diet, hormonal birth control, and antibiotics are all risk factors for vaginal yeast infections. Eliminating all of these, except for essential antibiotics, can help reduce the incidence of yeast infections. Using yogurt or probiotic ("friendly") bacterial supplements crowds out yeast organisms.

➤ Bacterial vaginosis may be prevented by good hygiene and nutrients aimed at healing the vaginal wall and promoting normal cervical mucus. There is some evidence that probiotics may also reduce the occurrence of vaginal bacterial infections.

➤ Bladder infections may be prevented with hygienic practices aimed at keeping harmful bacteria away from the urethra. Certain foods and drinks, such as those that contain caffeine, spices, and acid, have been found to contribute to inflammation of the bladder (interstitial cystitis) in some people. Reducing consumption of these may help reduce the risk of bladder infections as well.

➤ Low sexual desire may have a number of causes, including low levels of progesterone, low thyroid function, poor adrenal gland function, underweight, overweight, and lack of sleep. Postpartum changes, including breastfeeding, may cause a temporary drop in libido, which usually returns even as the mother continues nursing. Loss of libido during menopause may relate to low thyroid function, poor adrenal function, or lack of sleep, rather than to menopause in itself.

➤ Identifying and correcting the underlying causes can help to restore libido.

14

Increasing Your Energy & Decreasing Your Stress

A merry heart doeth good like medicine. — Proverbs 17:22 (KJV)

I have given talks on this topic at natural family planning (NFP) conferences and elsewhere, and it is one of my favorites. But how did I get from NFP and nutrition to energy and stress? As I counseled women on cycle irregularity, breastfeeding, or infertility, I gradually realized that many women who are seeking counseling for one problem — say cycle irregularity — are actually dealing with fatigue and stress as well. This topic does impact NFP, however. Fatigue and anxiety are common symptoms of PMS, as well as common symptoms of the perimenopausal "change of life." They reduce sexual desire. They are involved in postpartum blues. The adrenal hormones, which are altered by stress, affect the function of other hormones, including progesterone and the thyroid hormones.

Fatigue causes stress, and stress causes fatigue. Oppositely, high energy and calm nerves go hand in hand. Strategies that naturally increase your energy will tend to reduce stress, so the place to start is with increasing your energy.

— INCREASING YOUR ENERGY

Have you ever considered what it is that makes you feel energetic? For example, if right now you are feeling bright and chipper, can you explain why? If, on the other hand, you are feeling "wiped out," can you explain it to yourself? Four major factors underlie the subjective feelings of high energy or fatigue: sleep, exercise, stress, and blood sugar levels.

ADEQUATE SLEEP
The first element of high energy should be obvious — enough sleep. There is no substitute for it. But are you getting enough sleep? Many women believe that six or seven hours of sleep is enough, but it is possible that you need eight or nine hours, maybe more, to feel and do your best. This is particularly true if you are pregnant or breastfeeding. I have had women tell me that they are fatigued from morning to night, and then ask me if there is some nutritional way to increase their energy. Yet when I ask them how much sleep they get, they may reply that they go to bed at 10:30 and get up at 5:00! Improved nutrition simply cannot compensate.

There is a good chance that *when* you sleep makes a difference. For some people, seven hours of sleep at night and a one-hour nap is more restful than nine hours of sleep at night and no nap. For myself, I am convinced that eight hours of sleep from midnight to 8:00 does me more good than eight hours from 10:00 to 6:00. Other "night people" can understand this, while "morning people" might find exactly the opposite is true.

Giving sleep the priority it requires is often tricky with the fast pace of modern society. Can you go to bed earlier? Get up later? Take a morning, afternoon, or evening nap? Many people say that they do not have enough time for sleep, but you will find that getting the sleep you need will make your waking time far more productive and much, much more pleasant — for you and for those around you.

APPROPRIATE EXERCISE

The second element that contributes to high energy is the right amount of exercise. Too much leaves you exhausted; too little leaves you sluggish. The right amount is invigorating. Everyone has had the experience of too much physical exertion leaving you drained, even for the next day — spading and planting a garden on a hot day, over-enthusiastically undertaking a new exercise program, or driving around town running half a dozen errands. (Even though much of driving a vehicle is done automatically by habit, it requires a great deal of sensory and motor activity, and a high degree of alertness. The eyes keep the brain busy. No wonder it wears you out.)

The right amount of exercise contributes to your sense of well-being in a number of ways. Physically, regular moderate exercise is a powerful way of regulating blood sugar levels, which, as you will see, is a major factor in your energy level. Nevertheless, a big caution to those who know that they should be getting more exercise is to start gradually. Right from the start, your exercise program should be pleasant and invigorating. You are not likely to stick with it if too much too soon overtires you.

STRESS

Stress causes fatigue, and fatigue causes stress. No matter what the stress, it is well-established scientifically that the body reacts physically in the same way. The stress hormones epinephrine and norepinephrine (adrenaline) are released, and they cause the heart rate and blood pressure to rise. They affect the brain so that you feel nervous, anxious, afraid, irritated, or angry, depending on what is happening around you. The response to stress "revs up your engine," which sooner or later will cause you to crash in exhaustion.

The word "stress" usually conjures up situations such as financial problems, relationship problems, and negative events that happen to you. However, pain, an acute illness, chronic illness, allergies, lack of sleep, excess exercise, skipping meals, prescription medications, and poor nutrition are also stresses to the body, which reacts like it does to any other stress. Many people do not realize that the feelings of stress they experience are more related to physical factors such as allergies, illness, sleeplessness, and poor nutritional habits than to the ordinary pressures that every day inevitably brings. Dealing with these physical stresses will almost automatically increase your energy.

BLOOD SUGAR LEVELS

The fourth and most underrated contributor to high energy levels is blood sugar control. The blood sugar glucose is the preferred fuel of many body cells. The brain's cells have no choice; they can use only glucose. They are dependent on a steady supply of glucose brought to them by the blood. If they get the glucose they need, they can perform their activities efficiently, as can the other body cells. What happens at the cellular level determines what happens to the whole person, physiologically speaking.

The key to high energy, then, is to get the glucose into the cells, particularly the brain cells. This depends first on blood glucose levels that are high enough to carry sufficient glucose. But it is overly simplistic to believe that high blood glucose levels alone ensure the brain's nutrition. For example, in untreated diabetes, the blood sugar levels are much too high, yet most of the body's cells are starving because without insulin, the glucose they need cannot enter. This is an example of a disease state, but in all cases, a number of vitamins and minerals, especially the B vitamins and magnesium, are needed to enable glucose to enter cells efficiently and to be used as a fuel to drive cellular processes.

When the brain gets and uses the glucose it needs, there are two side benefits. The first is increased mental alertness and ability to concentrate. I am surprised at how frequently and casually a woman will remark, as if it is a normal experience: "I can't think straight when I'm pregnant." Childbearing is a natural life experience which does not damage memory or concentration. What most likely has happened is that such a woman has not met the increased nutritional needs of pregnancy, especially for B vitamins, and is experiencing minor blood sugar drops that affect her mental function. Pregnancy is a time when blood sugar control is more difficult, but even then blood glucose drops can be prevented or corrected with careful nutrition.

The second benefit of stable blood sugar levels is calm nerves. If the blood glucose levels drop, the fight-or-flight hormones epinephrine and norepinephrine must be secreted to restore them. The side effects of nervousness, anxiety, irritability and so forth explain why some people (not you or me!) get grouchy when dinner is late. The role of stable blood glucose levels forms the closest link between energy and stress.

HOW THE BODY MAINTAINS BLOOD GLUCOSE LEVELS. Before reviewing practical ways of maintaining blood glucose levels, it is useful to understand that the body has two distinct metabolic states for blood sugar control. The first occurs right after you eat. During this time, called the "absorptive state," you use the fuel provided by the recent meal to maintain your blood glucose levels. The hormone insulin from the pancreas is secreted; its job is to keep the blood sugar levels from rising too high. It does so by enabling glucose to move out of the blood and into the cells for their energy needs. Insulin promotes storage of excess glucose in the liver, where it can be released later. Within the fat cells, insulin promotes storage of excess fuel as fat. Interestingly, the brain does not require insulin to get its glucose.

The second state, the fasting or "postabsorptive" state, occurs after a meal is digested and absorbed. During this phase, you maintain your blood glucose levels by releasing fuel from its storage locations within the liver and fat cells. A number of hormones stimulate this. Glucagon, a second pancreatic hormone; cortisol from the adrenal glands; and, if necessary, epinephrine and norepinephrine from the adrenals all maintain blood glucose levels by stimulating the liver to release its stored fuel. Notice the glands involved: pancreas, adrenals, and liver.

When the postabsorptive processes function well, you feel energetic and alert between meals, and, as a beneficial side effect, weight control is easier since you do not need to boost your blood sugar levels with another snack or meal. If you wake up tired or experience afternoon slumps which are noticeably helped by eating dinner, most likely the postabsorptive processes are not working as well as they might. Migraine headaches at these times are yet another symptom of poor postabsorptive blood sugar maintenance.

PRACTICAL STRATEGIES FOR MAINTAINING BLOOD SUGAR LEVELS. Below is a list of practical ways to maintain adequate blood glucose levels around the clock. The underlying strategy is first to eat in such a way that your absorptive state is prolonged. I like to put it this way: When you eat, you want to your food to raise blood glucose levels, but only moderately so that your blood sugar "flies under the radar" of excessive insulin release, which would cause a reactive drop in your blood glucose levels. The second goal is to provide the body with the vitamins and minerals that make the postabsorptive processes more effective.

1) EAT REGULARLY. Avoid long periods of fasting. Do not skip breakfast. Even under the best of conditions, there is a limit to how long and how well your postabsorptive processes can maintain adequate blood sugar levels.

2) AVOID SUGARS AND REFINED STARCHES ON AN EMPTY STOMACH. A sudden load of carbohydrates (sugars and starches, which are quickly digested to sugars) will rapidly raise the blood glucose, boosting your energy temporarily. However, high blood glucose triggers insulin, which can overcorrect the high blood sugar and leave you with a fatigue-producing drop in blood glucose called "reactive hypoglycemia." Even healthy foods, such as fruits and whole grain breads and cereal, can trigger reactive hypoglycemia if they are eaten alone.

3) MAKE EVERY MEAL AND EVERY SNACK A COMBINATION OF PROTEIN, CARBOHYDRATES (FRUITS, VEGETABLES, GRAINS), AND FATS. Carbohydrates alone raise blood glucose levels rapidly, as noted above. However, proteins and fats slow the digestive processes and the release of glucose into the blood. All

three together create a long-lasting absorptive state with steady blood sugar levels. The old expression is that such a meal "sticks to your ribs." Eggs, toast with butter, and an orange for breakfast; cheese and crackers for a snack; and any typical dinner menu with meat or fish, starchy vegetables and salad are examples of such combinations.

4) BE SURE TO GET ENOUGH OF THE HEALTHY FATS, SATURATED AND UNSATURATED. Your body must have essential fatty acids, which are neither vitamins nor minerals, but are building molecules for cell membranes and prostaglandins. All cells require them, but gland cells need them in particularly high amounts. They are unsaturated "good" fats found in nuts, seeds, and expeller-pressed salad oils. Moderate amounts of natural saturated fats, such as those found in meat and dairy products, provide the benefit of stabilizing blood sugar levels, since fats inhibit the emptying of the stomach.

5) CAFFEINE IS A GOOD SLAVE BUT A BAD MASTER. It raises blood glucose, giving you a boost. But it causes a reactive drop in blood glucose and stresses the adrenals, creating a roller coaster of blood sugar fluctuations that make you crave sugar or more caffeine.

6) AVOID THE ARTIFICIAL SWEETENER ASPARTAME (NUTRASWEET) which causes the body to release insulin, decreasing blood glucose levels. On an empty stomach this is responsible for a major side effect of aspartame consumption: headaches. Avoid other artificial sweeteners as well.

7) CONSIDER SUPPLEMENTS THAT SUPPORT NORMAL POSTABSORPTIVE BLOOD GLUCOSE LEVELS. I've listed the following in order of priority. (For specific amounts, see Table 7, Chapter 3):

Vitamin C is used in large amounts by the adrenal glands, especially under stress conditions.

B vitamins, including folic acid. These enable the liver to release glucose during fasting and the brain to use glucose efficiently. The B vitamin pantothenic acid is especially valuable to the adrenal glands.

Magnesium enables the body to use certain B vitamins. Dr. Guy Abraham, who carried out double-blind studies relating nutrition to PMS, noted that if the body is deficient in B vitamins and magnesium, the brain cannot efficiently metabolize glucose, and even small drops in blood glucose affect the brain's function, making the individual feel like a large drop has occurred.[1] This could explain why you feel as if you have the symptoms of low blood glucose, even though tests may show that you do not.

Essential fatty acids are essential to all glands, including the liver, adrenal glands, and pancreas, each of which is involved in raising fasting blood glucose levels. Good quality "expeller pressed" salad oils (such as canola oil) are available at health food shops, but I also recommend supplementing flax oil (five to ten 1 g capsules daily) or fish oil (1 teaspoon daily or five 1 g capsules).

Vitamin E prevents destruction of essential fatty acids.

Zinc is necessary to adrenal function.

— DECREASING YOUR STRESS

The term "stress" can mean a number of different things, but most people understand what you mean when you say you are stressed. To feel overwhelmed, to feel like you are not coping, to feel overburdened by circumstances or responsibilities, to feel worried or anxious — all these can be summarized in the expression, "I'm stressed out."

What causes stress? Financial worries, difficult children, too much work and not enough time, concerns about aging or sick loved ones, and broken relationships are all examples of situations that cause emotional stress. But allergies, infections, pain, sleeplessness, and low blood glucose also stress the body, and these physical stresses can trigger the same unpleasant emotional state that people call being "stressed out."

How do you deal with stress? The most common suggestion is to cut down on your activities in order to reduce stress or avoid stressful situations. Of course that is not always possible. For example, if you are caring for a chronically sick or high-needs child, you simply cannot decide not to do so any more. Perhaps your job is the stressful activity, but given the options, you feel you have no other satisfactory alternative. Maybe it is all the chauffeuring you do, but then again, you value the opportunities you are making for your children.

As most women have learned, talking about your stress is helpful. A sympathetic friend can be a real comfort when you feel down. When we adopted our seventh child, Vahn, from overseas, I felt anxious for a couple of months afterward, even though everything about the adoption and our baby's health, personality, and adjustment turned out better than we ever hoped. It really helped for listening friends to explain it for me, "You've just had a major life change. Look at all the unknowns you've been dealing with. No wonder you're stressed. Who wouldn't be?"

Prayer is a great consolation in stressful times. I love the prayer that Catholics use at each Mass: "...Protect us from all anxiety as we wait in joyful hope for the coming of our Savior, Jesus Christ." Christians believe that the Lord is the Prince of Peace, and the fruits of His Spirit include peace. Who has not had comfort in prayer?

Yet sometimes none of the above seems to help. You can see that you ought to be happy and at peace, yet even little things continually bother you. You see others coping better with bigger burdens than you are doing with smaller ones. You question yourself, your commitments, your relationships with others, and even your relationship with God. What is the missing link?

THE PHYSICAL ASPECTS OF STRESS

Human beings are not disembodied spirits, nor disembodied emotions. People are integrated physical, emotional, and spiritual beings. While it is common to recognize the emotional and even the spiritual aspects of stress, all too frequently the *physical* component is completely ignored.

The late, great nutritionist Adelle Davis, wrote extensively about stress and nutritional strategies for combating it. She emphasized the physical component — the role of the adrenal glands in the stress response.

The adrenal glands do so much that every one should be aware of them and what they do. They are two small glands that sit atop each kidney, above the waist near the back of the abdomen. Each adrenal gland is actually two separate glands, one inside the other. The inner adrenal medulla produces the fight-or-flight hormones epinephrine and norepinephrine (formerly called "adrenaline"). These hormones are the ones that cause the stress and anxiety of stage fright, or the bad reaction you may experience when flashing lights and a siren zero in behind your car as you are cruising along! They cause the classic fight-or-flight reaction — increased heart rate, elevated blood pressure, emotional anxiety or anger, and a flood of glucose into the blood.

The outer part of each adrenal gland is called the adrenal cortex. Each adrenal cortex produces a large number of steroid hormones. One of these hormones, aldosterone, is essential for life — it enables the kidneys to conserve the right amount of sodium for the body, and it causes the kidneys to secrete excess potassium. "Male" hormones are synthesized by the adrenal cortex; in women, these hormones contribute to sexual desire. Another key hormone, cortisol, raises the blood glucose by stimulating the liver to generate glucose. Hormones from the adrenal cortex stimulate and regulate the function of the immune system. Importantly, adrenal cortical hormones respond to stress — for example, cortisol rises sharply in response to stress.

STAGES OF STRESS. Davis cited Canadian physician Hans Selye, who detailed the response of the adrenal glands to acute and chronic stress into three stages. The first, the stage of alarm, is the acute reaction to a sudden stress. An example of such a stress might be a nasty skid on an icy road. The sudden flood of anxiety is caused by the adrenal medullae releasing the hormones epinephrine and norepinephrine, but cortisol is also released.

The second stage, the stage of resistance, occurs when a stress is prolonged. For example, if for a significant period of time you are uncertain about a loved one's life or health, you may experience prolonged stress. During this second stage, the adrenal cortices produce increased amounts of some hormones, including cortisol. Blood sugar is increased, insulin rises to correct the blood glucose levels, and other hormonal changes occur. You feel a sense of ongoing dread or worry. Subjectively, you would probably say, "I feel stressed, but I'm still hanging in there."

The third stage, which may occur if stress is prolonged, is the stage of exhaustion. The adrenals no longer can produce the hormones which enable the body to compensate, and the body is prone to illness. Subjectively, the person at this stage would say, "I'm on the brink. I just can't deal with anything anymore."

Adelle Davis emphasized several important conclusions from Dr. Selye's work. First, she pointed out, *physical* stresses as well as emotional stresses could put the body into any of the three stages of stress. The physical stresses of allergy, acute pain, chronic pain, acute illness, chronic illness, lack of sleep, excess exercise, toxins such as nicotine or even therapeutic drugs, or nutritional deficiencies can cause or contribute to the same stages of stress that emotional trauma can. Second, she wrote that major stresses such as surgery or being in a bad car accident could put the body into the third stage, the stage of exhaustion, in a matter of hours. Third, and most important, she stated that if the adrenal glands were nourished well enough to meet their increased needs during times of stress, the third and perhaps even the other stages of the stress response could be avoided.[2]

Understanding the physical causes of stress, the response of the adrenals to stress, and the nutritional needs of the adrenal glands during stress is a powerful way of dealing with stresses.

CHECKLIST FOR CAUSES OF ANXIETY. First, when the feelings of anxiety or worries come on, ask yourself what physical factors may be the actual cause, or a contributing cause. Here's a checklist: Lack of sleep? Low blood glucose? Too much exercise? Caffeine (which overstimulates the adrenals)? Poor diet recently? Allergies acting up? The pain of a headache or some other pain? An infection? Medications? Anything else? I once experienced two or three days of mild anxiety after donating blood. I remember telling my husband: "Honestly, nothing is bothering me. I just feel anxious. I think that giving the blood on an empty stomach and eating their junk food before I left must have stressed me physically — maybe really lowered my blood sugar." I had a similar response after passing a kidney stone several years ago; it was helpful to realize that the pain of the ordeal was causing the anxiety.

One day in late August I got my hair cut by a lady who kept saying she was having a terrible day. "I should be happy," she said. "My husband loves me and I have two wonderful sons. But I just feel so stressed lately! Especially today." It was a Monday, and she mentioned that the day before she had accompanied her two young sons on a Boy Scout hike into the woods. "My allergies just went crazy," she said. I explained that the adrenal glands respond to allergies by putting out stress hormones. Hers were probably exhausted by the exposure she had experienced hiking through a lush Indiana woodland in August. When your adrenal glands are exhausted, you feel like you cannot cope. I went home and lent her a copy of a previous edition of this book, to encourage her to look into nutrition. You can build your adrenals back up.

STRATEGIES TO COUNTERACT STRESS
Here are some ways to keep your stress levels down. Note that the second item overlaps with the strategies to keep your energy up through blood glucose control.

1) GET ENOUGH SLEEP, OR REST IN A DARK ROOM IF YOU SLEEP POORLY. Sleep rests the adrenals, allowing the stress hormones to decrease.

2) KEEP YOUR BLOOD GLUCOSE LEVELS STEADY BY EATING GOOD MEALS AND SNACKS REGULARLY. As outlined above, making every meal and every snack a combination of protein, carbohydrate, and fats is an excellent way to maintain steady blood glucose levels. When you do so, your adrenals are not stressed by the drop in blood glucose, and do not have to respond with their anxiety-producing hormones, epinephrine and norepinephrine.

3) ANTICIPATE KNOWN IMPENDING STRESSES WITH IMPROVED NUTRITION. If you know that you will be scheduled for surgery next month, plan to improve nutrition aimed at adrenal health a couple of weeks beforehand.

4) CONSIDER SUPPLEMENTS WHICH CAN MEET THE HIGHER NEEDS OF THE ADRENAL GLANDS DURING PERIODS OF EMOTIONAL OR PHYSICAL STRESS. The adrenal glands require vitamin A; B vitamins, especially pantothenic acid; vitamin C (more vitamin C is found in the adrenals than in any other body organ); essential fatty acids; vitamin E; and the minerals zinc and manganese. A high quality multivitamin/multimineral supplement, with additional vitamin C and about 5–10 grams of flax oil or 1 teaspoon of fish oil daily, is a good start. Additionally, vitamin B6 and the mineral magnesium are nerve calming and are well worth supplementing. Vitamin B12 (1,000 mcg/day) is beneficial to both energy and mood. Table 7 in Chapter 3 contains specific dose ranges for the other nutrients.

5) DO NOT RESTRICT SALT, UNLESS YOU ARE DIRECTED TO DO SO BY YOUR PHYSICIAN FOR OTHER REASONS. A lack of salt in the diet can stress exhausted adrenal glands by forcing them to manufacture the hormone aldosterone, which signals the kidneys to retain salt.

6) AS ALWAYS, SEEK THE APPROVAL OF YOUR HEALTH CARE PROFESSIONAL BEFORE SUPPLEMENTING.

THE ADRENAL GLANDS AND REPRODUCTIVE PROBLEMS

PMS. Premenstrual syndrome (PMS) often manifests itself with the symptoms of anxiety. PMS which does not respond to nutrition aimed at bolstering ovarian function, or PMS-like symptoms that are not related to the menstrual cycle, may indicate that the adrenal glands are involved. The adrenal stress hormone cortisol interferes with progesterone, and low progesterone is related to PMS.

MORNING SICKNESS. Low blood sugar levels can bring on nausea and vomiting in some women. Healthy adrenal glands are involved in the maintenance of blood sugar levels, and attention to adrenal support can lessen morning sickness.

POSTPARTUM BLUES. Postpartum mood problems may be related to adrenal function. A group of researchers from the National Institute of Child Health and Human Development has made this point and explained this connection. During pregnancy, the placenta produces a hormone that stimulates the adrenals to produce large amounts of their stress-reducing hormones. Once the placenta is passed after childbirth, the adrenals must be activated by the woman's own hormones from her hypothalamus. Failure of her body to produce adrenal hormones can result in postpartum depression. These researchers suggested that most women only need assurance that things are normal.[3]

I disagree only with their conclusion. The adrenals need vitamins, minerals, and essential fatty acids to do their job. The nutritional stress of pregnancy and the physical stress of childbirth can certainly contribute to adrenal burnout. *A Natural Guide to Pregnancy and Postpartum Health,* by Drs. Dean Raffelock and Robert Rountree, is an excellent book which deals specifically with nutrition for "pregnancy recovery," as they call it. I recommend it highly for anyone attempting to overcome stress-related mood problems. (See "Further Reading.")

MISCARRIAGE. Miscarriage is accompanied by a sense of loss, but all too often guilt also complicates the emotional response. I am frequently contacted after such a loss, and I counsel that adrenal burnout caused by blood loss as well as the emotional trauma may well be triggering the anxious feelings of guilt that so often illogically accompany miscarriage. I recommend the nutrition detailed in this chapter.

INFERTILITY. The stress of infertility can certainly be explained as an emotional stress. Paying attention to nutrition for adrenal support, as outlined above, is an excellent way to make it easier to take "one day at a time." On the other hand, do not let anyone try to convince you that you need only to "relax" to get pregnant. To suggest that an infertile couple just "relax" is an unkind and counterproductive counsel.

MENOPAUSE. As the hormones of fertility decline, the adrenal glands must produce their sex hormones to compensate. Healthy adrenals smooth the way to menopause.

For more detailed information on the link between stress and nutrition, read *Depression-Free Naturally,* by Joan Mathews Larson, Ph.D. (See "Further Reading.") In addition to recommendations of vitamin and mineral supplements, she reviews the use of amino acid supplements to enable the body to make its own beneficial neurotransmitters. In particular, she explains the use of 5-hydroxytryptophan (5-HTP) or tryptophan to enable the body to increase the neurotransmitter serotonin.

ANOTHER "DIETARY" APPROACH TO STRESS

Fast and Feast in Lent
Author unknown

Fast from judging others; feast on the Christ dwelling in them.

Fast from emphasis on differences; feast on the unity of life.

Fast from apparent darkness; feast on the reality of light.

Fast from thoughts of illness; feast on the healing power of God.

Fast from words that pollute; feast on phrases that purify.

Fast from discontent; feast on gratitude.

Fast from anger; feast on patience.

Fast from pessimism; feast on optimism.

Fast from worry; feast on divine order.

Fast from complaining; feast on appreciation.

Fast from negatives; feast on affirmatives.

Fast from unrelenting pressures; feast on unceasing prayer.

Fast from hostility; feast on non-resistance.

Fast from bitterness; feast on forgiveness.

Fast from self-concern; feast on compassion for others.

Fast from personal anxiety; feast on eternal truth.

Fast from discouragements; feast on hope.

Fast from facts that depress; feast on verities that uplift.

Fast from lethargy; feast on enthusiasm.

Fast from thoughts that weaken; feast on promises that inspire.

Fast from shadows of sorrow; feast on the sunlight of serenity.

Fast from idle gossip; feast on purposeful silence.

Fast from problems that overwhelm; feast on prayer that undergirds.

(*The Marist Messenger*, March 2003. Used with permission.)

Summary — Chapter 14

➤ The underlying causes of low energy and a sense of high stress are related, and the opposite is also true — high energy and calm nerves go hand in hand.

➤ The factors that contribute to high energy are adequate sleep, moderate exercise, and blood glucose control.

➤ Strategies to stabilize blood glucose levels, including regular meals of protein, carbohydrates, and healthy natural fats, increase your energy and decrease your stress.

➤ Vitamin, mineral, and essential fatty acid supplements, especially B vitamins, vitamin C, magnesium, and flax oil or fish oil, are also useful to aid the adrenal glands, which manage stress.

➤ Better adrenal health helps you cope with the stresses of PMS problems, morning sickness, postpartum blues, miscarriage, infertility, and menopausal changes.

15

Men's Fertility &
Reproductive Health

Enjoy life with the wife whom you love, all the days of the fleeting life that is granted you under the sun. — Ecclesiastes 9:9

The title *Fertility, Cycles & Nutrition* of course emphasizes the woman's reproductive health, but when it comes to fertility, the man's reproductive function is equally as important. About 20 percent of infertility is due to male factors only; and about 27 percent of infertility involves both members of the couple, so that almost 50 percent of infertility involves the man.[1] Fertility, overall reproductive health, and nutrition are closely related in men. Ongoing research shows more and more of a connection between vitamins, minerals, essential fatty acids and male fertility and reproductive health.

That is why the Couple to Couple League recommends that both spouses work together to improve their nutrition and other lifestyle factors as part of their self-help to overcome infertility. This is true even if charting or medical diagnosis indicates a problem only with the woman's fertility. Let me restate this vital point: If you are having difficulty conceiving, both of you should strive to improve your nutrition and overall health, whether or not you have reason to believe the infertility is due to only one of you. The infertility could involve both of you, but even if it does not, improved nutrition by one spouse can help compensate for subfertility in the other.

—— MALE INFERTILITY

"Quality and quantity" is the expression used by reproductive physiologists to summarize the essentials of male fertility. It refers to the male reproductive cells, the sperm. The quality of the sperm refers to their ability to move forward, to digest away the tissue surrounding the ovum, and to engage in actual fertilization. Quality can be judged by microscopically observing the shape (morphology) of the sperm as well as their movements (motility). Normal sperm have an oval head and a long, single tail; abnormalities such as double heads or short, twisted tails should be relatively few. Most sperm should be capable of forward movement by the whipping motion of the tail, and clumping of the sperm, called spermagglutination, should not occur in more than a fourth of the sperm cells. Sperm quality also includes the genetic material in the head of the sperm, the all-important DNA.

The quantity of sperm necessary for normal fertility is one of those numbers that human physiology instructors — including me! — love to use to awe their students. Each of the three to five milliliters of ejaculated semen typically contains from 60–120 *million* sperm. When the sperm count drops to "only" twenty million per milliliter, the man is usually infertile. These numbers seem to be necessary to overcome the acidic environment of the vagina, to compensate for loss as sperm migrate through the female reproductive tract, and to provide for adequate numbers if ovulation occurs two or three days after intercourse. Hundreds of sperm must arrive in the vicinity of the ovum to chemically digest its covering before the nucleus of a single sperm can fuse to the nucleus of the ovum, the event that begins the life of a new individual.

You may be aware that for more than a generation, average sperm counts in men have been falling significantly. Among the probable culprits in this decline are exposure to environmental estrogens, pesticides, industrial chemicals, and heavy metals such as lead and cadmium.[2] Overweight and poor nutrition are also factors.

OXIDATIVE STRESS. Research has led to the conclusion that "oxidative stress" underlies many if not most factors that reduce male fertility. What is oxidative stress? In laymen's terms, it refers to damage to cells by reactive by-products of their normal oxygen usage. These by-products can be neutralized by cellular enzymes and by non-enzyme "antioxidant" vitamins, minerals, and other molecules. For several reasons, sperm are more susceptible to oxidative stress than are most other cells. For example, they have a high rate of oxygen usage, but they have very little cellular material around their nuclei to offer protective antioxidant activity.[3]

The negative effects of heat exposure, smoking, infection, and aging are all related to oxidative stress. Even functions of sperm that cannot be easily measured are harmed by oxidative stress. Their ability to digest away the covering of an ovum and to fuse with the ovum are reduced by oxidative stress. The DNA itself is damaged by oxidative stress.[4]

Oxidative stress decreases to the extent that exposure to industrial chemicals, cigarette smoke, pesticides, heavy metals, and even household chemicals can be avoided. Meanwhile, improved nutrition provides antioxidants that counteract oxidative stress,[5] as well as other nutrients needed for sperm production and for the production of male hormones.

DIET AND LIFESTYLE FACTORS
OVERALL NUTRITION FOR MALE FERTILITY. Nutritional research has concentrated mostly on vitamins, minerals, and essential fatty acid supplements needed for healthy sperm, rather than on the overall diet. However, a diet rich in a variety of whole natural foods provides many antioxidant vitamins and minerals as well as other nutrients, including the wonderful "phytonutrients" plentiful in colorful fruits and vegetables. Trans fats should be generally avoided, and certainly by men hoping to improve their fertility. The dietary recommendations in Part I are a sensible starting point for improved nutrition.

OVERWEIGHT. Overweight and obesity can reduce fertility in men. They can be related to lower sperm counts, higher levels of estrogens in the body, and lower levels of testosterone.[6] Losing weight is a challenge, but finding a diet and exercise plan that suits your lifestyle and attempting to lose at least a moderate amount of weight can improve the levels of male hormones.[7] You of course will reap many other health benefits as well.

UNDERWEIGHT. Extreme weight loss in men progressively reduces sexual libido, testosterone levels, sperm motility, and sperm production, all of which can be restored when the man regains his weight.[8] Men are far less sensitive to underweight compared to women, but very vigorous exercise does increase oxidative stress on the body.[9]

ALCOHOL AND NICOTINE. Excess alcohol intake reduces testosterone levels and depletes protective antioxidants.[10] Smoking causes negative effects on all aspects of sperm health — motility, morphology, and the DNA.[11] It also contributes to erectile dysfunction and loss of libido.

SOY FOODS. Soy foods such as soy milk, soy nuts, and tofu contain weak estrogens called isoflavones. Eating significant amounts of such foods has been implicated in reduced sperm concentrations, according to Harvard School of Public Health researchers, who studied ninety-nine men who were the male members of infertile couples. Soy foods reduced sperm concentrations in a "dose-related" fashion. That is, higher soy food intake lowered sperm concentrations more, and men with the very highest intake of soy foods actually had 41 million fewer sperm per millimeter than men who did not use soy foods. The effect of soy foods on sperm concentrations was especially pronounced in overweight and obese men. (Total sperm counts were not reduced, however, as semen volume increased slightly among soy users.)[12] If you consume soy foods or soy milk frequently, you should consider cutting back. However, consumption of soy oil, such as is commonly found in salad dressings, was not investigated in this study, as it is not a protein food rich in isoflavones.[13]

CAFFEINE. Despite the fact that a number of studies exist linking caffeine consumption in women to delays in achieving pregnancy and to increased risk of miscarriage, caffeine has not been shown to be a cause of infertility in men. However, stress and poor diet are linked to oxidative stress in sperm,[14] so it seems prudent to use caffeine in pleasant moderation, and to rely more on adequate sleep and improved nutrition for a natural, overall boost in energy.

VITAMINS, MINERALS, AND ESSENTIAL FATTY ACIDS
ANDROVITE FOR MEN. Before detailing the benefits that various vitamins and minerals have on male fertility, I would like to jump ahead to the conclusion, and recommend the multivitamin/multimineral Androvite for Men. (See "Resources.") It "covers all the bases" so well that most men who are hoping to overcome infertility or other reproductive problems need only to supplement with Androvite to meet their vitamin and mineral needs. Androvite contains 1,000 mg of vitamin C, 50 mg of zinc, 400 mcg of folic acid, 400 IU of

vitamin E, and 200 mcg of selenium per full dose. See Appendix A, "Labeled Contents of Recommended Supplements," for the complete vitamin and mineral amounts in Androvite. Research that supports the ingredients in this supplement is summarized below.

In addition to Androvite, flax oil and fish oil are also valuable to male fertility. Also, a powerful natural antioxidant supplement, called astaxanthin, has markedly improved male fertility. These are also detailed below, and I also recommend them for overcoming male infertility.

VITAMIN C. In one of the most dramatic studies ever published on the effect of nutrition on reproductive function, twenty-seven men with infertility apparently due to spermagglutination (sperm which stick together and thus cannot move forward) were divided into two groups. Twenty received supplemental vitamin C (1,000 mg/day) plus calcium, magnesium, and manganese. At the end of two months, the wives of each of the twenty men who received supplemental vitamin C had become pregnant. In contrast, no wife of any subject in the group which did not receive supplemental doses had become pregnant. This program of supplementation significantly improved sperm quantity, morphology and motility, and reduced spermagglutination.[15]

A follow-up study used pure vitamin C (200 or 1,000 mg/day) and confirmed the beneficial effect of this nutrient on the same measures of fertility in men with spermagglutination. In only one week, sperm counts for those receiving 1,000 mg/day of vitamin C rose an average of 140 percent.[16] Similar results have been found when vitamin C has been supplemented in men who smoke.[17]

Vitamin C is ten times more concentrated in semen than in blood. A new study shows that this antioxidant vitamin also plays a major role in preventing damage to the DNA of the sperm. Importantly, damaged sperm DNA can be responsible for male infertility even when sperm count, motility and morphology are normal.[18] Testosterone production also depends on the presence of vitamin C.

ZINC AND FOLIC ACID. Zinc is another nutrient which is absolutely essential for sperm production and for synthesis of testosterone by the testes. The highest concentrations of zinc in the body are found in the sperm cells and in the prostate gland, and the prostate contributes importantly to male reproductive capability. Zinc works together with folate (folic acid) in the synthesis of DNA molecules, which sperm produce at a rapid rate. In a controlled, double-blind study, both fertile and infertile men were given supplements of zinc (66 mg) and folic acid (5,000 mcg) daily for six months. After six months, infertile men with low sperm counts had a 74 percent increase in sperm quantity.[19]

The richest source of zinc is red meat; fish, poultry, and dairy products do not contain as much, and a strictly vegetarian diet may lead to zinc deficiency.[20] Folic acid is plentiful in dark green leafy vegetables. Supplements which include both are valuable to male as well as to female fertility.

SELENIUM AND VITAMIN E. Selenium has a number of roles in the body, and it is highly concentrated in the testes. It is needed by the sperm to make their midpieces,[21] which is the middle part where energy production takes place to allow for their forward movement. Vitamin E is a major antioxidant that works together with selenium. Infertile men who supplemented both of these nutrients (225 mcg selenium and 400 mg vitamin E daily) for three months had improved sperm motility.[22]

More important, selenium, either alone or with other antioxidants (vitamins A, C, and E), given to infertile men with poor sperm motility resulted in an 11 percent pregnancy rate within three months of taking the supplements, as compared to no pregnancies in the control group.[23] Vitamin E supplemented along with other nutrients, including vitamin A and essential fatty acids, has resulted in increased pregnancy rates among men with very low sperm counts.[24] Vitamin E alone (300 mg twice daily) resulted in a 21 percent rate of pregnancy achievement within six months in men with poor sperm mobility compared to no pregnancies in control subjects.[25]

VITAMIN A. Vitamin A, which aids the lining membranes throughout the body, similarly benefits the lining cells of the testes' seminiferous tubules — and these cells are the developing sperm! Men have a higher need than women for vitamin A, and it affects men's reproductive organs significantly. Vitamin A deficiency results in shrinkage of the epididymides [plural], seminal vesicles, and prostate gland. Severe deficiency causes degeneration of the seminiferous tubules, resulting in decrease of semen volume, sperm count, and sperm motility.[26] Vitamin A is abundant in cod liver oil, whole milk, cheese, butter, eggs, and meat.

B VITAMINS. A damaging metabolite, homocysteine, creates oxidative stress on the body. Homocysteine levels are decreased by the B vitamins folic acid, B6, and B12. Australian infertility researcher Kelton Tremellen recommends daily supplements of 5,000 mcg folic acid, 100 mg B6, and 100 mcg of B12 to reduce the oxidative stress caused by homocysteine in infertile men.[27] The B vitamins are also involved in producing LH and FSH from the pituitary gland, and these two hormones stimulate sperm production and testosterone secretion in men.

ESSENTIAL FATTY ACIDS. The essential fatty acids linoleic and alpha-linolenic acid are required for male reproductive function. Long-time male fertility researcher Frank Comhaire of Belgium recommends supplements of flax oil, noting that it contains the hard-to-get essential fatty acid alpha-linolenic acid, which is low in subfertile men. This "omega-3" essential fatty acid is converted to the healthy fatty acids EPA and DHA, and these help the sperm to digest away the covering of the ovum and to bind to the ovum in fertilization. According to Dr. Comhaire, flax oil also contains several plant phytonutrients called lignans, which in the intestines are converted to weak, short-lived estrogens. These weak estrogens actually act opposite to what the name would cause you to expect. They inhibit the conversion of male hormone into estrogen, thus decreasing the amount of estrogen in men, which has a beneficial effect on sperm production.[28]

Several B vitamins, vitamin C, and zinc are required to convert the alpha-linolenic acid of flax oil into EPA and DHA. As an alternative to flax oil, Dr. Comhaire recommends fish oil, which contains EPA and DHA. Because EPA and DHA are highly unsaturated, he notes that it is mandatory to provide antioxidants along with fish oil.[29]

How much flax oil or fish oil should you supplement? About 5–10 grams daily of flax oil, and/or 5 g (1 teaspoon) of cod liver oil is my recommendation. Cod liver oil has "ready-made" DHA and EPA, and it provides some vitamin A and D, but does not provide the lignans mentioned above. Supplemental vitamin E in the range of 400 IU protects fish oil and flax oil from oxidative damage, and is valuable to male fertility as well.

ASTAXANTHIN. In a promising pilot study, a potent antioxidant found in algae, astaxanthin, was given in amounts of 16 mg daily to Swedish men being treated medically for infertility. This resulted in an amazing 54 percent pregnancy rate in three months, compared to an 11 percent pregnancy rate among untreated controls.[30] The astaxanthin was in a proprietary preparation called Astacarox, (AstaReal AB, Sweden). There are several proprietary preparations of astaxanthin available. If you chose to try it, and I suggest that you do, use the same amount as in this study (16 mg/day), and as always, seek the counsel of your health professional.

OTHER SUPPLEMENTS FOR MALE FERTILITY. L-carnitine, acetyl-L-carnitine, and co-enzyme Q10 are neither vitamins nor minerals, but are factors that are used by cells to produce energy. Studies of the effect of these on male fertility have been performed using a proprietary product called Proxeed, which contains all three. (Available at *www.proxeed.com*.) In the case of the carnitines, doses in the range of 2 g/day of L-carnitine plus 1 g/day of acetyl-L-carnitine have improved sperm quality and modestly increased pregnancy rates to 6.7 percent in three months.[31]

WORKING TOGETHER TO IMPROVE MALE FERTILITY

Sperm require over two months to mature from start to finish. Improvement of male fertility through nutrition may not occur immediately, except possibly in the case of spermagglutination. Please remember that whenever infertility is a problem, the first step is for both spouses to improve their nutrition and to employ all the fertility techniques taught by the Couple to Couple League. You may incorrectly assume that one spouse's subfertility is the cause, but often it is both spouses'.

Timing of intercourse based on the NFP chart, following a few days of abstinence, can help to compensate for a low sperm count in the husband as well as for poor mucus patterns in the wife. Attempting to optimize reproductive health through nutrition may also enable one spouse to compensate for the other's subfertility. For example, the wife's attempting to increase her cervical mucus with vitamin A may help to overcome infertility due to low sperm count or low sperm motility in the husband, and if excellent nutrition raises a man's sperm count to higher levels or better motility, it could aid the problem of partially blocked uterine tubes in the wife. But most of all, when the two of you form a team, in the kitchen as well as in the bedroom, you encourage each other. (See Appendix B, "Focus on Infertility.")

— MALE REPRODUCTIVE HEALTH —

LOW LIBIDO OR ERECTILE DYSFUNCTION

These two topics are not the same, and they may or may not be related. Low libido refers to low sexual desire, and the term erectile dysfunction has replaced the older term "impotence." The hormone testosterone is responsible for the physical basis of male libido, but actual sexual function depends on the levels of testosterone as well as on other factors.

NUTRITIONAL FACTORS. Dietary factors that affect fertility may also affect libido and erectile function. Obesity and overweight may also cause loss of libido, as excess body fat reduces the levels of testosterone.[32] Both zinc and vitamin C raise testosterone levels. Some medical doctors recommend as much as 100 mg of zinc daily to improve testosterone levels and sexual libido in men. I suspect that all of the above-mentioned vitamins, minerals, and essential fatty acids that improve semen quality would also be helpful to male desire and function. Since nutrients work together, it is better to supplement all of them rather than to rely on just one or two.

LOW THYROID FUNCTION. Low thyroid function (hypothyroidism) is several times more common in women, but it does occur in men. When it does, it can cause a decrease in testosterone levels. Not surprisingly, erectile dysfunction and loss of libido may result; however, the effect of hypothyroidism on actual male fertility is not well established.[33] The more subtle situation, called "subclinical" hypothyroidism, may also result in low levels of testosterone.[34]

If you are interested in judging your own thyroid function, you can try the "Barnes basal temperature test" discussed in Chapter 7 under the topic "Low Thyroid Function." In brief, you take your oral or underarm basal body temperature for several days, and then consider the results. According to Dr. Barnes, a man's underarm (equivalent to oral) basal temperature should be in the range of 97.8° F to 98.2° F. While I have noted in Chapter 7 that I consider this standard somewhat too high for women, I have no reason to doubt its accuracy for men.

The multivitamin/multimineral Androvite for Men contains nutrients that are ideal to support thyroid function — iodine, zinc, selenium, B vitamins, and vitamins C, A, and E. In addition, flax oil or fish oil should be supplemented to nourish the thyroid gland. As in women, not all low thyroid function responds to nutrition. If you believe that low thyroid function might be the cause of low libido, sexual dysfunction, or infertility, medical diagnosis and treatment is the next step if nutrition does not make a difference. Again, refer to "Low Thyroid Function" in Chapter 7 for further information.

PROSTATE HEALTH. The health of the prostate gland importantly affects the ability to maintain an erection. Therefore, the following sections should also be considered.

PROSTATITIS

A large number of urologists' patients are men with acute or chronic prostatitis. Prostatitis refers to infection or inflammation of the prostate gland, which is a disorder completely different from the benign prostatic hypertrophy (enlargement) that commonly causes problems in men over age fifty. The symptoms of prostatitis include pain between the legs or in the rectal area and sometimes pain with intercourse. More severe infection causes pain in the urethra and frequency of urination. Flare-ups can cause temporary erectile dysfunction. It is also possible for a man to have a chronic low-level prostate infection without being aware of it.

The usual medical treatment for prostatitis is antibiotic therapy. However, the infective microorganisms are notoriously difficult to eradicate and long-term treatment is often necessary. Many urologists routinely advise increased frequency of intercourse to "flush out" the gland, which empties its secretions into the urethra during intercourse. This obviously poses a problem to couples practicing chaste periodic abstinence as part of NFP. Fortunately, a number of natural strategies can immensely help the prostatitis-prone man to prevent the troublesome flare-ups.

AVOID FOODS THAT PRODUCE AN IRRITATING URINE. Spicy or acid foods can cause intense attacks of prostatitis within hours. Condiments such as mayonnaise, ketchup, mustard, relish and so forth should be avoided. Tomatoes, raw onions, sausages, pizza, tacos, soft drinks, tea, coffee and alcohol are other culprits. Sometimes food additives in processed items cause reactions that home-cooked equivalent dishes do not.

DRINK PLENTY OF WATER. Water dilutes the urine, and helps to avoid irritation to the prostate gland.

AVOID URINE BACKFLOW INTO THE PROSTATIC DUCTS. The bladder should be emptied regularly and not allowed to become overfull. "Shy bladder" is common among men with prostatitis, and relaxation, not straining, should be practiced when urine is voided.

IMPROVE BLOOD FLOW TO THE PROSTATE GLAND. Exercise such as running, boxer shorts instead of jockey briefs, and hot baths all aid circulation to this gland. Conversely, cigarette smoking, prolonged sitting, and constipation impede its blood flow. Avoid nasal sprays and other cold or allergy remedies which constrict nasal tissues — they do the same to prostate vessels, and infections thrive where blood flow is poor.[35]

NOURISH THE PROSTATE PROPERLY. Zinc is highly concentrated in this gland, and up 80 mg per day of supplemental zinc may be helpful, if it is balanced with 3 mg of copper.[36] Vitamin A, B vitamins, including B6 (50 mg twice daily), vitamin C, and selenium also contribute to prostate health.[37] Selenium is important to all of the male reproductive organs. The prostate gland has a high need for the essential fatty acids.

CONSIDER WHETHER YEAST OVERGROWTH MAY BE INVOLVED. See "Yeast Overgrowth" in Chapter 9 for further information on this subject. The anecdote below illustrates this possibility.

SELF-HELP FOR PROSTATITIS. An otherwise healthy 35-year-old man developed chronic prostatitis, and had taken "ten different courses of antibiotics within two and a half years." The bouts were occurring more and more frequently; longer treatment with antibiotics was required, and finally, a course of antibiotics did no good at all. During this time he gradually realized that certain foods triggered these attacks — soda pop, alcohol, processed meats, condiments, and most other processed foods. By strictly avoiding these, he could control the prostatitis, but he felt he was "always on the razor's edge" if he ate the wrong food.

He learned from Dr. William Crook's *The Yeast Connection* that chronic prostatitis is a possible symptom of yeast overgrowth, and he recalls that during his final few flare-ups his urologist could not culture bacteria from his prostatic fluid. He tried eating plain yogurt and noticed that it somewhat reduced the constant inflammation that troubled him. Reasoning that yogurt bacteria are largely killed off by the stomach's acid, he tried capsules of acidophilus, which are designed to release friendly bacteria into the intestine, where they combat yeast. They helped immensely.

He has not had a major recurrence nor used antibiotics for three years, and he considers the low-level inflammation virtually gone. Along with five capsules of probiotics daily, he takes vitamins and minerals and eats only low-sugar, unprocessed foods, except for occasional treats. Testing has confirmed that he is highly allergic to yeast, but he believes that medical treatment is unnecessary at this time. He reports that he feels better now than before the prostatitis started, and jokes that he is "forced to eat only healthy food," though his sensitivity to many of his former trigger foods has decreased markedly. One can only speculate about how his problem would have progressed had he not on his own found the yeast connection.

BENIGN PROSTATE ENLARGEMENT

Enlargement of the prostate gland (benign prostate hypertrophy) is a common condition in men over age fifty. Its symptoms include annoying frequency of urination and a poor stream of urine when voiding, and it can interfere with sexual functioning. Left untreated, it can ultimately damage the entire urinary system. Diet, vitamins, minerals, and particularly herbal remedies are helpful to this problem.

DIET. Eating fruits and vegetables that are rich in antioxidants, including the phytonutrients beta-carotene, lutein and vitamin C, decreases the risk of benign prostate hypertrophy, according to a very large study of American men.[38] Beta-carotene is found in orange and yellow plant foods such as carrots, and lutein is found abundantly in kale, collard greens, spinach, zucchini, and pumpkin. This is not to imply that a vegetarian diet is recommended for prostate health, but that the wonderful phytonutrients in plant foods truly should be eaten in abundance.

VITAMIN/MINERAL SUPPLEMENTS. The hormone prolactin rises as men age, and it contributes to prostate hypertrophy. The prolactin-inhibiting factor is the same in men as in women. The factor is dopamine, and levels of dopamine are increased by vitamin B6 and magnesium. These can be taken in the range of 50–100 mg B6 and 500–1,000 mg magnesium daily. Zinc also helps to reduce prolactin levels.

Androvite for Men, as mentioned previously, is an excellent multivitamin/ multimineral supplement for all aspects of male reproductive health. Flax oil (five to ten 1 g capsules, or 1–2 teaspoons of the liquid daily) or cod liver oil (1 teaspoon daily) provide fatty acids that are beneficial to the prostate gland. Androvite contains the vitamin E required as an antioxidant to protect these fatty acids.

HERBS. Extracts of the herb saw palmetto have been used successfully to reduce prostate enlargement, poor urine flow, and sexual dysfunction.[39] Saw palmetto is a source of the compound beta-sitosterol, which works by reducing the activity of an enzyme that changes testosterone into a more potent compound called dihydrotestosterone (abbreviated as DHT). DHT stimulates the growth of the prostate. There are many brands of saw palmetto available, and often they contain additional ingredients such as the herbs *Pygeum africanum*, stinging nettle, and pumpkin seed oil. All of these contain beta-sitosterol. Beta-sitosterol is also available in purified, more potent forms. The extract in the study cited above is called Permixon, and the men in the study used it in 160 mg amounts twice daily for two years. The positive results occurred within the first six months of use, except for the improvement of sexual function, which occurred after a year of use.[40]

It is prudent to discuss the use of herbs with your health care provider. You may also wish to visit a health food shop to compare various supplements of saw palmetto in terms of the amount of beta-sitosterol and for the addition of other herbs. Or, see ***www.drwhitaker.com*** for information on supplements for prostate health formulated by nutritionally-oriented medical doctor Julian Whitaker, M.D. Dr. Whitaker has updated and altered his formulations as new research or new products become available. (See "Resources.")

PREVENTING PROSTATE CANCER
Prostate cancer is a leading cancer killer among American men. Reducing the risk of this type of cancer is a topic of great research interest, and several large, long-term studies are underway to shed light on the link between nutrition

and prostate cancer. Both diet and supplements are being investigated for their role in preventing this disease, and there is much reason for optimism.

DIET. The incidence of prostate cancer is notably low in Asian countries, a fact that has been attributed to diet and lifestyle rather than to genetics. This is so because when Asian men move to North America, after a few years their risk of prostate cancer approaches that of Caucasian Americans.[41] Because of this, certain foods that are commonly used in Asia are being tested for their value in preventing prostate cancer. Such foods include soy products and green tea. Because of their effect on other aspects of male reproductive function, discussed previously, it is best to limit soy foods. Green tea, however, is very high in antioxidants, and new studies are adding evidence that drinking green tea frequently may reduce the incidence of prostate cancer.[42]

Intake of the phytonutrient lycopene, abundant in tomatoes, especially cooked tomatoes, has been found to reduce the risk of prostate cancer.[43] Other sources of this potent antioxidant include watermelon, pink grapefruit, apricots, and papaya.[44]

Consuming trans fats, which are found in hydrogenated and overheated vegetable oils, is a risk factor for the most common type of prostate cancer.[45]

Chapter 1 of this book, "Twelve Rules for Better Nutrition," suggests eating more plant foods, especially the brightly-colored ones (Rule I), and avoiding trans fats (Rule 3). These rules also encourage eating a greater variety of whole natural foods and avoiding sugary treats and refined starches. While the latter have not been examined in reference to prostate cancer, poor food choices certainly crowd out the healthy foods.

VITAMIN AND MINERAL SUPPLEMENTS. In a major placebo-controlled, long-term study, selenium supplements (200 mcg/day) reduced the death rate of many types of cancer by approximately half, and similarly reduced the risk of prostate cancer.[46] (Androvite for Men contains 200 mcg of selenium per full dose.) Supplementation with vitamin E and beta-carotene also significantly reduced the incidence of prostate cancer in a large study.[47] Stimulated by the encouraging results of these studies, other long-term studies on the value of selenium and vitamin E in preventing prostate cancer are currently in progress.

OTHER CONCERNS. Four large studies conducted in the 1990s showed that, for unknown reasons, the occurrence of prostate cancer is approximately doubled in vasectomized men.[48] Avoiding vasectomy is one sure way to reduce this risk.

AGE-RELATED CHANGES IN MEN
What can the two of you expect as time passes on? In men, there is no obvious "change of life" as there is in women. Whereas you can state confidently that all women become naturally infertile at menopause, no such statement can be made about men, and many older men with younger wives have fathered children. However, the male hormone testosterone gradually but steadily declines with age, which can affect both sexual desire and sexual function.

Sperm production on average decreases after age 55. Other changes in the function of the various reproductive organs can sometimes affect erection and ejaculation, even when sexual desire remains normal. The media have made us all too aware that there are drugs which can improve the age-related decline in sexual ability. Good nutrition, exercise, and weight control, as well as the remedies for prostate health just discussed, can naturally help with these issues while improving every other aspect of a man's overall health.

➤ Male infertility should be a consideration even when a couple believes that it is the woman who is infertile, and self-help should include both members of the couple.

➤ A man's fertility can be helped by decreasing exposure to environmental toxins, limiting alcohol, avoiding smoking, and losing weight if obesity is a factor.

➤ Sperm are very sensitive to "oxidative stress," and antioxidants can improve infertility. Supplements of vitamins C and E, folic acid, and the minerals zinc and selenium have been shown to improve sperm quantity or quality, and in some studies have increased pregnancy rates. The multivitamin/multimineral Androvite for Men is a good source of these nutrients. Flax oil or fish oil should also be supplemented, and supplements of the powerful antioxidant astaxanthin are also recommended.

➤ Male sexual desire and sexual function can be decreased by nutrient deficiencies, especially zinc and vitamin C, and by obesity. Low thyroid function may be involved, as well as prostatitis, a common infection or inflammation in men of all ages.

➤ A number of self-help strategies can reduce the incidence of prostatitis.

➤ Benign prostate hypertrophy (BPH), which increases as men age, causes annoying symptoms with urination and can impair sexual function. Antioxidant-rich plant foods reduce the incidence of BPH, and extracts of the herb saw palmetto provide beta-sitosterol, which can reduce the symptoms of BHT and improve sexual function.

➤ Ongoing research is also focusing on nutrition as a way of reducing the incidence of prostate cancer, a major cancer of men.

16

Questions & Answers, Part II:
Overcoming Reproductive Problems & Challenges

For I know well the plans I have in mind for you, says the Lord, plans for your welfare, not for woe! Plans to give you a future full of hope. — Jeremiah 29:11

MY BREASTS HURT SO MUCH SOMETIMES THAT I CAN'T EVEN HUG MY HUSBAND. OTHER TIMES THEY FEEL UNCOMFORTABLY FULL, BUT I'M NOT NURSING. PLEASE DON'T TELL ME IT'S MY COFFEE — I'LL GIVE UP ANYTHING ELSE!

It probably is caffeine, as you have no doubt suspected by the correlation between your coffee habit and your symptoms. Cutting down on caffeine is the primary dietary change that will help you. Flax oil (5–10 g/day; 1–2 teaspoons if you use the oil rather than capsules) and vitamin E (400–800 IU/day) are also useful for painful breasts. You may notice that sugar, salt, or starchy food binging causes water retention in a day or two, and retained fluid further aggravates breast tenderness.

Since mastalgia, as breast pain is technically called, is a common PMS symptom, the PMS nutritional strategy is well worth considering. If fact, new research shows that chasteberry (*Vitex agnus castus*), which helps some women with PMS, may also help with breast pain.[1] If you choose to try chasteberry extract, I suggest you use it in the form Fertility Blend, as recommended in Chapter 5.

I AM PRONE TO MIGRAINE HEADACHES. IS THERE A WAY OF HANDLING THEM WITHOUT MEDICATION?

Not all headaches are migraines, but migraine headaches are often throbbing headaches on only one side of the head. In about 10 percent of people who are prone to them, they begin with odd symptoms such as visual disturbances, speech disturbances, and sensitivity to light. The best approach is to prevent them, and diet and supplements are valuable for doing so. First, look for "triggers" and eliminate them whenever possible. Hypoglycemia is a major trigger for migraines in susceptible people, and avoiding blood sugar swings is a key strategy. Eat protein, fiber-rich plant foods, and natural fats at every meal and snack. Avoid alcohol and limit sugary treats. Even sweet fruits can cause a migraine, so all sweets should be eaten cautiously and on a full stomach only. Chapter 14 has further information about maintaining blood sugar levels.

The B vitamins and magnesium are helpful to maintaining normal blood glucose levels. Folic acid (2,000–4,000 mcg/day) is particularly valuable when taken with general supplements as suggested in Table 7 (Chapter 3).

Bright lights, chemical odors such as those from cleaning agents, gas stations, new carpets or cigarette smoke, can trigger migraines. Foods that contain the amino acid tyramine — aged cheeses, wine, beer — are possible culprits for precipitating migraines. So is MSG (monosodium glutamate), found in soy sauce. Reducing your caffeine intake is helpful, but do so gradually since sudden withdrawal may trigger a migraine.

If you experience symptoms that a migraine is coming on, there are certain things you can do to prevent it completely, or at least moderate the pain. First, get out of bright light and into dim light. Then, if you can, eat a hearty snack of protein, carbohydrate, and fat, such as cheese and crackers, or a hamburger on a bun. Take about 800–2,000 mcg of folic acid with it.

Most valuable of all, though, is to get uncomfortably cold for a little while. If it is winter, go outside without your coat on for five or ten minutes, but watch out if bright sunlight is reflecting off the snow. (If you live in northern Wisconsin, just go out *with* your coat on!) If it is warm out, take a cool shower in a dimly lit bathroom. The water does not have to be freezing, and you can alternate with warm water so that you are not miserably cold. Or, if you are caught where you cannot do either, try soaking your hands and feet in very cold water, or putting icy cold wash cloths on your forehead or the back of your neck. The chill causes blood vessels in your skin and elsewhere to constrict, rerouting more blood to your brain. That is why this is so helpful. When you are cold enough to get goose bumps, you are probably cold enough to make this very effective trick work for you. Just remember to stay in dim light while you do so.

I HAVE PMS, AND MY DOCTOR RECOMMENDED OPTIVITE THREE TIMES A DAY. BUT WHEN I FEEL GOOD I FORGET TO TAKE THEM, AND WHEN I FEEL BAD, IT'S TOO LATE! ANY SUGGESTIONS?

Yes, I do have one that works wonderfully. If you are married, ask your husband to take sincere responsibility for getting your vitamins out and reminding you to take them. If you are single, ask your mother, sister or roommate to help you in this way. This situation is very common among PMS sufferers, and those who live with you will probably be glad to help! For your part, respond maturely to their support.

If you live alone, place your vitamins where you will remember to take them — for example, in the bathroom so you can make them part of your after breakfast teeth-brushing routine. If you work outside the home, put them in your purse, and ask a trusted friend to remind you. Then, try not to let her down.

CAN I USE PROCYCLE AND FERTILITY BLEND TOGETHER? I AM HOPING TO GET PREGNANT.

Yes, use a three-fourths dose of ProCycle (three tablets daily) plus the full dose of Fertility Blend. You could also use a two-thirds dose of Optivite with Fertility Blend, or two-thirds dose of Professional Prenatal Formula with Fertility Blend. Check with your doctor, of course, and I recommend that you continue these if you get pregnant using them.

I HAVE BEEN HAVING TROUBLE GETTING PREGNANT, BUT MY CHARTS LOOK PRETTY NORMAL, LIKE I AM OVULATING. I HAVE NOT HAD ANY FERTILITY TESTING, BUT MY DOCTOR SAID THAT I PROBABLY AM HAVING A LUTEINIZED UNRUPTURED FOLLICLE EVERY MONTH, AND THAT IS WHY I AM NOT GETTING PREGNANT. COULD YOU EXPLAIN WHAT THIS IS?

A luteinized unruptured follicle is a rare event. It means that the follicle fails to release the ovum at the time when ovulation would normally occur, but then it begins to secrete progesterone, as if it were a corpus luteum. It can make the luteal phase longer than normal, but usually the cycle ends with a period. With no ovum released, the cycle is infertile, though you would not know it while you were in such a cycle.[2]

I suggest you look for other explanations for your infertility, as there are many more likely reasons that a woman can ovulate and still not get pregnant. Carefully evaluating your own charts with reference to the information in this book is a basic starting point. Refer also to Appendix B, "Focus on Infertility." In the event that fertility evaluation and ultrasounds confirm that you do have luteinized unruptured follicles, hormonal treatment can be used to stimulate the release of the ovum.

WE ARE POSTPONING A PREGNANCY FOR NOW USING NFP. BUT I'VE GOT MUCUS FROM THE TIME MY PERIOD ENDS UNTIL I OVULATE ON DAY 25 OR SO. WE WOULD NEED TO ABSTAIN A LOT LESS IF I DIDN'T HAVE SUCH A LONG PATCH OF MUCUS EVERY MONTH.

Improved nutrition can very possibly help you, and either a shorter mucus patch or a shorter cycle length will make a difference. I would like to provide you with a checklist to help you identify possible underlying causes of the long cycles or prolonged mucus. Then, you can refer to the appropriate sections of this book for specific nutritional aids. Keep in mind that more than one cause could apply to your situation. If so, do not "double up" on the suggested supplements. Just cover all the bases using Table 7 (Chapter 3) as a guide. Check into all of the following that might apply.

_____ 1. Are you nursing a baby? Have you discontinued nursing within your last three cycles? The cycle characteristics you describe are normal for cycling, nursing mothers, but classic cycle patterns are equally normal if you are nursing only a little. You can encourage your reproductive hormones to complete the transition from breastfeeding subfertility to full fertility with excellent diet and supplements. Table 13 (Chapter 10), "Suggested Food Goals for Pregnant and Nursing Women," will be helpful if you are nursing a great deal; see Table 1 (Chapter 1), "Suggested Daily Food Goals," if you are nursing very little or have weaned. Supplements as in Table 7 (Chapter 3) should be considered, and be very sure that vitamins A and E, the B vitamins, iodine and essential fatty acids are well-supplied. Professional Prenatal Formula by Life Time is excellent for both pregnant and nursing women, along with flax oil or fish oil supplements. (See "Resources.")

___ 2. Have you recently discontinued birth control pills or other hormonal birth control? If so, it is possible that their residual effects are still affecting you. It may take up to four cycles for mucus patterns to become normal after discontinuing hormonal birth control, and I have talked to women who believe that various negative effects have persisted for years after they went off the Pill. (See "Discontinuing Birth Control Pills or Other Hormonal Birth Control" in Chapter 9.)

___ 3. Are you in your late 40s? Perimenopausal cycle changes could account for this pattern. See Chapter 12, "Premenopause, Perimenopause, & Menopause" for nutritional suggestions for this time of life. If you are younger, look for other explanations besides age.

___ 4. Are you slender or underweight, even a little bit? Do you exercise vigorously? Have you dieted recently, even if you are still overweight? (See "Underweight or Inadequate Body Fat" in Chapter 7.)

___ 5. Are your pre-ovulatory basal temperatures around 97.2° F or lower? You may have a tendency to low thyroid function — maybe not enough to cause major symptoms, but enough to explain your prolonged mucus and delayed ovulation. (See "Low Thyroid Function" in Chapter 7.)

___ 6. Could you be vitamin A deficient? Another sign of this is heavy or prolonged menses. (See "Diet for Better Healing and Normal Blood Clotting" and "Supplements for Better Healing and Normal Blood Clotting" in Chapter 6). The recommendations to lighten heavy periods are helpful to prolonged mucus.

___ 7. Is your luteal phase usually less than twelve days from the first day of the temperature shift up to and including the last day before your period begins? (See "Luteal Phase Deficiency" in Chapter 7.)

___ 8. Are you obese or substantially overweight? (See Chapter 8.)

___ 9. Is there any light at all in your bedroom at night? Some women's mucus patterns improve when night lighting in their bedrooms is eliminated or controlled. (See "Sensitivity to Night Lighting" in Chapter 9.)

_____**10.** Do you drink more than two or three cups of coffee a day, or the equivalent in caffeinated soda pop? Are you eating chocolate almost daily? (See "Caffeine Consumption" in Chapter 9.) Do you use NutraSweet or other artificial sweeteners daily? (See the question and answer on this topic in Chapter 4.)

_____**11.** If none of the above applies, I recommend that you try the PMS nutritional plan as outlined in Chapter 5. If you are slender but not really underweight, try gaining just two or three pounds. Make sure that you are getting sufficient iodine (150 mcg/day) and vitamin E (400–800 IU/day). And finally, review the suggestions in Chapter 9 under the heading "Yeast Overgrowth."

If these suggestions will make a difference, they will do so within about three months.

DO YOU HAVE ANY ADVICE ABOUT ACNE? I WISH I COULD SAY I'M INTERESTED IN IT FOR MY TEENAGE DAUGHTER, BUT I ACTUALLY HAVE A PROBLEM WITH IT MYSELF, ESPECIALLY BEFORE MY PERIOD.

Yes, there is nutritional help for acne vulgaris, as pimples and blackheads are called. Acne vulgaris is caused by infection of the oil glands of the skin, the sebaceous glands. It is not the same as acne rosacea, or "adult acne," which has to do with excess proliferation of blood vessels in the skin of the face and neck. (I comment on rosacea below.)

Acne vulgaris may be related to high insulin levels, which in women trigger the production of "male" hormones and other factors that stimulate the skin to overproduce skin cells and sebum, the natural oil from the sebaceous glands. Really cutting down on foods that are sugary or high in refined starches (white flour) is very helpful.[3] Trans fats are also to be avoided, but the healthy oils such as olive oil and canola oil are beneficial. Milk is controversial when it comes to acne; some studies have found whole milk helpful, whereas some authors strongly advise against it. Chocolate is another controversial food; it is probably the sugar in it, not the chocolate itself, that makes so many teenagers reluctantly agree that yes, it is bad for their skin.

Fish oil (5 grams or 1 teaspoon daily) and/or flax oil (five to ten 1 g capsules or 1–2 teaspoons daily) are both beneficial when it comes to acne, as they have significant anti-inflammatory effects and also promote production of a more liquid sebum that is less likely to clog the sebaceous glands. You can use either or both together in the amounts just listed. The fat-soluble vitamins are also good for acne prevention: vitamin A, (8,000 IU of true vitamin A if pregnancy is a possibility; up to 25,000 if it is not; your doctor may prescribe higher levels); vitamin E (400–800 IU); and vitamin D (400–1,000 IU). Zinc works along with vitamin A, and 25–50 mg is helpful. Some nutritionally-oriented doctors specifically recommend higher amounts of zinc for acne, in the range of 100 mg, but you should certainly have your doctor's approval before using more than 25–50 mg. Acne vulgaris responds quite rapidly to improved nutrition, within a couple of weeks or a month.

If you are having symptoms that are consistent with polycystic ovary syndrome (PCOS), such as long, irregular cycles or evidence of elevated "male" hormones, please see Chapter 8, which deals with this topic. Chapter 8 discusses nutritional ways to decrease elevated insulin levels, which has many benefits, including benefits to acne vulgaris.

With reference to acne rosacea, the difficult-to-treat, progressive reddening of the skin of the face and neck, I believe that the same recommendations given here for acne vulgaris are advisable; that is, keep the sugary and starchy foods that increase insulin levels to a minimum. In addition, increasing the amount of acid in the stomach and increasing the digestive enzymes may help out with rosacea. It may be worth purchasing digestive enzyme tablets designed to supplement both stomach and small intestinal secretions. These are available in health food shops.

I QUIT NURSING MY BABY EIGHTEEN MONTHS AGO, BUT MY BREASTS HAVE STILL NOT COMPLETELY DRIED UP, AND MY LUTEAL PHASE IS STILL SHORT.

Galactorrhea, or milk in the breasts of non-nursing women, is not uncommon among those who have been pregnant. It most often indicates excessive prolactin secretion, or it can be a symptom of hypothyroidism, or, more rarely, hyperthyroidism. These topics are discussed in Chapter 7 under the headings "Luteal Phase Deficiency," "Low Thyroid Function," and "Hyperthyroidism." An evaluation by a doctor can and should be made to determine the cause of galactorrhea, but the temperature chart itself contributes to the diagnosis. Very low or very elevated waking temperatures suggest, respectively, low or elevated levels of thyroid hormone. A short luteal phase offers evidence of high prolactin levels when there is milk in your breasts.

The nutritional suggestions for lowering prolactin are listed as the subtopic "Abnormal Luteal Function (Luteal Phase Deficiency)" in Chapter 5. Vitamin B6 alone, in amounts of 300–600 mg/day, has eliminated both galactorrhea and amenorrhea caused by prolactin excess.[4] I once counseled a woman with secondary infertility who had a leakage of milk from one breast, even though her youngest child was six years old. She had received medical treatment for infertility without success. She tried the full dose of Optivite (300 mg vitamin B6; see Appendix A for complete contents), and within only a few days the leakage of milk stopped. In addition, she got pregnant without fertility treatment during her next cycle.

Fairly high amounts of vitamin B6 (200–300 mg/day) may be necessary to lower prolactin levels significantly, but magnesium in generous amounts (800–1,000 mg/day) may make less B6 necessary. Vitamins and minerals are natural substances that will get at the underlying cause, and are far preferable to the synthetic drug bromocriptine (Parlodel), which specifically lowers prolactin.

NutraSweet can raise prolactin levels and cause long cycles. Make sure you avoid it, and avoid other artificial sweeteners as well. (See the question and answer on this topic in Chapter 4.)

You may be surprised to learn that galactorrhea is frequently undetected by women who have this condition.[5] Careful expression of each breast, from edge to nipple, should be part your routine breast self-examination. Even a single drop of fluid should be reported to a doctor, unless you are pregnant or nursing has been discontinued recently.

IS CARPAL TUNNEL SYNDROME TREATABLE BY NUTRITION?

Carpal tunnel syndrome refers to pain, weakness, and numbness of the hands, wrists and sometimes elbows and shoulders. The usual advice it to avoid hyperextending the wrists by using removable splints. However, there is some evidence that vitamin B6 may be helpful for carpal tunnel syndrome, but it is not conclusive.[6] Dr. John Ellis noted that vitamin B6 and magnesium, which work together, were helpful for such symptoms in pregnant women. (See the subtitle, "Vitamin B6 and Magnesium for Edema" in Chapter 10 for more information.) If you wish to try nutrition for carpal tunnel syndrome, instead of vitamin B6 and magnesium only, use ProCycle as your multivitamin/multi-mineral. It contains both of these, as well as a good balance of other nutrients which enable vitamin B6 to work more effectively. (See "Appendix A.") The omega-3 fatty acids in flax oil or fish oil may be helpful, also, because of their strong anti-inflammatory effect.

IS THERE ANY EVIDENCE THAT NUTRITION CAN HELP PREVENT PREMATURE RUPTURE OF MEMBRANES?

Yes, there is. Premature rupture of membranes (PROM) means that the "bag of waters" breaks long before a woman is due to have the baby. It is one cause of premature delivery, because it may trigger premature labor, or labor may be induced because of the ruptured membranes. Smoking is a risk factor for PROM and for other causes of premature delivery. Good nutrition, especially enough dietary protein, generally helps to prevent prematurity, but there is evidence that vitamin C is low in women who have had PROM.[7] This makes sense, because the membranes are strengthened by collagen, a thread-like structural protein, and collagen cannot be made without vitamin C. The bio-flavinoids, which are nutrients found in the whitish rinds of citrus fruits, work along with vitamin C to do this job.

IS THERE ANY WAY TO DECREASE THE RISK OF GETTING FIBROID TUMORS? MY MOTHER, WHO IS 47, JUST GOT DIAGNOSED WITH ONE, AND I KNOW THEY RUN IN FAMILIES.

Fibroid tumors are stimulated by high levels of estrogen, and it is true that they may run in families. Avoiding overweight is perhaps the most effective way of preventing high estrogen levels, and overweight is a risk factor for fibroids. Nutrition aimed at raising progesterone and lowering estrogen is the next step. Vitamins and minerals that work together to do so are vitamin B6, other B vitamins, vitamin C, and magnesium. Optivite or ProCycle, each made to overcome PMS, contain these nutrients and others to help normalize your estrogen and progesterone. See Chapter 5 for complete information on PMS nutrition, which will be helpful to you.

I AM ONLY IN MY 30S, BUT I AM VERY CONCERNED ABOUT OSTEOPOROSIS. YET FROM WHAT I READ, CALCIUM ALONE DOESN'T SEEM TO BE THE ANSWER.

You are correct; studies on the effects of calcium supplementation on the bone loss disorder osteoporosis have not been especially promising. Both vitamin D and magnesium are necessary for the body to use calcium, and it is good to remember that sugar increases loss of magnesium.

Interestingly, correcting certain cycle irregularities may reduce your risk of osteoporosis. A study of athletic women published in the *New England Journal of Medicine* established that athletic women who experienced only one or more short luteal phase cycles or anovulatory cycles per year were losing bone mass at a time of life when other women were gaining bone. In this study, luteal phase was determined by basal temperatures, and elevated temperatures of less than ten days were considered a short luteal phase. The authors expressed concern that short luteal phase is a "silent" risk factor for osteoporosis, because women with short luteal phases usually have very regular menstrual periods.[8] It is certainly an obvious factor to women who chart, and based on research discussed in this book, a reversible one. The anovulatory cycles referred to above are less common than short luteal phase cycles. They may be an extreme form of the short luteal phase cycle, a consequence of underweight, or a manifestation of low thyroid function. These cycle irregularities often respond to proper nutrition; see the appropriate subtitles in Chapter 7 ("Luteal Phase Deficiency," "Underweight or Inadequate Body Fat," or "Low Thyroid Function") for nutrition to overcome them.

Incidentally, I believe that the short luteal phases seen during breastfeeding and during the perimenopause are natural fertility transitions and are not a cause for special concern.

I AM 35 YEARS OLD AND HAVE HAD SIX CHILDREN. I HAVE BREASTFED THEM ALL. I AM SMALL-BONED, AND MY GRANDMOTHER BROKE HER HIP WHEN SHE WAS SEVENTY. DOES HAVING MANY CHILDREN INCREASE THE RISK OF OSTEOPOROSIS?

This is a question that has interested a number of researchers, and some of the answers are coming from an ongoing study of women from the Old Order Amish religion. They are very family-oriented and have a tradition of large families and of breastfeeding their babies. Results of these studies actually show the reverse of what you might think: Bone mineral density is higher, and therefore risk of bone fracture of the hip is lower, in women who have had large numbers of children. Some of this effect, however, is due to the modest increase in weight that is common as women have many babies, and as women age the benefit is lost. However, having many children (and in this large study five to ten children was most common) had no negative effect on bone density whatever.[9]

You are probably aware that being small-boned and having a relative with a bone fracture are risk factors for osteoporosis. I encourage you to get a bone density test now, while you are still in your thirties. Diet, exercise, and vitamin and mineral supplements can enable you to maintain or restore your bone health at your age, and finding out what your bone status is now is a great motivator should you find your bones are less dense than you would like. See Chapter 12's topic "Maintaining Bone Health" for more information.

HOW DO YOU SEE THE ROLE OF STRESS IN INFERTILITY?

In general, I think that the role of "stress" as most people understand it is overrated as a cause of infertility. The emphasis on daily life stresses, such as constant deadlines, constant chauffeuring, or the constant need to have the house clean and the garden weeded, misses the point. I do not think that those stresses are the ones that contribute to infertility, at least not directly. It is *physical* stress, which many people seem to overlook completely, that truly can contribute to infertility.

The physical stresses that affect fertility are the chronic stress of poor nutrition, lack of sleep, and in some women, too much physical exertion, even if they enjoy their exercise routines or sports activities. All of these stresses can be involved even with cycles that show ovulation. The kind of modern stresses that we talk about so much — being too busy or striving for perfection — in my opinion affect fertility mostly insofar as they cause women to miss out on good nutrition and adequate sleep, or make them feel that they must exercise excessively. Improved nutrition, enough sleep, and moderate exercise are what I mean when I write about stress reduction.

That is why I take issue with that unsolicited advice to infertile couples, "Relax!" Yes, an episode of severe emotional stress, such as the death of a loved one, a major financial reversal, or an unwelcome, untimely move across country, can cause a delay in ovulation, sometimes for weeks. But once ovulation resumes, fertility will be restored. Please, if you are not infertile, do not suggest that your infertile friends relax. I have never spoken to a woman anxious to conceive who was not hurt and worried by that counterproductive advice. I facetiously encourage our infertility clients to "go ahead and be uptight!" Knowing that it does not matter is good for their peace of mind.

CAN WOMEN TAKE ANDROVITE FOR MEN? I DON'T HAVE PMS, AND IT LOOKS LIKE THREE OR FOUR TABLETS WOULD BE A GOOD GENERAL VITAMIN.

Yes, you can. You can take the full dose, which is six tablets, even if you become pregnant, assuming your doctor's approval. The labeling of the vitamin A confuses people, but if you read the label carefully you will see that it contains only 5,000 IU of retinyl palmitate (true vitamin A) per full dose; the rest is beta-carotene. Only true vitamin A, not beta-carotene, has been related to birth defects, in amounts beginning at 10,000 IU.[10]

The full dose of Androvite for Men is especially good, I think, for women who need adrenal support, as the adrenals produce steroid hormones and therefore have nutritional needs much like the testes'. I also consider it helpful for thyroid support, due to its substantial mix of minerals along with the vitamins. Because of this, it may be beneficial for hair loss,[11] especially when taken along with flax oil.

With my doctor's approval, I used the full dose of Androvite for Men as part of my prenatal supplementation when I was pregnant with our eighth child, but nevertheless, she turned out to be a girl!

I AM CONCERNED THAT MY 22-YEAR-OLD DAUGHTER IS EATING A VEGAN DIET. WHAT WORRIES ME MORE IS THAT SHE IS ENGAGED, AND I AM AFRAID OF WHAT MIGHT HAPPEN WHEN SHE GETS PREGNANT. SHOULD I BE CONCERNED?

It is important to open the lines of communication to discuss why your daughter has chosen a vegan diet. If it is for her own health, why not encourage her to check out your local food co-op or health food shop, where she can see that healthy organic milk, meat, and eggs are available? If it is because she wants to lose weight, there are healthier, easier ways to do so. If it has to do with ethical concerns for animals, you can point out that organic eggs and organic milk come from animals that are allowed normal access to pasture. Even if she will not eat meat or fish, eating eggs and milk products (ovolacto-vegetarianism) is much easier to implement, and it is much easier to remain healthy by eating animal protein and fat. Meanwhile, if she listens to Mom, you should at least suggest fresh whole plant foods, grains and beans, essential oils, and comprehensive supplements as described in Chapter 3. Vitamin B12, zinc, and a number of other nutrients are often deficient in those who eat no animal foods.

Done haphazardly, a vegan diet can contribute to infertility due to underweight, stress, or nutritional deficiencies. I believe that only those who get excellent nutritional counseling from an experienced midwife or obstetrician should attempt to become pregnant while eating a vegan diet. Once pregnancy occurs, the mother-to-be should be encouraged to at least eat eggs and milk, and take supplements tailored by a nutritional counselor.

I have observed that veganism, and to a lesser extent, ovolacto-vegetarianism, are often smokescreens for anorexia nervosa in young women. Anorexia nervosa is a psychological disorder, but my opinion is that in addition to good psychological and nutritional counseling, supplements aimed at adrenal support, as discussed in Chapter 14, are very helpful. When adrenal exhaustion is overcome, sometimes anxieties, including anorexia, are also overcome.

How can I find a good nutritional counselor?

You might be expecting me to give you a website as my response, but I think that the best way to find someone right in your community is to visit your local food co-op or health food shop and ask there for recommendations. Food co-ops in particular are often the unofficial local clearinghouse for information on every variety of alternative health care, including the names and reputations of nutritionally-oriented medical doctors, osteopaths, chiropractors, birth attendants, and so forth. Keep in mind that co-op employees are often members who work only a few hours per week, so if one person cannot help you, perhaps the next day's employees can!

What should I look for in selecting my nutritional counselor?

Here are some traits that I think form the ideal. To avoid awkward grammatical constructions, I have used the generic "he," though of course your counselor is equally likely to be a woman.

1. He is a qualified health professional, educated in the functions of the human body. He could be a medical doctor, an osteopathic doctor, a chiropractor, a nutritionist, or one of the less familiar naturopathic or homeopathic doctors. If you have serious health problems such as cardiovascular disease, kidney disease, or diabetes, make every effort to find a medical or osteopathic doctor who is aware of the benefits of nutrition for your particular condition.

2. He is enthusiastically interested in the role of nutrition in health and disease, and he stays informed about new research involving nutrition and health.

3. He directs you to appropriate laboratory tests of your nutritional status, and can prescribe nutrients in potencies and chemical forms that are not available over the counter.

4. He not only is open to your input, but also considers your awareness and participation in your health care indispensable. He sees health care as an equal partnership with his client, and he recognizes that ultimate decision-making rests with you. He directs you to websites, asks you to read pamphlets, and recommends whole books. He is unafraid to say, "I don't know," and he appreciates published information or anecdotes that you provide to help him help you more effectively.

5. He recognizes the role of the emotions in health and healing, and he is genuinely encouraging and uplifting about the healing power of the human body.

6. He is available by telephone or e-mail. After an initial visit or two, and any necessary laboratory assessments, he is prompt and gracious about answering brief questions by e-mail or phone. He knows you are not made of money.

MY DOCTOR IS OKAY WITH MY VITAMINS AND MINERALS, BUT HE IS NOT REALLY THAT KNOWLEDGEABLE. DO YOU THINK THAT I WOULD BE BETTER OFF LOOKING FOR ANOTHER ONE?

Not necessarily. If you have established a good relationship of mutual respect, it is absolutely worth keeping that relationship. If you have no serious health disorders and if you are willing to read in the field of nutrition, you may get along very well by simply letting your doctor know what you are doing. Your good health probably contributes to his openness to nutrition. If on the other hand you have serious health problems to deal with, you may have more to gain if you have the input of another nutritional advisor along with a supportive primary doctor. My experience is that this is a very workable situation as long as the doctor isn't "down on it because he's not up on it!"

Further Reading

CHAPTER 1

Get the Sugar Out: 501 Simple Ways to Cut the Sugar Out of Any Diet, 2nd ed., by Ann Louise Gittleman (New York: Three Rivers Press, 2008). Here is a book that will explain the problems with sweet additives to our foods. Sugar is only one of the additives that are discussed; high fructose corn syrup, sugar alcohols, aspartame, sucralose, and Stevia are also covered. It contains quite a bit of practical information on reading labels, and offers many tips and recipes to "get the sugar out!"

Breastfeeding and Natural Child Spacing: The Ecology of Natural Mothering, Classic Edition, by Sheila Kippley (2008). This book has the best information I know of on how to breastfeed, including long-term breastfeeding, and on feeding solids during later babyhood. I am very grateful to my dear friend, Sheila, that I read the original edition of this book before my first child was born. It has helped me with the next eight as well!

The Art of Breastfeeding: Empowering Women to Give Their Babies the Best Start, by Linda Kracht and Jackie Hilgert (The Couple to Couple League, 2008). Another good source of information on introducing solid foods to breastfed babies. Beyond that, however, this is an excellent resource to learn why extended breastfeeding is best for not only for babies, but for mothers, fathers, and families as well. Learn how to get breastfeeding off to a good start, how to navigate common obstacles, and how nursing will impact your fertility cycles.

CHAPTER 2

Saving Dinner: The Menus, Recipes, and Shopping Lists to Bring Your Family Back to the Table, by Leanne Ely (New York: Ballantine Books, 2003). If you are having trouble getting started with better nutrition, *Saving Dinner* has already anticipated what you need to be successful. The author knows that you need quick-to-cook dishes. She knows that shopping lists will save you time and frustration. She knows that your family wants everything to taste delicious. She even knows that you prefer not to use your oven during the summer! This cookbook contains no dessert menus, but with all the tasty foods to start with and the spices for added flavor, you won't miss dessert. You may wish to follow the menu plans closely, or you may just enjoy browsing through this book, picking up some good ideas to bring the family back to the table. Leanne Ely's website is ***www.savingdinner.com.***

Whole Foods for the Whole Family, by Roberta Bishop Johnson, ed. (Franklin Park, IL: La Leche League International, 1993). A user-friendly cookbook for those attempting to improve their home cooking using all natural ingredients. This book contains detailed sections on sprouting and bread baking, and even has a children's section. Many recipes offer options to improve nutrition, accommodate food allergies, add variety, or make meals "quick-n-easy!" I consider this an ideal cookbook, at least for those who are trying to improve their diet while still "cooking American."

CHAPTER 3

Nutrition Almanac, 6th ed., by John D. Kirschman and Nutrition Search, Inc. (New York: McGraw-Hill, 2007). The best use of this book is as a reference to find out what is in your food. How many calories are in a cup of almonds? How much fiber is in a cup of kidney beans? Are sunflowers a good source of protein? It contains useful information on every vitamin and mineral, and features many charts of the nutrients found in particular foods. It even has a section on phytonutrients, including names and functions of a dozen or so of these newly discovered plant nutrients.

Gardening Without Work: For the Aging, the Busy and the Indolent, 3rd ed., by Ruth Stout (The Lyons Press, 1988). Describes the easiest way imaginable to garden organically. You need enough fall leaves, grass clippings, spoiled hay or straw to cover your garden deeply — and this book.

Prescription for Nutritional Healing: A Practical A-Z Reference to Drug-free Remedies Using Vitamins, Minerals, Herbs & Food Supplements, 4th ed., by Phyllis A. Balch, C.N.C. (New York: Avery Press, 2006). This is a thick but easy-to-use reference which lives up to its name. Use it as the family "medical" guide. It is a comprehensive book that contains descriptions of the ailments you are interested in, followed by priority lists of vitamins, minerals, essential fatty acids, amino acids, herbs, and other supplements particular to that ailment.

CHAPTER 4

Aspartame (NutraSweet): Is It Safe? by H.J. Roberts, M.D. (Philadephia: The Charles Press, 1990). Dr. Roberts wrote this book because of the unexpected challenges to his specialty, difficult diagnoses, that occurred after NutraSweet became popular. While the book is not focused on women's health, it nevertheless covers a number of menstrual cycle irregularities that may relate to use of this artificial sweetener. It explains the mechanisms by which it does so; for example, by increasing insulin levels and prolactin levels. It discusses the biochemistry of aspartame and facts regarding its testing for safety.

CHAPTER 5

Optivite PMT® and Gynovite® Plus Total Dietary Programs for Women With Answers to the Most Commonly Asked Questions by Susan A. Beck, B.S.N., R.N., M.A., and Guy Abraham, M.D., (Torrance, CA: Optimox Corp., 1992). This booklet is primarily a guide to taking the vitamin supplement Optivite, which is the multivitamin/multimineral supplement that Dr. Abraham formulated and tested for PMS. In the first few pages, the book summarizes the symptoms and risk factors of PMS. It explains how much

Optivite to take based on the Menstrual Symptom Diary, which is included as the centerfold in the booklet. Depending on the improvement in symptoms, it advises adjustment in the total dosage. It also explains the possible side effects of upset stomach, nausea, and loose stools that occasionally occur in women taking Optivite.

The most useful part is the third section, "Common Questions Asked by Our Customers about Optivite." Can you take it when pregnant? (Yes, with your physician's approval.) Can a teenage girl take it? (Yes, the full dose if she is over 100 pounds and menstruating regularly.) Is it okay for men to take Optivite? (Yes, but Optimox Corporation has a product available for men called Androvite for Men.) All in all, there are sixty questions and answers. One question and answer even covers the topic of Optivite and luteal phase deficiency and infertility.

By the way, this pamphlet, as the title implies, devotes a couple of pages to the postmenopausal time and the supplement Gynovite Plus, which is aimed at protecting women's bone health in the time after the fertile years.

Often when I write about vitamin and mineral supplements, I remind the reader to discuss the topic with a nutritionally-aware physician. This little booklet is an excellent resource to have in hand when you do so.

CHAPTER 6

Endometriosis: A Key to Healing and Fertility through Nutrition, by Dian Shepperson Mills, M.A., and Michael Vernon, Ph.D. (London: Thorsons, 2002). A thick book with small print, *Endometriosis* is like a Bible — open it to any page and you will learn, be encouraged, and be motivated. It contains an amazing array of detailed recommendations for improved nutrition, and always includes the rationale behind the recommendations. It proposes a diet that includes animal products but emphasizes whole fresh fruits, vegetables, grains, and legumes, with moderate use of dairy products. Its recommendation to find and eliminate food intolerances, such as wheat products, is very valuable. Though scientific at its core, it is compassionate in its tone. Recommended by Mary Lou Ballweg, president of the International Endometriosis Association.

CHAPTER 7

Dr. John Lee's Hormone Balance Made Simple: The Essential How-to Guide to Symptoms, Dosage, Timing, and More by John R. Lee, M.D., and Virginia Hopkins (New York: Warner Wellness, 2006). Finally, here is a relatively short handbook that guides you (and ideally, your health care professional) in the use of natural hormones, especially progesterone, but also estrogen and testosterone. Why, when, which one, and how much are all easily answered.

However, there is one important correction: The sidebar, "The Best Way to Calculate When to Use Progesterone Cream if You're Having Periods," (p. 129–130) is flawed. It uses an outdated "rhythm" approach, recommending that women start using progesterone cream two weeks before they expect their next period. No! Women with cycles who choose to use natural progesterone cream should start it after ovulation is confirmed by the third day of temperature rise, so that the progesterone does not interfere with the pre-ovulatory hormones. In many women who have estrogen dominance, the luteal phase is so short that this recommendation will result in progesterone usage well before ovulation, interfering with the natural hormone processes at that time. According to the Foreword of the book, one of the three major causes of poor results with natural hormones is using them at the wrong time (p. xii). The underlying assumption that women cannot or will not ascertain their ovulation time through NFP charting is simply that — an assumption.

The author frequently refers the reader to the late Dr. Lee's previous books, *What Your Doctor May Not Tell You about Menopause*, and *What Your Doctor May Not Tell You About Premenopause*. These two books have much more information about nutrition, but if you need only the practical help of using hormone creams, they are entirely optional.

While *Dr. Lee's Hormone Balance* points out that estrogen dominance may cause low thyroid function, the book is not particularly aimed at assisting women with low thyroid function from other causes. And with reference to polycystic ovary syndrome, it states that "PCOS disappears rapidly in most women when they cut sugar and refined carbohydrates from their diets," an optimistic assertion that defies the experience of the many women who have struggled with this ongoing metabolic imbalance. Still, it is a worthwhile book for those interested in natural hormone replacement.

The Thyroid Hormone Breakthrough: Overcoming Sexual and Hormonal Problems at Every Age, by Mary J. Shomon (New York: Collins, 2006). Mary Shomon is herself a woman who has low thyroid function. Spurred on originally by her own search for effective treatment, she has become a patient advocate and tireless writer on the topic of thyroid dysfunction. In this book, she looks particularly at the effects that both hypothyroidism and hyperthyroidism have on all aspects of female reproduction: menstrual pain, heavy menses, PMS, postpartum thyroiditis, infertility, and perimenopausal symptoms. The book is very comprehensive, covering medications for hypothyroidism, treatment for hyperthyroidism, and the link between other hormone dysfunctions and thyroid disorders. If you are troubled by symptoms that may fit thyroid disease, you will get far better medical care if you are informed by this book. While it covers technical topics, it is divided into easy-to-find subtopics, and is written for an intelligent layperson. It recommends charting your cycle to better understand it.

Female Fertility and the Body Fat Connection, by Rose E. Frisch, Ph.D. (Chicago: University of Chicago Press, 2002). As a Harvard School of Public Health professor, Dr. Frisch did the groundbreaking research on the link between women's athletic endeavor, body weight, body fat, and menstrual cycles. In this book, she approaches the topic autobiographically rather than through a strictly scientific approach. Yet the science is always present, as she explains the physiology behind the phenomenon of amenorrhea caused by excessive exercise. *Female Fertility and the Body Fat Connection* is not written as a self-help book, but it is fascinating reading about how scientific inquiry progresses once the basic scientific tool — the questioning mind — is engaged.

Dr. David Reuben's Quick Weight-Gain Program: Safe, Easy Weight Gain for Every Age and Situation, by David Reuben, M.D. (New York: Crown Publishers, 1996). As far as I can tell, there is no other book available like this one, perhaps because so many people are trying to do exactly the opposite of Dr. Reuben's topic! Most underweight women do not need a book to explain to them how to exercise less and eat more, but if you are having a hard time gaining weight, this book will show you strategies that work. The chatty style is very motivational, though the book emphasizes a sexy body more than a healthy body. It is a good book for men, women, or children, the elderly, and the chronically ill.

CHAPTER 8

The Fertility Diet: Groundbreaking Research Reveals Natural Ways to Boost Ovulation and Improve Your Chances of Getting Pregnant, by Jorge E. Chavarro, M.D., Sc.D.; Walter C. Willett, M.D., D.P.H.; and Patrick J. Skerrett (New York: McGraw-Hill, 2008). An important book based on the huge Nurses' Health Study, particularly involving nurses who were trying to get pregnant during the study. Based on analysis of thousands of nurses' reports of diet, exercise, body weight, and so forth, the authors make numerous recommendations for improved diet. It covers the problems with sugary foods and trans fats. It has a chapter on celiac disease. It covers ovulatory infertility, including polycystic ovary syndrome (PCOS). A very nice feature related to PCOS is a chapter that includes evaluation of various weight-loss diets. Please note that *The Fertility Diet* is not a resource for those looking for help with endometriosis, male infertility, PMS, menopause, or cycle irregularities related to low thyroid function, short luteal phase, or age.

Dr. Atkins' New Diet Revolution: The Low-Carb Approach That Has Helped Millions Lose Weight and Keep It Off, by Robert C. Atkins, M.D. (New York: Quill, an imprint of HarperCollins, 2002). This is the update of Dr. Atkins' famous book, published shortly before his death in 2003. It is a valuable reference for anyone with polycystic ovary syndrome (PCOS). If you are interested in losing weight, you may find it far too strict, but it is full of many good ideas regarding weight loss. For example, his contention that protein and fat satisfy the appetite, while low fat, high carbohydrate diets promote cravings rings true with many women. It contains an excellent chapter on "vita-nutrients" to supplement while you are trying to lose weight or keep it off. The book is actually fun to read; Dr. Atkins' style is witty and often endearing.

CHAPTER 9

The Yeast Connection and Women's Health by William G. Crook, M.D., with Carolyn Dean, M.D., N.D.; and Elizabeth B. Crook (Jackson, TN:

Professional Books, 2005). This book is the latest edition of the original, *The Yeast Connection*. Part 2, "Yeast Related Problems That Affect Women," includes chapters entitled "PMS," "Vaginitis," "Endometriosis," and "Vulvodynia." Other chapters for both men and women include "Interstitial Cystitis," "Infertility," and "Sexual Dysfunction." Even if you do not have yeast overgrowth, the whole foods, low sugar diet that Dr. Crook advocates will certainly improve your health.

Chronic Candidiasis: Your Natural Guide to Healing with Diet, Vitamins, Minerals, Herbs, Exercise, and Other Natural Methods, by Michael T. Murray, N.D. (Roseville, CA: Prima, 1997). The voracious researcher Dr. Murray has provided an excellent resource for men, women, or children with yeast overgrowth, also called candidiasis. Despite the biology involved with this topic, it is clearly and concisely explained. Among the many helpful features of this book is information on natural alternatives to antibiotics for various infections. Dr. Murray's dietary approach emphasizes an overall vegetarian approach, though it does not completely exclude animal products.

The Schwarzbein Principle II, by Diana Schwarzbein, M.D., with Marilyn Brown (Deerfield Beach, FL: Health Communications, Inc., 2002). The unwieldy name makes it difficult to recommend this book friend to friend, especially when you go to write down the title, but it is a very good book! Dr. Schwarzbein is a nutritionally-aware endocrinologist. Her book covers adrenal burnout, thyroid problems, and elevated insulin levels, always with a nutritional approach. Unlike so many health books written for women by medical doctors, she does not ignore "the elephant in the living room" — birth control pills. She is firmly against these artificial steroid hormones. In Chapter 13, "Step Three: Tapering Off or Avoiding Toxic Chemicals," she includes birth control pills, stating that "....you can never achieve complete hormonal balance while taking BCPs because they disrupt the sex hormone system, and, because all hormones are connected, the body's entire hormone system is disrupted, too." My favorite chapter in the book, however, is Chapter 12: "Step 2: Managing Stress and Getting Enough Sleep." She is right as rain about the need for sleep.

The Effects of Light on the Menstrual Cycle: Also Infertility, Clinical Observations, by Joy DeFelice, R.N. (Spokane, WA: The Natural Family Planning Program of the Sacred Heart Medical Center, 2003). Mrs. DeFelice, a natural family planning professional, observed the effect of eliminating night lighting on the regularity of the menstrual cycle beginning in 1976. The research community is now able to explain this phenomenon through the effect of light on the pineal gland and its secretion of melatonin, which affects reproductive hormones. This booklet is a practical guide that explains why and how to eliminate night lighting in order to have more regular cycles and improved fertility. Her advice is no substitute for improved nutrition, but she herself reminds the reader of the necessity of good nutrition, exercise, and stress reduction. If you are having difficulty sleeping, this booklet will help you also.

CHAPTER 10

Preventing Eclampsia: An Interview with Tom Brewer, M.D. by C.J. Puotinen (Townsend Letter for Doctors and Patients, Nov., 2004). This article, easily available through the Internet, concisely summarizes Dr. Brewer's life work, which involved clinical experience with thousands of pregnant women. It details the diet he developed, and compares the medical approach to eclampsia to the nutritional approach. It is completely referenced with 83 citations, all of them annotated by the author. In addition to preventing eclampsia, Dr. Brewer relates his pregnancy diet to better birth weights, more full-term births, and better mental development in children born to mothers who followed his diet.

What Every Pregnant Woman Should Know: The Truth About Diet and Drugs in Pregnancy, by Gail Sforza Brewer and Tom Brewer, M.D. (New York: Penguin Books, 1985). Extensively researched but built on Dr. Tom Brewer's experience with several thousand pregnant women, this is the classic book that describes the details of pregnancy nutrition, especially the role of diet in preventing metabolic toxemia of late pregnancy. Though it explains the consequences of poor diet to mother and baby, it is a very reassuring book that shows how a good diet dramatically reduces the incidence of a number of pregnancy-related problems, not just toxemia of pregnancy. There are more than enough books that have been written on pregnancy, but this is the one I place at the top of the list.

Managing Morning Sickness, 2nd ed., by Marilyn M. Shannon (Cincinnati: The Couple to Couple League, 1998). This short booklet promotes the hypothesis that overcoming low blood sugar is an important factor in overcoming morning sickness. It includes practical dietary strategies aimed at stabilizing your blood glucose, settling your tender stomach, and preventing low blood pressure. There are suggestions for supplements to discuss with your doctor. As you can guess, I seldom disagree with the author.

A Natural Guide to Pregnancy and Postpartum Health, by Dean Raffelock, D.C., Robert Rountree, M.D., and Virginia Hopkins (New York: Avery, 2002). Here is an excellent book with information to help you have a wonderfully healthy pregnancy, and equally as important, a wonderfully healthy and joyous postpartum time with your new baby. As the authors point out, many women are overstressed, anxious or depressed during the postpartum time, and much of that can be helped by better nutrition. The authors note again and again that your baby is made from the food you eat, and nutritional deficiencies often catch up with mothers after the birth. They propose good, preferably organic, whole plant and animal foods. Moreover, they make the case that nutritional deficiencies are very difficult to overcome with improved diet alone, and they are strong proponents of supplementing.

When it comes to the supplements that they recommend, the authors give the amounts that are safe for pregnant women and their unborn babies, and for mothers with nursing babies (though in some cases higher amounts are known to be safe, as in the case of folic acid).

In no other book have I seen the role of supplements in overcoming the toxins in the body or in the environment so well explained. That in itself is very encouraging, as it is easy to get discouraged when you find out about "indoor air pollution," pesticide residues on your fresh produce, and so forth. The book also includes an easy-to-understand chapter on the digestive system, explaining leaky gut syndrome and offering practical solutions for it. I highly recommend this book.

Let's Have Healthy Children, by Adelle Davis, revised by Marshall Mandell, M.D. (New York: Signet Books, 1981). This is the last edition of the original book on diet and supplements for pregnancy. Adelle Davis was far ahead of her time on this topic, though she drew her conclusions and recommendations from the available research literature. The book is still an immense help both for pregnancy and for nutritional care of babies and children. Adelle Davis strongly believed that even the minor complaints of pregnancy — nausea, headache, fatigue, varicose veins, "mask" of pregnancy — are abnormalities that can be prevented or reversed with proper diet and supplements. The book is out of print, but is available via the Internet.

CHAPTER 12

Before the Change: Taking Charge of Your Perimenopause, 2nd ed., by Ann Louise Gittleman (San Francisco: HarperSanFrancisco, 2004). Here is the book that will be your most thorough yet readable guide to the changes in your hormones and moods as your fertile years pass. It emphasizes improved diet, vitamins, minerals, healthy oils, natural progesterone, exercise, stress reduction, and adrenal gland support. I consider this the best book available on premenopause, perimenopause, and menopause. It is much easier and more enjoyable to use than the late Dr. Lee's book, *What Your Doctor May Not Tell You about Menopause* (see below), but Ms. Gittleman refers to and includes Dr. Lee's recommendations.

What Your Doctor May Not Tell You about Menopause: The Breakthrough Book on Natural Hormone Balance, by John R. Lee, M.D., and Virginia Hopkins (New York: Warner Wellness, 2004). This is the update of the book that made the phrase "estrogen dominance" a household term, and through it Dr. Lee popularized the use of over-the-counter natural progesterone cream. The book is thick and covers many other hormonal problems and hormone interactions that affect women's health. It is not a page-by-page read, but is a reference that takes some time to absorb. In addition to his advocacy for natural hormones, Dr. Lee was a firm advocate of holistic nutrition and comprehensive supplements.

What Your Doctor May Not Tell You About Premenopause: Balance Your Hormones and Your Life from Thirty to Fifty, by John R. Lee, M.D., Jesse Hanley, M.D., and Virginia Hopkins (New York: Warner Books, 1999). There is considerable overlap between Dr. Lee's premenopause book and the other one on menopause. I personally prefer the *Menopause* book, but this one covers infertility and contains sobering information about the health risks associated with oral contraceptives.

The Myth of Osteoporosis: What Every Woman Should Know about Creating Bone Health, by Gillian Sanson (Ann Arbor, MI: MCD Century, 2003). The unfortunate title of this book might discourage a sensible person from opening it, but I have found it to be helpful and reassuring. Mrs. Sanson is part of a family that has a genetic disorder that causes the bone loss disease osteoporosis at a young age, and so she has lived with the information gathering and decision making that such a serious problem requires. She recommends good nutrition, maintenance of normal weight (as opposed to underweight), exercise, and — very important — prevention of fractures as the basis of bone health. She explains the problems with the drug therapies for osteoporosis. She is critical of bone density measurement, a point on which I disagree. Nevertheless, you will learn more practical information about maintaining bone health through this book than through many longer ones.

CHAPTER 14

Depression-free, Naturally: 7 Weeks to Eliminating Anxiety, Despair, Fatigue, and Anger from Your Life by Joan Mathews Larson, Ph.D., (New York: Ballantine Wellspring, 2001). Dr. Larson works from the hypothesis that the disorders listed in the title result from biochemical imbalances that are correctable through targeted nutrition. She presents a large amount of information which can be somewhat confusing. However, used as a reference, this book can help you to identify what might be out of balance in your body. It has many specific suggestions for help. In addition to recommending vitamins and minerals, Dr. Larson is a proponent of the use of free amino acids to provide the body with the building blocks to make beneficial neurotransmitters — for example, serotonin.

Resources

GENERAL
The Couple to Couple League International
for Natural Family Planning

P.O. Box 111184
Cincinnati, Ohio 45211
Telephone: 513-471-2000
Website: ***www.ccli.org***
Email: ccli@ccli.org

As a volunteer instructor for this organization, along with my husband, I am very partial to it. But I think that I am being completely objective to call it the world's best organization for learning the world's best method of birth control. CCL currently has over 600 teaching couples in the United States and in several foreign countries; find the ones nearest you by checking their website or calling the office.

The professionally trained teaching couples hold series of three monthly classes at local hospitals or churches. They cover all aspects of modern "sympto-thermal" natural family planning (NFP):

➤ health benefits of NFP

➤ effectiveness of NFP in preventing pregnancy, NFP during breastfeeding, and cycle irregularity

➤ achieving pregnancy through fertility awareness and other natural fertility aids

➤ NFP as a way of love and life.

Supplemental classes on how to use NFP during the transition times of postpartum and premenopause are also available.

Teaching couples also provide telephone counseling if cycle irregularities occur, or for any additional questions or consultation needed by new users. A home study course is available for those who do not live in an area where the classes are taught. Whether you are having difficulty achieving pregnancy or are attempting to act in harmony with your body as you avoid a pregnancy, you will gain much from these professionally prepared, practical classes.

CCL's motto is "Natural Family Planning — It's Safe, Healthy and Effective ... and it can change your hearts in surprising ways!"

Women's Health America
1289 Deming Way
Madison, WI 53717
Telephone: 1-800-558-7046
Website: *www.womenshealth.com*

Women's Health America provides information, education, and products related to women's reproductive health, from premenstrual syndrome (PMS) to perimenopause to menopause. They maintain a referral list of physicians who treat PMS, and a catalog of books, cassettes, and articles on this topic. They promote self-care first, in the form of improved diet and targeted supplements, exercise, and stress management. WHA manufactures ProCycle PMS, the multivitamin/multimineral that I recommend for PMS as well as for certain types of cycle irregularity and infertility. They also carry Optivite PMT, which is similar to ProCycle.

However, natural, "bio-identical" hormone replacement tailored to the need of each individual woman is their specialty, and they can help you with testing your hormones and finding a like-minded physician in your area. I consider this one of the best sites on the internet for women's health.

CHAPTER 2

Saving Dinner
Website: *www.savingdinner.com*

Practical, warm-hearted, and health-oriented, this is a delightful website if you are trying to improve your home cooking. It covers topics such as snack foods, freezer foods, preparing meals with a tight budget, and packing your kids' school lunches. It provides lists to help you to shop and cook for your family. You can select from the low carbohydrate diet, the gluten-free diet, the vegetarian diet, or just the family-friendly healthy diet. It is a browser's delight, but you need to subscribe to get the weekly Menu-Mailer, with its detailed shopping list, menus, and recipes for the week.

Local Harvest
Website: *www.localharvest.org*

Another browser's delight, localharvest.org puts you in touch with your local organic farms and farmers. More than that, it shows you how to get started eating local. For example, their February 2009 newsletter makes the point that many families are convinced of the *why*, but are uncertain as to the *how* when it comes to improved nutrition. Here's the summary of that article, just to give you the flavor of this top-notch website:

> Start with whole foods. Don't make it too hard. Study your region's agricultural strengths, and play up to them. Look for ways to be creative with your budget. Be gentle with your self and your family as you try out new habits. Do these things, and you will set yourself up for a highly satisfying adventure in local eating, and a deeper connection to your food.

CHAPTER 3

American Pro Life Enterprise
P.O. Box 1281
Powell, OH 43065
Telephone: 1-800-227-8359
Website: *www.kuhar.com*
Email: order@kuhar.com
Bogomir M. Kuhar, Pharm.D.

The vitamin and mineral supplements recommended in this book are available from American Pro Life Enterprise, which will send your order anywhere in the continental U.S. for a nominal shipping charge. Besides stocking Optivite, Androvite, ProCycle, Professional Prenatal Formula, and other food supplements, American Pro Life Enterprise stocks a complete line of prescription drugs, health and beauty aids. For an extra "Group Discount" identify yourself as a reader of this book. American Pro Life Enterprise does not sell any contraceptives or abortifacient drugs or devices. It also donates a portion of the proceeds of pro-life generated sales back to the movement. For information or to place your order for any item mentioned above, call the above toll-free number.

LifeTime / Nutritional Specialties, Inc.
1967 N. Glassell St.
Orange, CA 92865
Telephone:1-800-333-6168
Website: *www.lifetimevitamins.com*

LifeTime produces Professional Prenatal Formula, an excellent nonprescription supplement which contains vitamins and minerals in amounts very similar to Table 7 (Chapter 3). It is ideal for pregnant and breastfeeding women and for women preparing to conceive. Professional Prenatal Formula is far better balanced and far more potent than prescription prenatal vitamins — I suggest you compare labels. Women (or men) who are attempting to overcome anemia or fatigue will also find it an excellent supplement. If your local health food shop does not stock these vitamins, you can order them through American Pro Life Enterprise, listed above. See *www.iHerb.com* for listed ingredients.

CHAPTER 5

Optimox Corporation
P.O. Box 3378
Torrance, CA 90510
Telephone: 1-800-223-1601
Website: *www.optimox.com*

Optimox Corporation developed Optivite PMT, the multi-vitamin/multi-mineral supplement which has been shown to alleviate PMS symptoms even under double-blind conditions. Some physicians also support the use of

Optivite for pregnant women (six tablets/day plus 500 mg magnesium/day plus folic acid) and for breastfeeding women (four tablets/day plus 500 mg magnesium).

Optimox Corporation also makes a complete vitamin/mineral supplement, Androvite for Men. I consider Androvite an excellent supplement for men who are trying to overcome infertility or other reproductive health problems.

You can phone or visit the website for more information on these supplements or PMS. These supplements may also be ordered from your local pharmacy or from American Pro Life Enterprise, listed above.

CHAPTER 6

The Endometriosis Association
8585 N. 76th Place
Milwaukee, Wisconsin 53223
Telephone: 1-414-355-2200
Website: *www.endometriosisassn.org*

Founded in 1980 by Mary Lou Ballweg, who herself has endometriosis, and Carolyn Keith, the purpose of The Endometriosis Association is to assist women with endometriosis to find the best and most current answers to their particular situation. They cover all aspects of this disease, and are not particularly focused on nutritional approaches.

CHAPTER 7

The Broda O. Barnes, M.D., Research Foundation, Inc.
P.O Box 110098
Trumbull, CT 06611
Telephone: 1-203-261-2101
Website: *www.brodabarnes.org*

The Broda O. Barnes, M.D., Research Foundation, Inc., is a not-for-profit organization dedicated to education, research and training in the field of thyroid and metabolic balance. They have been longtime advocates for better testing for thyroid function, including the use of the basal temperature chart, and they also advocate for natural thyroid replacement rather than synthetic thyroid hormone. They carry the late Dr. Barnes' original book, *Hypothyroidism: The Unsuspected Illness*, and also recommend books on other hormonal dysfunctions, including one on replacement of testosterone in men.

Fertility Blend for Women/Fertility Blend for Men
The Daily Wellness Company
1946 Young Street Suite 360
Honolulu, HI 96826
Telephone: 1-866-222-9862
Website: *www.fertilityblend.com*

Learn more about Fertility Blend, the supplement which has been tested under double-blind conditions for its effect in increasing the pregnancy rate for women, especially those with low progesterone levels. This supplement has also significantly increased the number of days of elevated temperatures in women who have charted their basal temperatures. It contains chasteberry extract, green tea extract, and a number of vitamins and minerals. This is the wave of the future — compounding several nutrients, not just one, and testing them in a scientifically acceptable way.

CHAPTER 9
Celiac Disease Foundation
13251 Ventura Blvd. #1
Studio City, CA 91604
Telephone: 1-818-990-2354
Website: *www.celiac.org*

The Celiac Disease Foundation (CDF) is an organization recognized throughout the world. CDF strives to promote awareness and build a supportive community for patients, families and health care professionals. CDF is actively involved in advocating for patient concerns and networking with other national and international organizations.

The Celiac Disease Foundation's website is a good way to get better acquainted with this disease of gluten intolerance, but it is not a substitute for the care of a doctor and dietitian.

The Celiac Sprue Association
P.O. Box 31700
Omaha, NE 68131
Telephone: 1-877-CSA-4CSA
Website: *www.csaceliacs.org*

The Celiac Sprue Association remains the largest non-profit celiac support group in America, with over 125 chapters and resource units across the country, and over 9,000 members worldwide. A dedicated force of volunteer officers and committee members serve as the organization's strong backbone, affectionately calling themselves "Celiacs Helping Celiacs."

CHAPTER 10
Blue Ribbon Baby
Website: *www.blueribbonbaby.org*

This is the website for those hoping to become pregnant soon, or those already expecting. It is dedicated to continuing the work of obstetrician Tom Brewer, M.D., whose long career centered on promoting healthy, adequate nutrition as the means of preventing pre-eclampsia, or metabolic toxemia of late pregnancy, as it is also called. The website contains detailed charts on what foods and how much of them to eat, and also contains alternatives for expectant mothers who are vegetarians, are intolerant of milk, or need other alternative recommendations. If you have had pre-eclampsia or a premature baby, please get acquainted with this website — especially if you have been told that your situation is not explainable. This is the best on the web for how to eat during pregnancy.

La Leche League International
P.O. Box 4079
Schaumburg, IL 60168-4079
Telephone: 1-800-525-3243
Website: *www.lalecheleague.org*

Breastfeeding involves your baby's nutrition as well as your own. This wonderful organization is dedicated to helping mothers breastfeed successfully, no matter what adverse circumstances may be present. A series of four meetings is held at a leader's home to instruct and encourage you, and your leader provides non-medical telephone counseling also. By all means take the class before your baby is born if possible. You will also meet other like-minded mothers through "The League." If you cannot locate a League leader through your food co-op or white pages of the telephone directory, check their website or contact the central office above.

CHAPTER 11

Genetics & Disabilities Diagnostic Care Center
P.O Box 4548
Virginia Beach, VA 23454
Telephone: 1-757-425-1969
Website: www.*lleichtman.org*

To gain a fuller understanding of the metabolic challenges that people with Down syndrome face, as well as the promising possibility for improving their health through nutrition, see the website of pediatrician and geneticist Lawrence Leichtman, M.D., of Virginia Beach, Virginia. He treats children with Down syndrome using targeted nutritional therapy as well as other approaches. The article titled "Targeted Nutritional Intervention (TNI) in the Treatment of Children and Adults with Down Syndrome" is of particular interest (*www.lleichtman.org/tni*).

Trisomy 21 Research Foundation
Telephone: 1-800-899-3413
Website: *www.nutrivene.com*

Pediatrician and geneticist Dr. Lawrence Leichtman, is the founder of Trisomy 21 Research Foundation. This website provides information about Nutrivene-D, the targeted supplement for children and adults with Down syndrome. If you learn that you are going to have a child with Down syndrome, or if you already have a child with DS, you will find this website full of encouragement and practical suggestions.

CHAPTER 12
Women's Wellness Today
Susan M. Lark, M.D.
Telephone: 1-877-437-5275
Website: *www.drlark.com*

I have subscribed to Dr. Lark's newsletter for several years and have found it informative and up-to-date. It has excellent new information for perimeno-pausal and menopausal women, and covers many other female problems not related to pregnancy or breastfeeding. For example, a recent issue covered urinary incontinence, and another one covered low sexual desire. Other topics are not specifically related to the reproductive system, such as natural cures for psoriasis, or natural beauty products. While most of her articles make a link between new scientific studies and practical applications, she has a slight new-age bent. For example, she includes insert articles on various types of meditation. Still, I would not be without this newsletter, and I have a great respect for the contributions to women's health that Dr. Lark has made through her writing.

CHAPTER 15
Health and Healing
Julian Whitaker, M.D.
Telephone: 1-800-539-8219
Website: *www.drwhitaker.com*

This newsletter is excellent for keeping up on new research related to general nutrition and health. It is not written specifically for men, but nevertheless, Dr. Whitaker has a great interest in the problems of men as they age. Heart disease, hypertension, cancer, diabetes, arthritis, depression, prostate prob-lems, vision problems and many other common health concerns are topics that he addresses regularly. Dr. Whitaker also comments on the political aspects of nutrition and nutritional supplementation, a particularly enlighten-ing topic.

The website provides much information, links to research publications, and provides access to his multivitamin/multimineral, named Forward, which is an excellent supplement that covers all the bases quite well. Other supple-ments which he has formulated for particular problems, such as prostate health, joint health, or vision health, are also available by phone or via the website.

APPENDIX B
Apex Medical Technologies, Inc.
10064 Mesa Ridge Court, Suite 202
San Diego, CA 92121
Telephone: 1-800-345-3208
Website: *apexfertility.com*

This company sells special kits to ethically obtain a semen sample for analysis.

Appendix A:

Labeled Contents of Recommended Supplements

— ANDROVITE FOR MEN —

Ingredient	Amount per 6 tablets		%DV*
Vitamin A	25,000	IU	500%
(as retinyl palmitate and 80% as beta-carotene)			
Vitamin C	1000	mg	1667%
Vitamin D (as cholecalciferol)	400	IU	100%
Vitamin E (as d-alpha tocopheryl succinate)	400	IU	1333%
Thiamin (as thiamine mononitrate)	50	mg	3333%
Riboflavin	50	mg	2941%
Niacin (as niacinamide)	50	mg	250%
Vitamin B6 (as pyridoxine HCl)	100	mg	5000%
Folic Acid	400	mcg	100%
Vitamin B12 (as hydroxocobalamin)	125	mcg	2084%
Biotin	125	mcg	42%
Pantothenic Acid (as Ca Pantothenate)	100	mg	1000%
Iron (as amino acid chelate)	18	mg	100%
Iodine (as hydrolyzed protein complex)	150	mcg	100%
Magnesium (as magnesium oxide)	500	mg	125%
Zinc (as amino acid chelate)	50	mg	333%
Selenium (as hydrolyzed protein complex)	200	mcg	286%
Copper (as amino acid chelate)	2	mg	100%
Manganese (as amino acid chelate)	10	mg	500%
Chromium (as hydrolyzed protein complex)	200	mcg	167%
p-Aminobenzioc Acid (PABA)	25	mg	*
Betaine HCl	100	mg	*
Pancreatin 4X	75	mg	*
Inositol	36	mg	*
Hesperidin	35	mg	*
Rutin	25	mg	*
Boron (Hydrolzed Protein Complex)	3	mg	*

* Daily Value (DV) not established.
Other ingredients: Micosolle®, a silica-based excipient containing a non-ionic surfactant, cellulose and modified cellulose, silica, stearic acid, pharmaceutical glaze, magnesium stearate, natural flavor and annatto as natural source of color.

— OPTIVITE PMT —

Ingredient	Amount per 6 tablets		%DV*
Vitamin A	12500	IU	250%
(as retinyl palmitate and 60% as beta-carotene)			
Vitamin C	1500	mg	2500%
Vitamin D (as cholecalciferol)	100	IU	25%
Vitamin E (as d-alpha tocopheryl succinate)	100	IU	333%
Thiamin (as thiamine mononitrate)	25	mg	1666%
Riboflavin	25	mg	1471%
Niacin (as niacinamide)	25	mg	125%
Vitamin B6 (as pyridoxine HCl)	300	mg	15000%
Folic Acid	200	mcg	50%
Vitamin B12 (as hydroxocobalamin)	60	mcg	1000%
Biotin	60	mcg	20%
Pantothenic Acid (as Ca Pantothenate)	25	mg	250%
Iron (as amino acid chelate)	15	mg	83%
Iodine (as hydrolyzed protein complex)	75	mcg	50%
Calcium (as amino acid chelate)	125	mg	12.5%
Magnesium (as amino acid chelate)	250	mg	63%
Zinc (as amino acid chelate)	25	mcg	167%
Selenium (as hydrolyzed protein complex)	100	mg	143%
Manganese (as amino acid chelate)	10	mg	500%
Chromium (as hydrolyzed protein complex)	100	mcg	83%
Potassium (as hydrolyzed protein complex)	48	mg	1%
Choline (from choline bitartrate)	313	mg	*
Citrus Bioflavonoids	250	mg	*
Betaine HCl	100	mg	*
Pancreatin 4X	93	mg	*
Inositol	24	mg	*
p-Aminobenzioc Acid (PABA)	25	mg	*
Rutlin	25	mg	*

* Daily Value (DV) not established.
Other ingredients: Stearic acid, carnauba wax, hydroxypropyl methlcellu-
lose, silica, magnesium stearate, pharmaceutical glaze, titanium dioxide, and
natural flavors.

— PROCYCLE PMS —

Ingredient.	Amount per 4 tablets	%DV*
Vitamin A	12500 IU	250%
(as Palmitate and 60% as beta-carotene)		
Vitamin C (ascorbic acid)	1500 mg	2500%
Vitamin D₃ (cholecalciferol)	400 IU	100%
Vitamin E (natural d-alpha tocopherol succinate)	200 IU	666%
Vitamin B₁ (thiamin HCl)	25 mg	1666%
Vitamin B₂ (riboflavin)	25 mg	1470%
Niacinamide	25 mg	125%
Vitamin B₆ (pyridozine HCl)	300 mg	15000%
Folic Acid	800 mcg	200%
Vitamin B₁₂a (hydroxocobalamin)	62.5 mcg	1041%
Biotin	62.5 mcg	20%
Pantothenic Acid (D-calcium pantothenate)	25 mg	250%
Calcium (amino acid chelate)	250 mg	25%
Iodine (from kelp)	75 mcg	50%
Magnesium (amino acid chelate)	500 mg	175%
Zinc (amino acid chelate)	25 mg	166%
Selenium (amino acid chelate)	200 mcg	285%
Copper (amino acid chelate)	5 mg	25%
Manganese (amino acid chelate)	10 mg	500%
Chromium (amino acid chelate)	200 mcg	166%
Potassium (citrate)	48 mg	1%
Propietary Blend	830.8 mg	*

Choline (bitartrate), Citrus Bioflavonoids, Betaine HCI, Pancreatin 4X (provides Protease, amylase and lipase), PABA (Para-Aminobenzoic Acid), Rutin and Inositol.

---

* Daily Value (DV) not established.
Other ingredients: Special Plant Cellulose, Vegetable Stearate, Natural Silica and Magnesium Stearate.

— FERTILITY BLEND FOR WOMEN —

Ingredient	Amount per 3 capsules		%DV*
Vitamin E (as d-alpha tocopherol)	150	IU	500%
Vitamin B6 (as pyridoxine hydrochloride)	6	mg	300%
Vitamin B12 (as cyanocobalamin)	12	mcg	200%
Folate (as folic acid)	400	mcg	100%
Iron (as gluconate)	18	mg	100%
Magnesium (as oxide)	400	mg	100%
Zinc (as gluconate)	15	mcg	100%
Selenium (as soduim selenate)	70	mcg	100%
Proprietary Blend	1080	mg	**

L-arginine
Green Tea (Camelia sinensis)-standardized (50% phenols)
Chasteberry (Vitex agnus-castus)-standardized (0.5% agnusides)

* Percent Daily Values (%DV) are based on a 2000-calorie diet.
** Daily Value (DV) not established.
Other ingredients: Rice Flour Powder, Silica, Magnesium Stearate.

— LIFETIME PROFESSIONAL PRENATAL FORMULA —

See *www.iherb.com* for ingredients.

Appendix B

Focus on Infertility

I will say to the north: Give them up! and to the south: Hold not back! Bring back my sons from afar, and my daughters from the ends of the earth. — Isaiah 43:6

The Couple to Couple League offers a systematic self-help approach to infertility that may help you to achieve pregnancy. Even if it does not help you directly, it will certainly tip the balance in favor of pregnancy as you seek medical care.

For six to nine months, implement all of the self-care options outlined below as a couple: charting and timing of intercourse, improved diet and nutritional supplementation for both spouses, and self-help targeted to the particular situation that seems to fit — weight gain if you are underweight, weight loss if you are overweight, and so forth. If in those six to nine months you do not become pregnant, continue the self-help strategies, but seek ethical medical intervention from a physician who is supportive of your moral values and is knowledgeable about or at least open to nutrition and nutritional supplements.

A. FOR 6–9 MONTHS, BOTH SPOUSES SHOULD IMPLEMENT ALL OF THE SELF-HELP OPTIONS THAT SEEM TO APPLY.

1. Take the CCL course, learn Natural Family Planning, and chart your cycles.

2. Time marital relations to the most fertile days of the cycle.

    a. Abstain for a few days before ovulation is expected.

    b. Have relations in an every-other-day pattern during the fertile time.

    c. Remain lying down for a short time after relations.

    d. If the mucus pattern is poor, the wife can use an over-the-counter product called Robitussin to improve her mucus secretion.

3. Make positive lifestyle changes.

    a. The husband should switch to wearing boxer shorts if his fertility status is unknown, or if he lives or works in a hot environment.

    b. Both spouses should quit smoking and avoid second-hand smoke.

    c. Alcoholic beverages should be used only in moderation.

d. At least the wife should limit caffeine to the equivalent of two cups of coffee daily.

e. The wife should try to lose or gain weight as needed.

f. For men, weight is not so critical, unless significant overweight or obesity is involved.

g. Get enough sleep, which along with better nutrition is a key to good health. A dark bedroom improves sleep and may improve the woman's reproductive hormones.

4. Both spouses should improve their diet as explained in Chapter 1.

5. Both spouses should take basic supplements as explained in Chapter 3.

a. For men: The vitamin Androvite for Men and flax oil and/or fish oil "covers all the bases."

b. For women, use a good multivitamin/multimineral, flax oil and/or fish oil, and other supplements as indicated by your chart and symptoms.

6. Use the NFP chart and other symptoms as detailed in Part II to make an educated guess as to what might be contributing to your infertility.

7. Men, consider Chapter 15 to improve your fertility if there is any doubt.

If you get pregnant within those six to nine months of self-help — wonderful! You won't be able to say exactly what might have helped, but you won't care! Your self-care will have been the best preparation for a healthy pregnancy, so continue the good nutrition and vitamins, minerals, and flax oil or fish oil, with the approval of your health care professional.

B. IF YOU ARE UNSUCCESSFUL IN THOSE SIX TO NINE MONTHS, CONTINUE YOUR SELF-HELP STRATEGIES, BUT ALSO LOOK FOR ETHICAL, PRUDENT MEDICAL INTERVENTION.

1. Do not wait longer than 12 months to do so.

2. Consult a fertility specialist rather than a family doctor or an obstetrician/gynecologist. A specialist who works with infertile couples on a daily basis is better able to offer you specific options based on your particular situation.

a. Choose a specialist who respects your moral beliefs.

b. Get a complete physical and hormonal evaluation.

c. Make sure the doctor can understand chart problems.

d. If at all possible, employ a doctor who uses a holistic approach that includes attention to nutrition, body weight, and lifestyle factors.

3. Proceed in a conservative, stair-step fashion.

a. Many doctors will start with a trial of Clomid or metformin before extensive testing. This can be a prudent starting point.

b. If you have had children or have miscarried previously, make sure there is a good reason if the doctor suggests semen evaluation or a test to see if your tubes are open. Request ethical semen collection, if necessary.

c. Be sure that ultrasounds and hormone tests are done at times consistent with what your NFP chart shows rather than with arbitrary cycle days.

If you get pregnant with such care, wonderful! Who knows how much of a difference all your self-help contributed!

C. IF YOU ARE STILL UNSUCCESSFUL, MAKE A DECISION AS TO HOW LONG YOU WILL CONTINUE, HOW MUCH MONEY YOU WILL SPEND ON INFERTILITY CARE, AND HOW MUCH ETHICAL INTERVENTION YOU WILL UNDERTAKE.

1. Consider your age, your finances, your own feelings about having another child, and whether or not it would still be possible or likely for you to conceive without medical care.

2. If you are Catholic, recognize that not all expensive and high-tech fertility care is immoral or forbidden by the Church. Make sure you know what is and what is not approved.

D. IF YOUR INFERTILITY PERSISTS AND YOU CONTINUE TO LONG FOR A CHILD, FOLLOW YOUR HEART AND CONSIDER ADOPTING A CHILD OR CHILDREN.

1. Infertility with longing for a child may be a call from God to place a homeless child into your family.

2. Adopting a child is not identical to giving birth, but it has a wonder and charm all its own that many people do not appreciate until they do adopt a child.

3. If it is a baby that is your heart's desire, you are most likely not too old to adopt a child from a country where adoptive parents are in short supply.

E. IN ANY CASE, PRAY ALWAYS FOR YOUR FAMILY AND FOR THE GRACE OF GOD TO MAKE PRUDENT DECISIONS AND TO LIVE WITH THOSE DECISIONS.

—— QUESTIONS AND ANSWERS ——

WHAT IS ROBITUSSIN? HOW DO I USE IT?

Robitussin is actually a cough medicine that makes nasal mucus more fluid. It also makes cervical mucus more fluid. Use the plain kind which contains the ingredient "guaifenesin" only. Any other variations of Robitussin, which contain other ingredients, may dry up mucus. Use plain Robitussin according to labeled directions on days of marital relations. While this recommendation may seem odd, it has helped many couples to conceive.

MY HUSBAND NEEDS A SEMEN ANALYSIS AND WE ARE TRYING TO DO THIS ETHICALLY. WHERE CAN WE OBTAIN A PERFORATED CONDOM?

A special type of condom is available from Apex Medical Technologies, Inc. The condom is thin, non-spermicidal and non-latex, and is only handled by the couple at home, who perforate it before having normal relations. Instructions are included for collecting the sample. (See "Resources.")

WHEN SHOULD COUPLES WHO HAVE ALREADY HAD CHILDREN SEEK FERTILITY CARE?

Answering the question of when to seek fertility care is not so hard for a couple in their fertile years who have never had children. Once 12 months of regular intercourse have passed without conceiving, most couples strongly suspect that something is wrong. Their friends, family, and doctor will assure them that that is not the ordinary way things happen. (If you are over 35, consider seeking fertility care after six months of infertility.)

It is for couples who have already had children that the question is harder to answer. The birth of a previous child or children reassures both of them that they are fertile, that having had a baby before is evidence that they can do it again. Yet all too often I meet couples in their fertile years who truly desire more children, but have not sought out fertility help after three, four, or five or more years of infertility. Do not wait more than 12 months.

I ALREADY HAVE [THREE, FOUR, FIVE, SIX] CHILDREN; HOW CAN I CALL THIS INFERTILITY?

Are you in your fertile years? The limit of human female fertility is about age 48; on average it declines sharply after age 45. Have you tried without success to conceive for at least six months to a year? Have you been able to rule out reversible causes such as underweight? If you answer yes to the above questions, your situation is called secondary infertility, which means difficulty in conceiving after having had children. The number of children you have already had is not part of the definition.

I ALREADY HAVE [THREE, FOUR, FIVE, SIX] CHILDREN; WILL THE DOCTOR LAUGH ME OUT OF THE OFFICE IF I GO THERE FOR INFERTILITY?

An NFP user with six children went through menopause at age 41. She was given the diagnosis in the office of a fertility specialist. She phoned me to ask about nutritional approaches. True menopause, with no periods and constant high levels of FSH and LH, is irreversible, both nutritionally and medically.

But I asked her a question: What did the doctor think of you, with six children, including preschoolers, seeking infertility treatment? Her answer was striking: The doctor had lived in Salt Lake City, Utah, where there is a high proportion of residents who are practicing Mormons, a faith which highly respects large families. He said that it was not uncommon for a Mormon woman to come to him in her early forties for fertility treatment, even though she might already have seven or eight children! So he was quite compassionate. By the way, this family dealt with this diagnosis in a wonderful way — they adopted a baby with special needs.

SHOULD I THINK THAT MAYBE GOD DOES NOT WANT US TO HAVE ANOTHER CHILD?

May I share my Catholic beliefs with you? God is the Lord of LIFE, and a soul for him in eternity procreated by a husband and wife is in keeping with His will! "Be fruitful and multiply" is a quote from Him.

All too often it seems to me that couples experiencing secondary infertility wonder if God is withholding children from them. I think the explanation is this: In most cases secondary infertility is hormonal in nature; it cannot be visualized like, for example, a fibroid tumor which is blocking the tubes. I do not imagine a woman who finds that she has a fibroid tumor that is causing her infertility would say that the fibroid tumor is evidence that "God does not want us to have another child." No, she most likely will have the surgery to remove the tumor. Hormonal imbalances and other less obvious factors may be more difficult to diagnose, but just because they cannot be seen does not mean that it is God preventing conception.

Let me use an analogy. If a young woman changes physically so that she notices very low basal temperatures, hair loss, coldness, fatigue, weight gain, and sluggish reflexes, yet nothing hurts and she still can tend to her home duties, should she conclude that God desires her to be a tired, low energy person? Of course not. If she is prudent she will go to considerable trouble to find the source of her problem. If it turns out to be a thyroid dysfunction, should she not be encouraged to take the thyroid hormone that can correct her problems and restore her good health?

WHAT IF MY FAMILY DOCTOR SAYS JUST TO WAIT?

Again, CCL advises six to nine months of charting, timing, weight gain or loss, and the vitamins and minerals which make the greatest difference to fertility. I am distressed to find that couples will wait longer than a year to seek help, having done all the self-care without success. If the wife is in her prime fertile years — say, up to age 35 — perhaps only time is lost. But if the wife is older than that, delay while waiting for another pregnancy could mean the difference between giving birth to more children or not.

Is it necessary to treat a physical disorder that doesn't hurt?

No, it is not, as long as the disorder is not life-threatening. Infertility is not life-threatening, and one could argue that it does not hurt like arthritis or a bad back. But it hurts one's heart in a way that those who have not suffered from it can hardly appreciate.

I just want to do things naturally.

The Catholic Church admonishes that when it comes to having children, we must do things naturally. That is, we may only conceive children by intercourse between husband and wife. As is obvious from this book, I am a strong advocate of natural self-help ways of improving fertility. Better diet, weight gain or loss, vitamin and mineral supplements, and timing of intercourse are all ways of improving the chances. However, if these measures do not work in six to nine months, CCL is wise to suggest that you seek medical assistance for diagnosis and treatment.

Let me repeat my previous analogy: If you have symptoms of low thyroid function, it is wise to look at your intake of iodine, essential fatty acids, and other vitamins and minerals. But, what if attention to good nutrition makes no difference? Wouldn't a prudent person seek medical help for proper diagnosis? Would he or she not take thyroid hormone as a medication in an attempt to correct overall health?

Fertility treatment takes injections, ultrasounds, and constant doctor visits. It's just too high-tech and expensive.

May I continue the analogy with thyroid function one more time? If a woman is diagnosed with low thyroid function, after a period of testing and adjustment, she can take a pill every day that can correct her hormonal problems. Why? Thyroid hormone is naturally secreted in a constant fashion, so one day's dose is the same as the next. Thyroid hormone, a small molecule derived from an amino acid, is not destroyed by the stomach or intestinal secretions, and it can be readily absorbed into the blood. Yes, it does take diagnosis and adjustment, but in theory and in practice, replacing thyroid hormone is relatively easy. Either synthetic thyroid hormone or hormones from slaughterhouse animals can be used, and the expense is modest.

In some cases, fertility treatment may just require oral supplements of thyroid medication, or the oral drugs Clomid or metformin. But there are reasons that some ethical fertility treatments involve injections and ultrasounds as well as significant expense. The fertility hormones FSH and LH are secreted in a manner that varies markedly throughout the cycle. Because they are protein hormones, they must be injected; otherwise the digestive system will destroy them. Progesterone may need to be injected in some cases, though other routes can also be used. In order to inject the right amount of hormone at the right time, ultrasounds of the developing follicles are essential.

Furthermore, if FSH and LH are required, they must come from human beings. It is very expensive to purify these hormones from huge quantities of urine from postmenopausal women. The changing pattern of hormone secretion and the nature of the hormones certainly makes hormone therapy for infertility more complicated than replacement of thyroid hormone, as in the example above.

SO YOU WOULD RECOMMEND SOME OF THESE HIGH-TECH FERTILITY PROCEDURES?

Let me restate CCL's recommendation for infertility: For six to nine months, try all of the self-help options in this book that are generally useful or are specific to your situation. If after that time you are still not pregnant, continue the self-care, but seek ethical medical care from a physician who is respectful of your moral beliefs and at least open to the role of nutrition.

Yes, this is a book that emphasizes nutrition for fertility. But ethical medical treatments are not incompatible with nutritional self-care, and the two together may make the difference.

I wish you all the children that your hearts desire.

Appendix C

Uterine Fibroids:
How I Kept my Uterus

by Kristine M. Severyn, R.Ph., Ph.D.

From *Family Foundations*, November-December 2004

Like many healthy women who practice and teach Natural Family Planning, I always thought hysterectomies were for other, older women … never for me. I planned to take my uterus with me to the grave. Thus, I was stunned to be diagnosed a month before my 50th birthday with the most common reason to surgically remove a uterus in the United States — uterine fibroids. In fifty percent of these operations, women also lose their ovaries.

Fibroids had enlarged my uterus to the size of an 18-week pregnancy, with the largest tumor the size of a softball. More than one-third of the 600,000 hysterectomies performed each year in this country are due to these benign growths.

Combining the diagnosis with my age, I became a target for gynecologists and general surgeons, who routinely view removal of the uterus and ovaries as a rite of passage for women in their 40s and 50s. Indeed, about one-third of American women will lose their uterus to surgery by the time they reach 60 years of age.

Since I did not relish castration as my 50th birthday present, and I wanted to keep my uterus, I spent five months researching non-hysterectomy options in medical and consumer sources. This research, along with my successful fibroid surgery, set me upon a mission to inform other women to be wary of pro-hysterectomy physicians.

The Lord truly blessed me with numerous resources, especially an experienced and understanding ob-gyn surgeon who never ridiculed my decision to keep my uterus, despite a diagnosis of large uterine fibroids. If you are diagnosed with uterine fibroids, in some cases hysterectomy may end up being the best option, but I've learned it should not be inevitable.

DOUBLE STANDARD
A general surgeon and a gynecologist told me that since I was too old to have more children, it was silly to have surgery to remove only the fibroids, called a myomectomy. Instead, they felt I should have my uterus, ovaries, and fallopian tubes all removed and go on estrogen replacement.

The surgeon even commented, "If you were my wife, that's what I would advise." By removing my healthy organs, he asserted that I would be spared future fears of cancer. With more research I found these claims unfounded, due to my lack of risk factors for such cancers (I was not overweight, never took hormones, was a virgin when I married, am monogamous, and gave birth to babies which I breastfed). When I asked the surgeon why men are not advised to have their testicles and prostates removed when their wives reach menopause, he retorted, "Well, men are different."

These physicians' medical advice seemed drastic and unnecessary to me, especially since fibroids virtually never become cancerous. Only a few months later my instincts were supported by new medical studies revealing the perils of long-term estrogen use in women (heart disease, breast cancer, dementia), leading women across the country to abandon their hormone prescriptions. In addition, I found that the standard practice of removing women's ovaries during hysterectomy for the purpose of cancer prevention is no guarantee against future ovarian cancer. The medical literature cites numerous examples of this cancer occurring in women who had their non-cancerous ovaries removed, i.e., ovarian cancer was found in other organs. And lastly, keeping one's ovaries facilitates a smoother transition to menopause, due to their ability to produce various hormones, even after menopause.

ADVERSE EFFECTS OF HYSTERECTOMY
Hysterectomy can be fraught with adverse physical, sexual, and psychological consequences, including urinary incontinence, vaginal prolapse, loss of sexual desire, inability to achieve orgasm, and depression. Medical studies reveal that urinary incontinence due to hysterectomy can manifest several years after the surgery. Sadly, mainstream medicine dismisses these problems as unrelated to hysterectomy.

An especially tragic case of potential dangers of hysterectomy involved a woman in my local community who wrongly trusted her gynecologist that hysterectomy was her only option for fibroids. The gynecologist damaged the woman's ureters (the tubes which carry urine from the kidneys to the bladder), leaving the woman with urine leaking out of her vagina. A second, temporary surgery fitted the woman with an external tube to collect urine outside her body. A third lengthy surgery attempted to permanently repair her problem. Last I heard, the woman left her job on disability and was in a nursing home.

Fortunately, a number of books and websites can help educate women about non-hysterectomy options, noted at the end of this article.

HOW COMMON ARE FIBROIDS?
About 50 percent of women have uterine fibroids, although most are unaware of their presence. An estimated 20 percent of white women and 50 percent of black women develop fibroids. The tumors also tend to run in families. (My older sister had them.)

Through my research I found two other CCL teachers affected by large fibroids. One woman chose no medical intervention, opting to wait for menopause, when the tumors tend to shrink. Two of us chose myomectomy, surgical removal of the fibroids, and were happy with the results. Living in different cities, we were both fortunate to find ob-gyn surgeons skilled in removing fibroids while retaining the uterus.

WHAT ARE THE SYMPTOMS OF FIBROIDS?

Most women have no symptoms with their fibroids. If symptoms occur, they usually affect menstruation, causing it to be more painful, with longer and/or heavier flow. With larger fibroids, pressure on the bladder may cause urinary frequency, or pressure on the rectum may cause constipation.

If painful or heavier periods begin to follow years of less painful periods, you may suspect fibroids. The ability to feel the largest tumor through my abdomen caused me to consult a gynecologist. Expansion of a woman's girth, without accompanying weight gain (more noticeable in thinner women), may also indicate the presence of uterine fibroids.

WHAT IS THE TREATMENT FOR FIBROIDS?

Because nearly 100 percent of fibroids will never become cancerous, they can be left alone, unless they are bothersome. Fibroids can also occur in younger women, but their time of most rapid growth is when a woman is aged 40–50. After menopause, when estrogen levels decrease, fibroids tend to shrink, but they may or may not totally disappear.

Depending on the size and location of the fibroids, combined with a woman's age, her desire to bear children, and how much trouble the tumors cause her, fibroid treatment varies. Treatment options include wait-and-see, estrogen antagonist injections (usually ineffective), uterine artery embolization, or surgery (myomectomy or hysterectomy).

Since the time of my surgery, **uterine artery embolization (UAE)** has become more prominent as a method to treat fibroids. Instead of a surgeon, the woman consults an interventional radiologist who, with the help of x-ray imaging, guides a catheter through a large groin blood vessel into the uterine blood vessels feeding the fibroids. Plastic spheres are injected into these vessels, and the fibroids shrink over a few months due to lack of blood supply. While some women have found success with this procedure, I am cautious about radiation and the injection of these spheres. This procedure can also eliminate a woman's ability to achieve orgasm.

WHAT ABOUT "ALTERNATIVE MEDICINE?"

While "alternative medicine," including diet, can be helpful for a variety of medical conditions, there is no evidence that it helps shrink uterine fibroids. Being an outspoken critic of mainstream medicine, I humbly admit that I am grateful for what surgery had to offer in the resolution of my fibroids. Even alternative medicine advocate and ob-gyn physician Dr. Christine Northrup, author of *Women's Bodies, Women's Wisdom,* finally agreed to surgery for her own large uterine fibroid. Despite unsuccessfully trying multiple alternative medicine modalities for four years, her fibroid continued to grow to the size of a large cantaloupe.

John Lee, M.D., saw success in slight shrinkage or preventing further growth of fibroids in his patients through the use of natural progesterone cream. This may be all that is needed to help a woman reach menopause, when fibroid symptoms usually decrease and tumors likely shrink. Natural progesterone cream is not the same as oral progestins, e.g., Provera. These latter products should be avoided due to their unpleasant side effects. Specifics on the use of natural progesterone cream are described in Dr. Lee's book, *What Your Doctor May Not Tell You About Premenopause.* (See "Further Reading.")

FIBROID SURGERY
In advanced western European countries, the surgical treatment for fibroids more routinely involves myomectomy, i.e., removing the tumor(s) while retaining the uterus. In contrast, the American surgical strategy is often hysterectomy. Ob-gyn physician Ivan Strausz, M.D., author of *You Don't Need a Hysterectomy,* calls hysterectomy "the ultimate failure in the care of fibroids," and feels it is "often...unjustified."

The medical controversy between the suitability of myomectomy vs. hysterectomy involves difficulties encountered in the two operations. For the experienced gynecological surgeon, hysterectomy is routine "cookbook" surgery. In contrast, myomectomy requires a surgeon with patience, who must think on his or her feet, making myomectomy less routine and often more tedious than hysterectomy. Thus, American physicians tend to prefer removing the uterus as opposed to repairing it. The risk of blood loss can be more significant with myomectomy than hysterectomy, but if handled correctly by a skilled surgeon, myomectomy can be very safe. Stanley West, M.D., author of *The Hysterectomy Hoax,* emphatically states: "There is no such thing as an impossible myomectomy."

One cited disadvantage of myomectomy is the approximately 30 percent chance of tumor recurrence in women who have the surgery in their 20s or early 30s. Ten percent of this group will require another myomectomy due to symptoms from their new fibroids. According to Lynn Payer, author of *How To Avoid A Hysterectomy,* the chance of fibroid regrowth should not, by itself, discourage a younger woman from seeking myomectomy instead of hysterectomy.

Tumor recurrence is much less of a problem, however, if myomectomy is performed in women closer to menopause, age mid- to late-forties. Despite the pressure many physicians place on women this age to undergo hysterectomy, Drs. Strausz and West believe these women are actually excellent candidates for myomectomy. Dr. West asserts, "There is no age limit to myomectomy."

Two years ago I underwent myomectomy by laparotomy, surgical removal of my fibroids through a 4 1/2-inch, horizontal, C-section-type incision. My carefully chosen ob-gyn surgeon knew I did not want blood transfusions or a hysterectomy. Prior to surgery, he assured me he would do nothing and sew me up with parts intact if things appeared more complicated than the ultrasounds suggested. In the end I hit the jackpot. All tumors were removed; I still have my uterus, tubes, and ovaries; and had minimal blood loss. After an overnight hospital stay I was discharged the next morning.

During the week following surgery I rested at home, taking only 600 mg of ibuprofen once or twice per day for pain. By three weeks post-op, I had returned to my daily 1.3-mile dog walks, twice-per-week lap swimming, and part-time hospital pharmacy job. Bike-riding soon followed.

WHAT HAVE I LEARNED?

1. Seek and ye shall find (Matthew 7:7). Plenty of good information is available for those who wish to resolve their fibroids without hysterectomy. While research takes time, it's worth it. Hysterectomy is permanent and often regretted.

2. If your doctor *only* encourages hysterectomy for your fibroids, run, don't walk, to find a second or even third opinion. There are good physicians out there who can fix your fibroids without resorting to hysterectomy. You may need to ask around, or travel to another town, but they're there.

— Dr. Severyn has a Ph.D. in biopharmaceutics and is a registered pharmacist. She and her husband, Tom, have been certified CCL Natural Family Planning teachers in Dayton, Ohio for 23 years.

Books and contacts that helped me learn more about fibroids and avoid hysterectomy:

1. *The Hysterectomy Hoax*, by Stanley West, M.D.

2. *You Don't Need a Hysterectomy*, by Ivan K. Strausz, M.D.

3. *The No-Hysterectomy Option*, by Herbert A. Goldfarb, M.D.

4. *How to Avoid a Hysterectomy*, by Lynn Payer

5. *Sex, Lies & the Truth About Uterine Fibroids*, by Carla Dionne (Founder and Executive Director, National Uterine Fibroids Foundation, ***www.uterinefibroids.com***)

6. Hysterectomy Educational Resources and Services (***www.HERSfoundation.com***)

7. *Fibroids*, by Johanna Skilling

8. *Women's Bodies, Women's Wisdom*, by Christine Northrup, M.D.

9. *What Your Doctor May Not Tell You about Premenopause*, by John R. Lee, M.D.

Endnotes

CHAPTER 1

1 Seeley, R., Stephens, T., and Tate, P. *Anatomy and Physiology* (New York: McGraw-Hill, 2008, p. 932). The essential amino acids are histidine, isoleucine, leucine, lysine, methionine, phenylalanine, threonine, tryptophan, and valine.

2 Chavarro, J., Willett, W., and Skerrett, P. *The Fertility Diet* (New York: McGraw-Hill, 2008, p. 81). If a "serving" of a food contains less than 0.5 grams of trans-saturated fat, it may be labeled "0 trans fats." Essentially no amount of trans fat is healthy, but 2.0 grams per day is considered acceptable by the United States Food and Drug Administration. This labeling policy makes it necessary to check for the presence of the term "partially hydrogenated," or "fully hydrogenated," whether or not a product advertises "0 trans fat" per serving.

3 Chavarro, J., Rich-Edwards, J., Rosner, B., et al. "Dietary fatty acids and the risk of ovulatory infertility" (*Am. J. Clin. Nutr.* 2007, 85:231-237).

4 Chavarro, J., Rich-Edwards, J., Rosner, B., et al. "A prospective study of dairy foods intake and anovulatory infertility" (*Human Reprod.* 2007, 22:1340-1347).

5 Gittleman, A. *Get the Sugar Out!*, 2nd ed. (New York: Three Rivers Press, 2008, pp. 53-58).

6 Chavarro, J., Willett, W., and Skerrett, P. (2008, p.147).

7 Dhingra, R., Sullivan, L., Jacques, P., et al. "Soft drink consumption and the risk of developing cardiometabolic risk factors and the metabolic syndrome in middle-aged adults in the community" (*Circulation* 2007, 116:480-488).

8 Gold, E., Bair, Y., Block, G., et al. "Diet and lifestyle factors associated with premenstrual symptoms in a racially diverse community sample: Study of women's health across the nation (SWAN)" (*J. Women's Health* 2007,16:641-656); Rossignol, A., and Bonnlander, H. "Caffeine-containing beverages, total fluid consumption, and premenstrual syndrome" (*Am. J. Public Health* 1990, 80:1106-1109).

9 Derbyshire, E. "Dietary factors and fertility in women of childbearing age" (*Nutrition and Food Science* 2007, 37:100-104).

10 Weng, X., Odouli, R., and Li, D. "Maternal caffeine consumption during pregnancy and the risk of miscarriage: A prospective cohort study" (*J. Obst. Gynecol.*, January 2008, pp. 1e1-1e8).

CHAPTER 2

1 Reinagle, M. *The Inflammation-Free Diet Plan* (New York: McGraw-Hill, 2006, p. 32).

2 Dickson, D. "Eating Sustainably" (3 *Rivers Food Co-op Currents*, Ft. Wayne, IN, Feb., 2008, p. 7).

3 Jemmott, J. "Chemicals, Contaminants, Pollution, Price: New Reasons to Rethink What You Drink" (*Reader's Digest Special Report*, Feb., 2008, pp. 118-125).

4 Keogh, J. "Nonstick Cookware Safety: Are There Alternatives to Teflon®?" (Revolution Health Group, *www.revolutionhealth.com/healthy-living*, updated 2/11/2008).

5 It is now possible to obtain non-stick cookware coated with natural ceramic powder. Starfrit® Alternative Eco-friendly Cookware is available at Amazon. com. It is recommended by Julian Whitaker, M.D., author of *Health and Healing* (Supplement to *Health and Healing*, May, 2008).

CHAPTER 3

1 Erasmus, U. *Fats That Heal, Fats That Kill* (Burnaby, BC, Canada: Alive Books, 1993, p. 282).

2 Saldeen, P., and Saldeen, T. "Women and omega-3 fatty acids" (*Obstet. Gynecol. Survey 2004*, 59:722-733).

3 Gittleman, A. *Get the Sugar Out!*, 2nd ed. (New York: Three Rivers Press, 2008, p. 239).

4 For a discussion of this topic in laymen's terms, see Raffelock, D., Rountree, R., and Hopkins, V. *A Natural Guide to Pregnancy and Postpartum Health* (New York: Avery, 2002, pp. 43-51).

5 See Appendix A, "Labeled Contents of Recommended Supplements." Guy Abraham, M.D., formulated both Optivite PMT and Androvite for Men.

6 Crook, W., Dean, C., and Crook, E. *The Yeast Connection and Women's Health* (Jackson, TN: Professional Books, 2005, p. 240).

7 Balch, P. *Prescription for Nutritional Healing*, 4th ed. (New York: Avery, 2006, p. 6).

8 "Introducing Dr. Whitaker's New and Updated Forward Plus Daily Regimen" *www.drwhitaker.com* (November, 2005). Complete listing of nutrients in Forward Plus, a multivitamin/multi-mineral/essential fatty acid supplement regimen formulated by Dr. Julian Whitaker.

9 Lee, J., with Hopkins, V. *What Your Doctor May Not Tell You About Menopause* (New York: Warner Books, 2004, pp. 418-424).

10 Raffelock, D., Rountree, R., and Hopkins, V. *A Natural Guide to Pregnancy and Postpartum Health* (New York: Avery, 2002, pp. 129-149).

11 Lark, S. "Daily Answer." Supplement to *The Lark Letter* (Potomac, MD: Healthy Directions, December, 2005, p. 3).

12   Seibel, M. "The role of nutrition and nutritional supplements in women's health" (*Fertil. Steril* 1999, 72:579-591).

CHAPTER 4

1   Gittleman, A. "Along Came Soy" in *Before the Change: Taking Charge of Your Perimenopause* (HarperSanFrancisco, a division of HarperCollins Publishers 2004, pp.137–141).

2   Chavarro, J., Willett, W., and Skerrett, P. *The Fertility Diet* (New York: McGraw-Hill, 2008, p. 99).

3   Chavarro, J., Toth, T., Sadio, S., et al. "Soy food and isoflavone intake in relation to semen quality parameters among men from an infertility clinic" (*Human Reprod.* 2008, 11:2584-2590).

4   Atkins, Robert C., *M.D. Dr. Atkins' New Diet Revolution* (New York: Quill, an Imprint of HarperCollins, 2002, p. 219).

5   Roberts, H., *Aspartame (NutraSweet): Is It Safe?* (Philadelphia: The Charles Press, 1990, pp. 168-172).

6   Gittleman, A. *Get the Sugar Out!* 2nd ed. (New York: Three Rivers Press, 2008, p. 69).

7   Hibbeln, J., Davis, J., Steer, C., et al. "Maternal seafood consumption in pregnancy and neurodevelopment outcomes in childhood (ALSPAC study: an observational cohort study)" (*The Lancet* 2007, 369:578-585).

8   Davis, A. *Let's Cook It Right* (New York: Signet Books, 1970, p. 15).

9   Whitaker, Julian, M.D. "Why Children Should Take Supplements" (*Health and Healing* 2001 11(9), 1-3).

10   Patel,. S., Malhotra, A., White, D., et al. "Association between reduced sleep and weight gain in women" (*Am. J. Epidemiology* 2007, 164: 947-954).

11   Whitaker, J. "Marvelous Melatonin" (*Health and Healing* 2008, 18 (2) 7-8).

12   Raffelock, D., Rountree, R., and Hopkins, V. (2002, p. 221).

13   Lee, J., and Hopkins, V. *Dr. John Lee's Hormone Balance Made Simple* (New York: Wellness Central, 2006, pp. 166-167).

CHAPTER 5

1   Harrison, M., and Ahlgrimm, M. *Self-Help for Premenstrual Syndrome*, 3rd ed. (New York: Random House, 1998, p. xiii).

2   Beck, S., and Abraham, G. *Optivite PMT and Gynovite Plus Total Dietary Programs for Premenstrual Syndrome and Menopause with Answers to the Most Commonly Asked Questions* (Torrance, CA: Optimox Corp., 1992, p. 26).

3   If you are bothered by acne, see the question and answer that covers this topic in Chapter 16.

4 Abraham, G. "Nutritional factors in the etiology of the premenstrual tension syndromes" (*J. Reprod. Med.* 1983, 28:446-464).

5 Abraham, G., and Rumley, R. "Role of nutrition in managing the premenstrual tension syndromes" (*J. Reprod. Med.* 1987, 32:405-422).

6 Goei, G., Ralston, J., and Abraham, G. "Dietary patterns of patients with premenstrual tension" (*J. Appl. Nutr.* 1982, 34:9-17).

7 Abraham, G. (1983).

8 Goei, G., Ralston, J., and Abraham, G. (1982).

9 Abraham, G., and Rumley, R. (1987).

10 Delitala, G., Masala, A., Alagna, S.,et al. "Effect of pyridoxine on human hypophyseal trophic hormone release: A possible stimulation of hypothalamic dopaminergic pathway" (*J. Clin. Endocrinol. Metab.* 1976, 42:603ff); Abraham, G. "Nutrition and the premenstrual tension syndromes" (*J. Appl. Nutr.* 1984, 36:103-124).

11 Abraham, G., and Rumley, R. (1987).

12 Hargrove, J., and Abraham, G. "Effect of vitamin B6 on infertility in women with the premenstrual tension syndrome." (*Infertility* 1979, 2:315ff).

13 Abraham, G., and Hargrove, J., "Effect of vitamin B6 on premenstrual symptomatology in women with premenstrual tension syndromes: A double blind crossover study" (*Infertility* 1980, 3:155ff); Williams, M., Harris, R., and Dean, B., "Controlled trial of pyridoxine in the premenstrual syndrome" (*J. Int. Med. Res.* 1985,13:174ff); Wyatt, K., Dimmock, P., Jones, P., et al. "Efficacy of vitamin B-6 in the treatment of premenstrual syndrome: systematic review" (*Br. Med. J.* 1999, 318:1375-1381); Canning, S., Waterman, M., and Dye, L. "Dietary supplements and herbal remedies for premenstrual syndrome (PMS): A systematic research review of the evidence for their efficacy" (*J. Reprod. And Infant Psychol.* 2007, 24:363-378); Kashanian, M., Mazinani, R., and Jalalmanesh, S. "Pyridoxine (vitamin B6) therapy for premenstrual syndrome" (*Int. J. Obstet. Gynecol.* 2007, 96:43-44).

14 Henmi, H., Endo, T., Kitajima, Y., et al. "Effect of ascorbic acid supplementation on serum progesterone levels in patients with a luteal phase defect" (*Fertil. Steril.* 2003, 80: 459-461).

15 Fuchs, N., Hakim, M., and Abraham, G. "The effect of a nutritional supplement, Optivite for Women, on premenstrual tension syndromes: I. Effect on blood chemistry and serum steroid levels during the midluteal phase" (*J. Appl. Nutr.* 1985, 37:1-11).

16 Abraham, G., and Rumley, R. (1987).

17 Abraham, G. (1983).

18 Abraham, G., and Lubran, M. " Serum and red cell magnesium levels in patients

with premenstrual tension" (*Am. J. Clin. Nutr.* 1981, 34:2364-2366).

19 Goei, G., Ralston, J., and Abraham, G. (1982).

20 Bendich, A. "The potential for dietary supplements to reduce premenstrual syndrome (PMS) symptoms" (*J. Amer. Coll. Nutr.* 2000, 19:3-12); Girman, A., Lee, R., and Kligler, B. "An integrative medicine approach to premenstrual syndrome"(*Clin. J. Women's Health* 2002, 2:116-127); Quaranta, S., Buscaglia, M., Meroni, M., et al. "Pilot study of the efficacy and safety of a modified-release magnesium 250 mg tablet (Sincromag®) for the treatment of premenstrual syndrome" (*Clin. Drug. Invest.* 2007, 27:51-58).

21 Abraham, G., and Rumley, R. (1987).

22 Abraham, G. (1983).

23 Goei, G., Ralston, J., and Abraham, G. (1982).

24 Abraham, G. (1983).

25 Abraham, G., and Rumley, R. (1987).

26 Abraham, G. (1984).

27 Abraham, G., and Taylor, R. "Premenstrual Tension Syndromes" in *Current Therapy in Obstetrics and Gynecology*, edited by E. Quilligan, M.D., and F. Zuspan, M.D. (Philadelphia: W.B. Saunders Co., 1990, pp. 100-105).

28 "The monounsaturates and polyunsaturates should come predominantly from vegetables oils in order to emphasize oleic, cis-linoleic, and alpha-linolenic acid. Good sources of these unsaturated fatty acids are, respectively, olive, safflower, and flaxseed oil. The ingestion of animal fats and hydrogenated vegetables should be curtailed in order to minimize the intake of arachidonic acid, saturated fatty acids, and trans-unsaturated fatty acids." Abraham, G., and Taylor, R. (1990).

29 Abraham, G. (1983); Beck, S., and Abraham, G. (1992, p. 3).

30 Abraham, G., and Taylor, R. (1990).

31 Rossignol, A., and Bonnlander, H. "Caffeine-containing beverages, total fluid consumption, and premenstrual syndrome" (*Am. J. Public Health* 80:1106-1110, 1990).

32 Beck, S., and Abraham, G. (1992, p. 27).

33 Roberts, H., *Aspartame (NutraSweet): Is It Safe?* (Philadelphia: The Charles Press, 1990, pp. 168-172).

34 Goei, G., and Abraham, G. "Effect of a nutritional supplement, Optivite, on symptoms of premenstrual tension" (*J. Reprod. Med.* 1983, 28:527-531).

35 Abraham and Rumley (1987); Chakmakjian, Z., Higgins, C., and Abraham, G. "The effect of a nutritional supplement, Optivite for Women, on premenstrual

tension syndromes: II. Effect on symptomatology, using a double-blind crossover design" (*J. Appl. Nutr.* 1985, 37:12ff); Stewart, A., "Clinical and biochemical effects of nutritional supplementation on the premenstrual syndrome" (*J. Reprod. Med.* 1987, 32:435-441); London, R., Bradley, L., and Chiamori, N. "Effect of a nutritional supplement on premenstrual symptomatology in women with premenstrual syndrome: A double blind longitudinal study" (*J. Am. Coll. Nutr.* 1991, 10:494-499).

36 Kashanian, Mazinani, and Jalamanesh (2007).

37 Hemni, H., Endo, T., Kitajima, Y., et al. (2003).

38 Fuchs, N., Hakim, M., and Abraham, G. (1985).

39 Optimox Corp. (***www.Optimox.com***, March 24, 2009).

40 Abraham, G., and Rumley, R. (1987).

41 Beck, S., and Abraham, G. (1992, p. 18).

42 Ahlgrimm., M., in "In Step with Marla Ahlgrimm," by M. Shannon (*Family Foundations* 2008, 34(6):30-31).

43 Schellenberg, R. "Treatment for the premenstrual syndrome with Vitex agnus castus fruit extract: prospective, randomized, placebo controlled study" (*Br. Med. J.* 2001, 322:134-137).

44 Girman, A., Lee, R., and Kligler, B. (2002).

45 Wutteke, W. "Dopaminergic action of extracts of Vitex agnus castus" (*Forschende Komplementarmedizen* 1996, 6:329-330).

46 Westphal, L., Polan, M., and Trant, A. "Double-blind, placebo-controlled study of FertilityBlend: a nutritional supplement for improving fertility in women" (*Clin. Exp. Obst. & Gyn.* 2006, xxxiii:205-208).

47 Thys-Jacobs, S., McMahon, D., and Bilezikian, J. "Cyclical changes in calcium metabolism across the menstrual cycle in women with premenstrual dysphoric disorder" (*J. Clin. Endocrinol. Metab.* 2007, 92:2952-2959).

48 Bertone-Johnson, E., Hankinson, S., Benich, A., et al. "Calcium and vitamin D intake and risk of incident premenstrual syndrome" (*Arch. Intern. Med.* 2005, 165:124601252).

49 Thys-Jacobs, S., Starky, P., Bernstein, D., et al. " Micronutrients and the premenstrual syndrome: the case for calcium" (*J. Am. Coll. Nutr.* 2000, 19:220-227).

50 Lark, S. "The Celebrity's Edge" (*The Lark Letter*, July, 2004, pp. 1-5).

51 Ahlgrimm, M. (2008).

52 For an explanation of the value of salivary testing, see Lark, S. "The Salivary Hormone Test: Why It's Better Than the Rest" (*Women's Wellness Today* 14 (1):4-5; or ***www.drlark.com***).

53 Barron, M. "Light exposure, melatonin secretion, and menstrual cycle parameters: an integrative review" (*Biol. Res. Nursing* 2007, 9:49-69).

54 Bertone-Johnson, E., Hankinson, S., Bendich, A., et al. (2005).

55 Abraham, G. (1990, p. 105).

56 Bertone-Johnson, E., Hankinson, S., Bendich, A., et al. (2005).

57 2007-08 PMS: How Far Have We Really Come? (*Women's Health America Online Newsletter* (**www.womenshealth.com**, August, 2007).

58 Ahlgrimm, M. (2008).

59 Beck, S., and Abraham, G. (1992).

60 Shrim, A. Boskovic, C., Maltepe, Y., et al. "Pregnancy outcome following use of large doses of vitamin B6 in the first trimester" (*J. Obstet. Gynecol.* 2006, 26:749-751).

61 Ahlgrimm, M. (2008).

CHAPTER 6

1 Livdans, A., Harvey, P., and Larkin-Thier, S. "Menorrhagia: A synopsis of management focusing on herbal and nutritional supplements, and chiropractic" (*J. Can. Chiropr. Assoc* 2007, 51:235-246).

2 Livdans, A., Harvey, P., and Larkin-Thier, S. (2007).

3 Rothman, K., and Moore, L. "Teratogenicity of high vitamin A intake" (*NEJM* 1995, 333:1369-1373). Beta-carotene, which is not pre-formed vitamin A, can be taken in amounts far higher than the guideline given here.

4 Livdans, A., Harvey, P., and Larkin-Thier, S. (2007).

5 Hudson, T. "Using nutrition to relieve primary dysmenorrhea" (*Alt. & Comp. Therapies*, June 2007, pp. 125-128).

6 Proctor, M., and Farquhar, C. "Diagnosis and management of dysmenorrhea" (*Br. Med. J.* 2006, 332:1134-1138).

7 Visvanathan, N., and Wyshak, g. "Tubal ligation, menstrual changes, and menopausal symptoms" (*J. Women's Health and Gender-Based Medicine* 2000, 9:521-527); Kutlar, I., Ozkur, A., Balat, O., et al. "Effects of three different sterilization methods on utero-ovarian Doppler blood flow and serum levels of ovarian hormones" (*Euro. J. Obstet. Gynecol. and Reprod. Biol.* 2005, 122:112-117).

8 Livdans, A., Harvey, P., and Larkin-Thier, S. (2007).

9 Derman, O., Kanbur, N., Tokur, T., et al. "Premenstrual syndrome and associated symptoms in adolescent girls" (*Euro. J. Obstet. Gynecol. and Reprod. Biol.* 2004, 116:201-206).

10 Puder, J. , Blum, C., Mueller, B., et al. "Menstrual cycle symptoms are associated

with changes in low-grade inflammation" (*Euro. J. Clin. Invest.* 2006, 36:58-64).

11 Horrobin, D. "The role of essential fatty acids and prostaglandins in the premenstrual syndrome" (*J. Reprod. Med.* 1983, 28:465-468).

12 Proctor, M., and Farquhar, C. (2006).

13 Fjerbaek, A., and Knudsen, U. "Endometriosis, dysmenorrhea, and diet — What is the evidence?" (*Euro. J. Obstet. Gynecol.* 2007, 132:140-147).

14 Harel, Z., Biro, F., Kottenhahn, R., et al. "Supplementation with omega-3 polyunsaturated fatty acids in the managment of dysmenorrhea in adolescents" (*Am. J. Obstet. Gynecol.* 1996, 174:1335-1338).

15 Deutch, B., Jorgensen, E., and Hansen, J. "Menstrual discomfort in Danish women reduced by dietary supplements of omega-3 PUFA and B12" (*Nutr. Res.* 2000, 20:621-631).

16 Saldeen, P. and Saldeen, T. "Women and Omega-3 fatty acids" (*Obstet. Gynecol. Survey* 2004, 59:722-730).

17 Ziaei, S., Faghihzadeh, S., Sohrabvand, F., et al. "A randomised placebo-controlled trial to determine the effect of vitamin E in treatment of pimary dysmenorrhea" (*Br. J. Obstet. Gynecol.* 2001, 108:1181-1183); Dennehy, C. "The use of herbs and dietary supplements in gynecology: an evidenced-based review" (*J. Midwifery & Women's Health* 2006, 51:402-409).

18 Dennehy, C. (2006); Proctor, M., and Farquhar, C. (2006).

19 Witz, C., and Burn, W. "Endometriosis and infertility: Is there a cause and effect relationship?" (*Gyn. And Obstet. Invest.* 2002, 5(suppl:)2-11).

20 Osteen, K., Bruner-Tran, K., and Eisenberg, E. "Reduced progesterone action during endometrial maturation: a potential risk factor for the development of endometriosis" (*Fert. Steril.* 2005, 83:529-537); Bulun, S., Cheng, Y., Yin, P., et al. "Progesterone resistance in endometriosis: link to failure to metabolize estradiol" (*Molec. and Cell. Endocrinol* 2006, 248:94-103).

21 Cunha-Filio, J., Gross, J., Lemos, N., et al. "Hyperprolactinemia and luteal insufficiency in infertile patients with mild and minimal endometriosis" (*Horm. Metab. Res.* 2001, 33:216-220).

22 Hargrove, J., and Abraham, A. "The ubiquitousness of premenstrual tension in gynecologic practice" (*J. Reprod Med.* 1983, 28:435-437).

23 Hargrove, J., and Abraham, A. "Abnormal luteal function in women with endometriosis" (*Fertil. Steril.* 1983, 34:302).

24 Hargrove, J. Personal communication to Marilyn Shannon (April 6, 1990).

25 Sesta, F., Pietropolli, A., Capozzola, T., et al. "Hormonal suppression treatment of dietary therapy versus placebo in the control of painful symptoms after conservative surgery for endometriosis stage III-IV. A randomized comparative

trial" (*Fertil. Steril.* 2007, 88:1541-1547).

26 Lark, S. "End the Pain of Endometriosis" (*Women's Wellness Today,* June, 2008, pp. 6-7).

27 Kohama, T., Herai, K., and Inoue, M. "Effect of French maritime pine bark extract on endometriosis as compared with leuprorelin acetate" (*J. Reprod. Med.* 2007, 52:703-708).

28 Lark, S. (June, 2008).

29 Crook, W., Dean, C., and Crook, E. *The Yeast Connection and Women's Health* (Jackson, TN: Professional Books, 2005, p.74).

CHAPTER 7

1 De Souza, M. "Menstrual disturbances in athletes: A focus on luteal phase defects" (*Med. Sci. Sports Exer.* 2003, 35:1553-1563); De Souza, M., Van Heest, J., Demers, L., et al. "Luteal phase defects in recreational runners: Evidence for a hypometabolic state" (*J. Clin. Endocrinol Metab.* 2003, 88:337-346).

2 Bruchalski, J. (Personal communication to M. Shannon, October 6, 2008). John Bruchalski, M.D., is an NFP-only obstetrician/gyneoclogist at the Tepeyac Family Center in Fairfax, VA.

3 Roberts, C., and Murphy, A. "Endocrinopathies associated with recurrent pregnancy loss" (*Sem. in Reprod. Med.* 2000, 18:357-362).

4 Roberts, C., and Murphy, A. (2000).

5 Dudas, I., Rockenbauer, M., and Czeizel, A. "The effect of preconceptual multivitamin supplementation on the menstrual cycle" (*Arch. Gynecol. Obstet.* 1995, 256:115-123).

6 Check, J. "Ovulation defects despite regular menses: part III" (*Clin. Exp. Obst. & Gyn.* 2007, XXXIV: 133-136).

7 McIntosh, E. "Treatment of women with the galactorrhea-amenorrhea syndrome with pyridoxine (vitamin B6)" (*J. Clin. Endocrinol Metab.* 1976, 1192ff)

8 Hargrove, J., and Abraham, G. "Effect of vitamin B6 on infertility in women with the premenstrual tension syndrome" (*Infertility* 1979, 2:315-317).

9 Henmi, H., Endo, T., Kitajima, Y., et al. "Effect of ascorbic acid supplementation on serum progesterone levels in patients with a luteal phase defect" (*Fertil. Steril.* 2003, 80: 459-461).

10 Abraham, G. "Nutritional factors in the etiology of the premenstrual tension syndromes" (*J. Reprod. Med.* 1983, 28:446-464).

11 Fuchs, N., Hakim, M., and Abraham, G. "The effect of a nutritional supplement, Optivite for Women, on premenstrual tension syndromes: I. Effect on blood chemistry and serum steroid levels during the midluteal phase" (*J. Appl. Nutr.* 1985, 37:1-11).

12 Kasse-Annese, B., and Danzer, H. *The Complete Guide to the Treatment of Premenstrual Problems* (Santa Monica, CA: Patterns Publishing, 1984, p. 65).

13 Westphal, L., Polan, M., and Trant, A. "Double-blind, placebo-controlled study of FertilityBlend: a nutritional supplement for improving fertility in women" (*Clin. Exp. Obst. & Gyn.* 2006, xxxiii:205-208).

14 Westphal, L., Polan, M., and Trant, A. (2006).

15 Milewicz, A., Gejdel, E., Sworen, H., et al. "Vitex agnus castus-extrakt zur behandlung von regeltempoanomalien infolge latenter hyperprolaktinamie" (*Arzneimettel-Forschung* 1993, 43:752-756; reviewed in Fugh-Berman, A., and Kronenberg, F. "Complementary and alternative medicine (CAM) in reproductive-age women: a review of randomized controlled studies" (*Reproductive Toxicology* 2003, 17:137-152).

16 Poppe, K., Velkeniers, B., and Glinoert, D. "Thyroid disease and female reproduction" (*Clin. Endocrinol.* 2007, 66:309-321).

17 Shomon, M. *The Thyroid Hormone Breakthrough: Overcoming Sexual and Hormonal Problems at Every Age* (New York: Collins, an imprint of HarperCollins, 2006, pp. 33-34, 37).

18 Lark, S. "Solutions for a Healthy Thyroid" (*Women's Wellness Today* 2007, 14:1-5).

19 Shomon, M. (2006, pp. 82-86).

20 Shomon, M. (2006, p. 80).

21 Balch, P. *Prescription for Nutritional Healing*, 4th ed. (New York: Avery Press, 2006, p. 503).

22 Melotte-Athmer, A. "Iodine needed for proper thyroid function" (*CCL News* 1986, 12(5):3).

23 Whitaker, J. "Could It Be Your Thyroid?" (*Health and Healing* 2007, 17(6):1-7).

24 De Souza, M., Van Heest, J., Demers, L., et al. (2003).

25 Frisch, R. *Female Fertility and the Body Fat Connection* (Chicago: University of Chicago Press, 2002, p. 99).

26 Lark. S., (2007); Whitaker, J., (2007); Shomon, M., (2006, pp. 69-71).

27 Franklyn, J. "Subclinical thyroid disorders–Consequences and implications for treatment" (*Annales d'Endocrinologie* 2007, 68:229-230).

28 Barnes, B., and Galton, L. *Hypothyroidism: The Unsuspected Illness* (New York: Harper and Row, 1976, p. 136).

29 Puglio, P. "Hypothyroidism: The relationship to menstrual disorders." (*Women's Health Connections*, Complementary Issue II). Available through the Barnes

Foundation, P.O Box 110098, Trumbull, CT 06611. Telephone 203-261-2101; or *www.brodabarnes.org.*

30 Barnes, B., and Galton, L. (1976, p. 46).

31 *www.brodabarnes.org.*

32 Franklyn, J. (2007).

33 Frisch, R. (2002, pp. 75-78).

34 Frisch, R. (2002, p. 17).

35 Frisch, R. (2002, pp. 85-88).

36 Frisch, R., (2002, p. 141).

37 Manore, M. "Nutritional recommendations and athlete menstrual dysfunction" (*Int. Sports Med J.* 2004, 5:45-55).

38 Frisch, R. (2002, pp. 170-173).

39 De Souza, M., (2003); De Souza, M., Van Heest, J., Demers, L., et al. (2003).

40 Manore, M. (2004).

41 Manore, M. (2004).

CHAPTER 8

1 Rotterdam ESHRE/ASRM-Sponsored Consensus Workshop Group. "Revised 2003 consensus on diagnostic criteria and long-term health risks related to poly-cystic ovary syndrome" (*Fertil. Steril.* 2004, 81:19-25).

2 Norman, R., Dewailly, D., Legro, R., et al. "Polycystic ovary syndrome" (*The Lancet* 2007, 370:685-697).

3 Norman, R., Dewailly, D., Legro, R., et al. (2007).

4 Norman, R., Dewailly, D., Legro, R., et al. (2007).

5 Franks, S., Robinson, S., and Willis, D. "Nutrition, insulin, and polycystic ovary syndrome" (*Reviews of Reproduction* 1996, 1:47-53).

6 Franks, S., Robinson, S., and Willis, D. (1996).

7 Kasin-Karakas, S., Cunningham, W., and Tsodikov, A. "Relation of nutrients and hormones in polycystic ovary syndrome" (*Am. J. Clin.* 2007, 85:688-694).

8 Liepa, G., Sengapta, A., and Karsies, D. "Polycystic ovary syndrome (PCOS) and other androgen excess-related conditions: Can changes in dietary intake make a difference?" (*Nutrition in Clin. Prac.* 23:63–71, 2008).

9 Kasin-Karakas, S., Cunningham, W., and Tsodikov, A. (2007).

10 Atkins, R. "Atkins diet relieves ovarian-cyst problems." (*Dr. Atkins' Health*

Revelations, July, 2000, pp. 3-5).

11 Chavarro, J., Willett, W., and Skerrett, P. *The Fertility Diet* (New York: McGraw-Hill 2008, p. 183).

12 Chavarro, J., Rich-Edwards, J., Sosner, B., et al. "Dietary fatty acid intake and the risk of ovulatory infertility" (*Am. J. Clin. Nutr.* 2007, 85:231-237).

13 Chavarro, J. Personal communication to M. Shannon (Mar. 17, 2008) "In the overwhelming majority of cases the underlying condition affecting ovulation was PCOS although there were other conditions that we considered as accurate reports of 'ovulatory infertility' such as anovulation due to hyperprolactinemia, hypothyroidism, hypopituitarism and premature ovarian failure."

14 Chavarro, J., Willett, W., and Skerrett, P. (2008, pp. 147, 184).

15 Gittleman, A. *Get the Sugar Out!*, 2nd ed. (New York: Three Rivers Press, 2008, pp. 14-16).

16 Chavarro, J., Rich-Edwards, J., Rosner, B., and Willett, W. "A prospective study of dairy foods intake and anovulatory infertility" (*Human Reprod.* 2007, 22:1340-1347).

17 Dhingra, R., Sullivan, L., Jacques, P., et al. "Soft drink consumption and the risk of developing cardiometabolic risk factors and the metabolic syndrome in middle-aged adults in the community" (*Circulation* 2007, 116:480-488).

18 Roberts, H., *Aspartame (NutraSweet): Is It Safe?* (Philadelphia: The Charles Press, 1990, pp. 147-150).

19 Roberts (1990, pp. 194-195).

20 Chavarro, J., Rich-Edwards, J., Rosner, B., et al. "Use of multi-vitamins, intake of B vitamins, and risk of ovulatory infertility" (*Fertil. Steril.* 2008, 89:668-676).

21 Guzelmeric, K., Alkan, N., Pirimoglu, M., et al. "Chronic inflammation and elevated homocysteine levels are associated with increased body mass index in women with polycystic ovary syndrome" (*Gynecol. Endocrinol.* 2007, 23:505-510).

22 Kilicdag, E., Bagis, T., Tarim, E., et al. "Administration of B-group vitamins reduces circulating homocysteine in polycystic ovarian syndrome patients treated with metformin: a randomized trial" *Human Reprod.* 2005, 20:1521-1528).

23 Schachter, M., Raziel, A., Strassburger, D., et al. "Prospective, randomized trial of metformin and vitamins for the reduction of plasma homocysteine in insulin-resistant polycystic ovary syndrome" (*Fertil. Steril.* 2007, 88:227-230).

24 Hahn, S., Haselhorst, U., Tan, S., et al. "Low serum 2,5-hydroxyvitamin D concentrations are associated with insulin resistance and obesity in women with polycystic ovary syndrome" (*Exp. Clin. Endocrinol. Diabetes* 2006, 114:557-583).

25 Ingraham, B., Bragdon, B., and Nohe, A. "Molecular basis of the potential of vitamin D to prevent cancer" (*Cur. Med. Res. Opin.* 2008, 24:139-149).

26 Whitaker, J. "Weight Loss is Not Just About Fat" (*Health and Healing* 1997, 7:5-8).

27 Whitaker, J., Personal communication to M. Shannon (October 12, 1996) Dr. Whitaker stated that 400 mcg of chromium is safe during pregnancy.

28 Balch, P. *Prescription for Nutritional Healing*, 4th ed. (New York: Avery, 2006, pp. 33, 362).

29 Kasim-Karakas, S., Almario, R., Gregory, L., et al. "Metabolic and endocrine effects of a PUFA rich diet in PCOS (*J. Clin. Endocrinol. Metab.* 89:615–620, 2004).

30 Saldeen, P., and Saldeen, T. "Women and omega-3 fatty acids" [CME Review Article] (*Obstet. Gynecol. Survey* 2004, 59:722-730).

31 Moran, L. et al. "Exercise and lifestyle modification in PCOS [Symposium: Effects of lifestyle modification in PCOS]" (*Reprod. BioMedicine Online* 2002, pp. 573-578).

32 Randeva, H., Lewandowski, K., Drzewoski, J., et al. "Exercise decreases plasma total homocysteine in overweight young women with polycystic ovary syndrome" (*J. Clin. Endocrinol. Metab.* 2002, 87:4496-4501).

33 "Nutrition Information Leads to Much-Desired Pregnancy," Letter to the Editor (*Family Foundations*, Sept.-Oct. 2001, p. 25).

34 Shomon, M. *The Thyroid Hormone Breakthrough: Overcoming Sexual and Hormonal Problems at Every Age* (New York: Collins, an imprint of HarperCollins, 2006, pp. 33, 37).

35 Lee, J., and Hopkins, V. *Dr. John Lee's Hormone Balance Made Simple* (New York: Warner Wellness, 2006, pp. 102-103).

CHAPTER 9

1 Crook, W. *The Yeast Connection* (Jackson, TN: Professional Books, 1986, p. 1).

2 Galland, L. "Foreword" in *The Yeast Connection and Women's Health*, by William G. Crook, M.D., with Carolyn Dean, M.D. (Jackson, TN: Professional Books, 2005, pp. xi-xiv).

3 Murray, M. *Chronic Candidiasis* (Roseville, CA: Prima Publishing, 1997, pp. 14-16).

4 Crook, W. *The Yeast Connection and Women's Health* (Jackson, TN: Professional Books, 2005, pp. 12-13).

5 Smith, K. "Purging out the yeast: An informal study of yeast overgrowth" (An unpublished document provided by K. Smith to M. Shannon, June, 2004).

6 Trowbridge, J., and Walker, M. *The Yeast Syndrome* (New York: Bantam Books, 1986, p. 187).

7 Lark, S. "The Countless Pros of Probiotics" (*Women's Wellness Today*, March, 2008, pp.1-5).

8 Galland, L. "Nutrition and Candida Albicans" *in* Bland, J. *A Year in Nutritional Medicine*, 2nd ed. (New Canaan, CT: Keats Publishing, 1986, pp. 211-220).

9 Crook, W., (2005, p. 240); Murray, M., (1997, pp. 78-79); Trowbridge, J., and Walker, M., (1986, pp. 168-169).

10 Smith, K. (2004).

11 Schwarzbein, D. *The Schwarzbein Principle II: The Transition* (Deerfield Beach, FL: Health Communications 2002, p. 378).

12 Sutterlin, M., Bussen, S., Rieger, L., et al. "Serum folate and vitamin B12 levels in women using modern oral contraceptives (OC) containing 20 mg ethynyl estradiol" (*European J. Obstet. Gynecol. & Reprod. Biol.* 2003, 107:57-61).

13 Thane, C., Bates, C., and Prentice, A. "Oral contraceptives and nutritional status in adolescent British girls" (*Nutri. Res.* 2002, 22:449-462).

14 Berry, C., Montgomery, C., Sattar, N., et al. "Fatty acid status of women of reproductive age" (*European J. Clin. Nutr.* 2001, 55:518-524).

15 Thane, C., Bates, C., and Prentice, A. (2002).

16 Thane, C., Bates, C., and Prentice, A. (2002).

17 Grant, E. *Sexual Chemistry: Understanding Our Hormones, the Pill and HRT* (London: Cedar Press, 1994, pp. 12, 13, 103).

18 Barron, M. "Light exposure, melatonin secretion, and menstrual cycle parameters: An integrative review" (*Biological Research for Nursing* 2007, 9:49-69).

19 Barron, M. (2007).

20 Davis, S., Mirick, D., and Stevens, R. "Night shift work, light at night, and risk of breast cancer" (*J. National Cancer Institute* 2001, 93:1557-1562).

21 Barron, M. (2007).

22 DeFelice, J. "The Effects of Light on the Menstrual Cycle: Also Infertility, Clinical Observations" (Spokane, Washington: The Natural Family Planning Program of the Sacred Heart Medical Center, 2003).

23 Barron, M. (2007).

24 DeFelice, J. (2003).

25 DeFelice, J. (2003).

26 Barron, M. (2007).

27 Whitaker, J. "Reset Your Biological Clock" (*Health and Healing* 2003, 13(2), pp. 6-8).

28 Takasaki, A., Nakamura, Y., Tamura, H., et al. "Melatonin as a new drug for improving oocyte quality" (*Reprod. Med. and Biol.* 2003, 2:139-144).

29 Whitaker, J. (2003).

30 DeFelice, J. (2003, p. 23).

31 Wilcox, A., Weinburg, C., and Baird, D. "Caffeinated beverages and decreased fertility" (*The Lancet*, Dec. 24/31, 1988, pp. 1453-1455).

32 Christianson, R., Oechsli, F., and van den Berg, B. "Caffeinated beverages and decreased fertility" (*The Lancet*, Feb. 8, 1989, p. 378); Bolumar, F., Olsen, J., Rebagliato, M., et al. "Caffeine intake and delayed conception: A European multicenter study on infertiltiy and subfecundity" (*Am. J. Epidemiology* 1997, 145:324-334); Derbyshire, E. "Dietary factors and fertility in women of child-bearing age" (*Nutrition and Food Science* 2007, 37:100-104).

33 Caan, B., Quesenberry, C., and Coates, A. "Differences in fertility associated with caffeinated beverage consumption" (*Am. J. Public Health* 1998, 88:270-273).

34 Weng, X., Odouli, R., and Li, D. "Maternal caffeine consumption during pregnancy and the risk of miscarriage: a prospective cohort study" (*J. Obst. Gynecol.*, Jan. 2008, pp. 1e1-1e8).

35 Caan, B., Quesenberry, C., and Coates, A. (1998).

36 Pellicano, R., Astegiano, M., Bruno, M., et al. "Women and celiac disease: association with unexplained infertility" (*Minerva Medica* 2007, 98:217-219).

37 Lark, S. "Living Well with Celiac Disease" (*The Lark Letter*, Mar. 2006, pp. 5-8).

38 Hin, H., and Ford, F. "Celiac disease and infertility: making the connection and achieving a successful pregnancy" (*J. Family Health Care* 2002, 12:94-97).

39 Bradley, R., and Rosen, M. "Subfertility and gastrointestinal disease: 'Unexplained' is often undiagnosed" [CME review article] (*Obstet. Gynecol. Survey* 2004, 59:108-117).

40 Chavarro, J., Willett, W., and Skerrett, P. *The Fertility Diet* (New York: McGraw-Hill, 2008, pp. 129-131).

41 Shrim, A., Boskovic, R., Maltepe, C., et al. "Pregnancy outcome following use of large doses of vitamin B6 in the first trimester" (*J. Obstet. Gynecol.* 2006, 26: 749-751); Guy Abraham, M.D., also reports this upper level safe and beneficial during pregnancy when used as part of a multi-vitamin/multimineral containing other B vitamins and magnesium: Beck, S., Abraham, G. "Optivite PMT and Gynovite Plus Total Dietary Programs for Premenstrual Syndrome and Menopause" (Torrance, CA: Optimox Corp., 1992, p. 27).

42 Wilson, W. "Pre-conceptional vitamin/folic acid supplementation 2007: The use of folic acid in combination with a multi-vitamin supplement for the prevention of neural tube defects and other congenital anomalies." (Joint Society of Obstetricians and Gynaecologists of Canada-Motherisk Clinical Practice Guideline (*J. Obstetricians and Gynaecologists of Canada*, Dec. 2007, pp. 1003-1013) This organization recommends supplementing 5.0 mg (5,000 mcg) of folic acid for women with health risks, including epilepsy, insulin dependent diabetes, and obesity; Goh, Y., and Koren, G. "Folic acid in pregnancy and fetal outcomes" (*J. Obstet. & Gynaecol.* 2008, 28:3-13) Folic acid supplementation in amounts up to 5,000 mcg is recommended for all women to prevent neural tube defects. This amount does not mask vitamin B_{12} deficiency, according to these authors.

43 Raffelock, D., Rountree, R., and Hopkins, V. *A Natural Guide to Pregnancy and Postpartum Health* (New York: Avery Press, 2002, p.131) These authors, one a medical doctor and the other a chiropractor, consider as much as 5,000 mcg of vitamin B_{12} safe during pregnancy and breastfeeding.

44 Shannon, M. "Down Syndrome and Folic Acid, Adoption Update, and Surprise Pregnancies" (*Family Foundations*, Jan.-Feb. 2000, pp. 6–7).

45 The answer to this intriguing question was provided, correctly in my opinion, by older sister Regina, who helps care for our flock of chickens: "No, they have *elbows* on their legs."

CHAPTER 10

1 Weng, X., Odouli, R., and Li, D. "Maternal caffeine consumption during pregnancy and the risk of miscarriage: a prospective cohort study" (*J. Obst. Gynecol.*, Jan. 2008, pp. 1e1-1e8).

2 Glenville, M. "Nutritional supplements in pregnancy: commercial push or evidence based?" (*Curr. Opin. Obstet. Gynecol.* 2006, 18:642-647).

3 Fugh-Berman, A., and Kronenberg, F. "Complementary and alternative medicine (CAM) in reproductive-age women: a review of randomized controlled studies" (*Reprod. Toxicol.* 2003, 17:137-152).

4 Shrim, A. Boskovic, C., Maltepe, Y., et al. "Pregnancy outcome following use of large doses of vitamin B_6 in the first trimester" (*J. Obstet. Gynecol.* 2006, 26:749-751).

5 Fugh-Berman, A., and Kronenberg, F. (2003).

6 Puotinen, C. "Preventing eclampsia: an interview with Tom Brewer, M.D." (*Townsend Letter for Doctors and Patients*, Nov., 2004).

7 Brewer, T. "If You Are Pregnant" (***www.BlueRibbonBaby.org.*** *If You Are Pregnant Subpages*, c. 2007).

8 Puotinen, C. (2004, p. 6).

9 Davies, M. "Evidence for effects of weight on reproduction in women

[Symposium: Diet, nutrition, and exercise in reproduction]." (*Reprod. BioMed. Online* 2006, 12:552-561); Kiel, D., Dodson, E., Artal, R., et al. "Gestational weight gain and pregnancy outcomes in obese women" (*Obstet. Gynecol.* 2007, 110:752-758).

10   Oken, E., Ning, Y., Rifas-Shiman, S., et al. "Diet during pregnancy and risk of preeclampsia or gestational hypertension" (*AEP* 2007, 17:663-668).

11   Frederick, I., Williams, M., Dashow, E., et al. "Dietary fiber, potassium, magnesium and calcium in relation to the risk of preeclampsia" (*J. Reprod. Med.* 2005, 50:332-344).

12   Duvekot, E., de Groot, C., Bloemenkamp, K., et al. "Pregnant women with a low milk intake have an increased risk of developing preeclampsia" (*European J. Obstet. & Gynecol.* 2002, 105:11-14).

13   Duvekot, E., de Groot, C., Bloemenkamp, K., et al., (2002).

14   Ahlgrimm, M., in "In Step with Marla Ahlgrimm," by M. Shannon (*Family Foundations* 2008, 34(6):30-31).

15   Beck, S., and Abraham, G. *Optivite PMT and Gynovite Plus Total Dietary Programs for Premenstrual Syndrome and Menopause with Answers to the Most Commonly Asked Questions* (Torrance, CA: Optimox Corp., 1992).

16   Kwock, D., The Daily Wellness Co. "Upon a physician's evaluation and recommendation to do so, FertilityBlend for Women can be continued during pregnancy for the purpose of sustaining improved progesterone levels and overall health." (Personal communication to M. Shannon, Feb. 6, 2009).

17   De la Calle, M., Usandizaga, R., Sancah, M., et al. "Homocysteine, folic acid and B-group vitamins in obstetrics and gynaecology" (*European J. Obstet. & Gynaelcol.* 2003, 107:125-134).

18   Wen, S., Chen, X., Rodger, M., et al. "Folic acid supplementation in early second trimester and the risk of preeclampsia" (*Am. J. Obstet. Gynecol.* 2008, 198:45-e1–45-e7).

19   De la Calle, M., Usandizaga, R., Sancah, M., et al. (2003).

20   Makedos, G., Papanicolaou, A., Hitoglou, A., et al. "Homocysteine, folic acid and B12 serum levels in pregnancy complicated with preeclampsia" (*Arch. Gynecol. Obstet.* 2007, 275:121-124).

21   De la Calle, M., Usandizaga, R., Sancah, M., et al. (2003); Ray, J., and Laskin, C. "Folic acid and homocyst(e)ine metabolic defects and the risk of placental abruption, pre-eclampsia and spontaneous pregnancy loss: A systematic review" (*Placenta* 1999, 20:519-529).

22   Juarez-Vazquaz, J., Bonizzoni, E., and Scotti, A. "Iron plus folate is more effective than iron alone in the treatment of iron deficiency anaemia in pregnancy: a randomised, double-blind clinical trial" (*Br. J. Obstet. Gynaecol.* 2002, 109:1009-1014).

23 Lee, K., Zaffke, M., and Baratte-Beebe, K. "Restless legs syndrome and sleep disturbance during pregnancy: the role of folate and iron" (*J. Women's Health and Gender-Based Medicine* 2001, 10:335-341).

24 De la Calle, M., Usandizaga, R., Sancah, M., et al. (2003).

25 Goh, Y., and Koren, G. "Folic acid in pregnancy and fetal outcomes" (*J. Obstet. & Gynaecol.* 2008, 28:3-13).

26 Raffelock, D., Rountree, R., and Hopkins, V. *A Natural Guide to Pregnancy and Postpartum Health* (New York: Avery, 2002, p. 131).

27 Ellis, J., and Presley, J. "B6 and Pregnancy" in *Vitamin B6: The Doctor's Report* (New York: Harper and Row, 1973, pp.90, 96-97).

28 Ellis, J., and Presley, J. (1973, pp.112-113).

29 Scalf, R., personal communication to M. Shannon (March, 1990).

30 Hibbeln, J., Davis, J., Steer, C., et al. "Maternal seafood consumption in pregnancy and neuro-development outcomes in childhood (ALSPAC study: an observational cohort study)" (*The Lancet* 2007, 369:578-585).

31 Olsen, S., Secher, N., Tabor, A., et al. "Randomized clinical trials of fish oil supplementation in high risk pregnancies. Fish Oil Trials in Pregnancy [FOTIP] Team" (*Br. J. Obstet. Gynaecol.* 2000, 107:382-395).

32 Erasmus, U. *Fats That Heal, Fats That Kill* (Burnaby, BC, Canada: Alive Books, 1993, p. 263).

33 Raffelock, D., Rountree, R., and Hopkins, V. (2002, p. 146).

34 Rothman, K., and Moore, L. "Teratogenicity of high vitamin A intake" (*NEJM* 1995, 333:1369-1373).

35 Raffelock, D., Rountree, R., and Hopkins, V. (2002, p. 146).

36 Casey, B., and Leveno, K. "Thyroid disease in pregnancy" (*Obstet. Gynecol*, 2006, 108:1283-1292).

37 Casey, B., and Leveno., K. (2006).

38 Shomon, M. *The Thyroid Hormone Breakthrough* (New York: Collins, 2006, p. 231).

39 Raffelock, D., Rountree, R., and Hopkins, V. (2002, p. 221).

40 Lee, J., and Hopkins, V. *Dr. John Lee's Hormone Balance Made Simple* (New York: Wellness Central, 2006, pp. 139-140).

41 Raffelock, D., Rountree, R., and Hopkins, V. (2002, pp. 199-203).

CHAPTER 11

1 George, L., Granath, F., Johansson, A., et al. "Risks of repeated miscarriage" (*Paediatric and Perinatal Epidemiology* 2006, 20:119-126).

2 Roberts, C., and Murphy, A. "Endocrinopathies associated with recurrent pregnancy loss" (*Seminars in Reproductive Medicine* 2000, 18:357-362).

3 George, L., Granath, F., Johansson, A., et al. (2006).

4 Maconochie, N., Doyle, P., Prior, S., et al. "Risk factors for first trimester miscarriage — results from a UK-population-based case-control study" (*BJOG* 2007, 114:170-186).

5 Maconochie, N., Doyle, P., Prior, S., et al. (2007).

6 Maconochie, N., Doyle, P., Prior, S., et al. (2007).

7 Bennett, M., "Vitamin B12 deficiency, infertility and recurrent fetal loss" (*J. Reprod. Med.* 2001, 46:209-212).

8 Weng, X., Odouli, R., and Li, D. "Maternal caffeine consumption during pregnancy and the risk of miscarriage: a prospective cohort study" (*J. Obst. Gynecol.*, January 2008, pp. 1e1-1e8).

9 Rice, H., and Baker, B. "Workplace hazards to women's reproductive health" (*Minnesota Medicine*, Sept. 2007, **http://www.minnesotamedicine.com/ PastIssues/September2007/tabid/2209/Default.aspx**).

10 Nepomnaschy, P., Welch, K., McConnell, D., et al. "Cortisol and very early pregnancy loss" (*PNAS* 2006, 103:3938-3942).

11 Fritz, M., Adamson, G., Barnhart, K., et al. "Progesterone supplementation during the luteal phase and in early pregnancy in the treatment of infertility: an educational bulletin" (*Fertil. Steril.* 2008, 89:789-792); Dendrinos, S., Makrakis, E., Botsis, D., et al. "A study of pregnancy loss in 352 women with recurrent miscarriages" (*Arch. Gynecol. Obstet.* 2005, 271:235-239); Potdar, N., and Konje, J. "The endocrinological basis of recurrent miscarriage" (*Curr. Opin. Obstet. Gynecol.* 2005, 17:424-428); George, L., Granath, F., Johansson, A., et al. (2006).

12 Ohara, N., Tsujino, T., and Maruo, T. "The role of thyroid hormone in trophoblast function, early pregnancy maintenance, and fetal neurodevelopment" (*J. Obstet. Gynaecol. Can.* 2004, 26:982-990).

13 Abalovich, M., Gutierrez, S., Alcaraz, G., et al. "Overt and subclinical hypothyroidism complicating pregnancy" (Thyroid 2002, 12:63-68).

14 Potdar, N., and Konje, J. (2005).

15 Roberts, C., and Murphy, A. (2000).

16 Davies, M. "Evidence for effects of weight on reproduction in women [Symposium: Diet, nutrition and exercise in reproduction]" (*Reprod. BioMed. Online* 2006, 12:552-561).

17 Maconochie, N., Doyle, P., Prior, S., et al. (2007).

18 Martinelli, P., Troncone, R., Paparo, F., et al. "Celiac disease and unfavorable outcome of pregnancy" (*Gut* 2000, 46:332-335).

19 Rossi, E., and Costa, M. "Fish oil derivatives as a prophylaxis of recurrent miscarriage associated with antiphospholipid antibodies (APL): A pilot study" (*Lupus* 1993, 2, 319-323); Carla, G., Iovenitti., P., and Falciglia, K. "Recurrent miscarriage associated with antiphospholipid antibodies: prophylactic treatment with low-dose aspirin and fish oil derivatives" (*Clin. Exp. Obstet .Gynecol.* 2005, 32:49-51).

20 George, L., Granath, F., Johansson, A., et al. (2006).

21 Dendrinos, S., Makrakis, E., Botsis, D., et al. (2005).

22 Leridon, H. "A new estimate of permanent sterility by age: Sterility defined as the inability to conceive" (A paper presented at the Annual Meeting of the Population Association of America, Philadelphia, PA, Mar. 31-April 2, 2005, reviewed in Billari, F., Kohler, H., Andersson, G., et al. "Approaching the limit: Long-term trends in late and very late fertility." (*Population and Development Review* 2007, 33:149-170).

23 Maconochie, N., Doyle, P., Prior, S., et al. (2007).

24 Goh, Y., and Koren, G. "Folic acid in pregnancy and fetal outcomes" (*J. Obstet. Gynaecol.*, 2008, 28:3-13).

25 Goh, Y., and Koren, G. (2008); Wilson, W. "Pre-conceptional vitamin/folic acid supplementation 2007: The use of folic acid in combination with a multi-vitamin supplement for the prevention of neural tube defects and other congenital anomalies" [Joint Society of Obstetricians and Gynaecologists of Canada-Motherisk Clinical Practice Guideline] (*J. Obstetricians and Gynaecologists of Canada*, Dec. 2007, pp. 1003-1013).

26 De la Calle, M., Usandizaga, R., Sancah, M., et al. (2003).

27 Eskes, T. "Abnormal folate metabolism in mothers with Down syndrome offspring: Review of the literature" (*European J. Obstet. & Gynaelcol. And Reprod. Biol.* 2006, 124:130-133).

28 De la Calle, M., Usandizaga, R., Sancah, M., et al. "Homocysteine, folic acid and B-group vitamins in obstetrics and gynaecology" (*European J. Obstet. & Gynaelcol.* 2003, 107:125-134).

29 Goh, Y., and Koren, G. (2008).

30 Erickson, J., "Folic acid and prevention of spinal bifida and anencephaly: 10 years after the U.S. Public Health Service recommendation" (*MMWR Recommendations and Reports* 2002, RR13:1-3; *www.cdc.gov/mmwr/preview/mmwrhtml/rr5113al.htm*).

31 Rothman, K., and Moore, L. "Teratogenicity of high vitamin A intake" (*NEJM* 1995, 333:1369-1373).

32 Wilson, W. (2007).

33 Goh, Y., and Koren, G. (2008).

34 Czeizel, A., Metneki, J. And Dudas, I. "Higher rate of multiple births after peri-conceptional vitamin supplementation" (*NEJM* 1994, 330:1687-1688).

35 Bailey, L., and Berry, R. "Folic acid supplementation and the occurrence of congenital heart defects, orofacial clefts, multiple births, and miscarriage" (*Am. J. Clin. Nutr.* 2005, 81suppl.):1213S-1217S).

36 Li, Z., Gindler, J., Wang, H., et al. "Folic acid supplements during early preg-nancy and the likelihood of multiple births: a population-based cohort study" (*The Lancet* 2003, 361:380-384).

37 Kallen, B., "Use of folic acid supplementation and risk for dizygotic [fraternal] twinning" (*Early Human Development* 2004, 80:143-151).

38 Czeizel, A., and Vargha, P. "Periconceptual folic acid/multivitamin supplemen-tation and twin pregnancy" (*Am. J. Obstet. Gynecol.* 2004, 191:790–794).

39 Ray, J., and Laskin, C. "Folic acid and homocyst(e)ine metabolic defects and the risk of placental abruption, pre-eclampsia and spontaneous pregnancy loss: A systematic review" (*Placenta* 1999, 20:519-529).

40 Hook, E., and Czeizel, A. "Can terathanasia explain the protective effect of folic-acid supplementation on birth defects?" (*The Lancet* 1997, 350:513-515).

41 Windham, G., Shaw, G., Todoroff, K., et al. "Miscarriage and the use of multi-vitamins or folic acid" (*AM. J. Med. Genetics* 2000, 90:261-262).

42 Hook, E., and Czeizel, A. (2002).

43 Bailey, L., and Berry, R. (2005).

44 Maconochie, N., Doyle, P., Prior, S., et al. (2007).

45 Whitaker, J. "Down Syndrome Can Be Treated" (*Health and Healing* 2007, 17:1-3).

46 Leichtman, L. "Targeted nutritional intervention (TNI) in the treatment of children with Down syndrome: principles behind use, treatment protocols, and an expanded bibliography" (***www.lleichtman.org/tni 2002***).

47 Gueant, J., Gueant-Rodriguez, R., Anello, G, et al. "Genetic determinants of folate and vitamin B_{12} metabolsim: A common pathway in neural tube defect and Down syndrome?" (*Clin. Chem. Lab. Med.* 2003, 41:1473-1477).

48 James, S., Pogribna, M., Pobribny, I., et al. "Abnormal folate metabolism and mutation in the methylenetetrahydrofolate reductase gene may be maternal risk factors for Down syndrome" (*Am. J. Clin. Nutr.* 1999, 70:495-499). ["The nondisjunction event is maternal in ~95% of cases, occurring primarily during meiosis I in the maturing oocyte, before conception."]

49 James, S., Pogribna, M., Pobribny, I., et al. (1999); Hobb, C., Sherman, S., Yi, P., et al. "Polymorphisms in genes involved in folate metabolism as maternal risk factors for Down syndrome" (*Am. J. Hum. Genet.* 2000, 67:623-630); Sheth,

J., and Smeth, F. "Gene polymorphism and folate metabolism: a maternal risk factor for Down syndrome" (*Indian Pediatrics* 2003, 40:115-123); Eskes, T. "Abnormal folate metabolism in mothers with Down syndrome offspring: Review of the literature" (*European J. Obstet. Gynaecol. And Reprod. Biol.* 2006, 124:130-136); Coppede, F., Colognato, R., Bonelli, A., et al. "Polymorphisms in folate and homocysteine metabolizing genes and chromosome damage in mothers of Down syndrome children" (*Am. J. Med. Genetics* 2007, Part A 143A:2006-2015).

50 Takamura, N., Kondoh, T., Ohgi, S., et al. "Abnormal folic acid-homocysteine metabolism as maternal risk factors for Down syndrome in Japan" *European J. Nutrition* 2004, 43:285-287).

51 Ray, J., Meier, C., Vermeulen, M., et al. "Prevalence of trisomy 21 following folic acid food fortification" (*Am. J. Med. Genetics* 2003, 120A:309–313).

52 Whitaker, J. (Personal communication to M. Shannon, October 13, 1996).

53 Whitaker, J. (Personal communication to M. Shannon, October 29, 1996).

54 Slama, R., Bouyer, J., Windham, G., et al. "Influence of paternal age on the risk of spontaneous abortion" (*Am. J. Epidemiol.* 2005, 161:816-823).

55 Eskes, T. (2006).

56 Tremellen, K. "Oxidative, stress and male fertility-a clinical perspective" (*Human Reproduction Update*, pp. 1-16, 2008).

57 Tremellen, K. (2008).

CHAPTER 12

1 ACOG Committee Opinion, "Age-Related Fertility Decline" (*J. Obstet. Gynecol.* 112 [No. 2, Part 1 Aug 2008]: 409–411.

2 Shomon, M. *The Thyroid Hormone Breakthrough: Overcoming Sexual and Hormonal Problems at Every Age* (New York: Collins, an imprint of HarperCollins, 2006, p. 37).

3 Badawy, A., Ostate, O., and Sherief, S. "Can thyroid dysfunction explicate severe menopausal symptoms?" (*J. Obstet. Gynecol.* 2007, 27:503-505).

4 Lee, J., and Hopkins, V. *Dr. John Lee's Hormone Balance Made Simple: The Essential How-to Guide to Symptoms, Dosage, Timing, and More* (New York: Wellness Central, 2006, p. 30).

5 Franks, S., Robinson, S., and Willis, D. "Nutrition, insulin, and polycystic ovary syndrome" (*Reviews of Reproduction* 1996, 1:47-53).

6 Gittleman, A. *Before the Change: Taking Charge of Your Perimenopause* (San Francisco: HarperSanFrancisco, a division of HarperCollins Publishers, 2004, pp. 68-69).

7 Abraham, G. Personal communication to M. Shannon (1991).

8   Gittleman, A. (2004, pp. 78-79).

9   Lee, J. *What Your Doctor May Not Tell You About Menopause* (New York: Warner Wellness, 2004, p. 336).

10 Lee, J. (2004, pp. 81-82).

11 Lee J., and Hopkins, V. (2006, pp. 93-95).

12 Lark, S. "My Alkaline Power Plan for Healthy Bones" (*The Lark Letter*, July, 2006, pp. 1-6).

13 Lark, S. (2006).

14 Garland, C., Garland, F., Gorham, E., et al. "The role of vitamin D in cancer prevention." (*Am. J. Public Health* 2006, 96:252-261).

15 Lark, S. (2006).

16 Sanson, G. *The Myth of Osteoporosis: What Every Woman Should Know About Creating Bone Health* (Ann Arbor, MI: MCD Century, 2003, p. 153).

17 McIlwain, H., M.D, and Bruce, D., Ph.D., et al. *Reversing Osteopenia: The Definitive Guide to Recognizing and Treating Early Bone Loss in Women of All Ages* (New York: Owl Books, 2004, p. 7).

18 Lee, J. (2004, pp. 162-171).

19 Brandt, F. "Sugar: The Enemy Within" in *10 Minutes/10 Years* (New York: Free Press, a trademark of Simon and Schuster, Inc., 2007, pp. 35-51).

CHAPTER 13

1   Horowitz, B., Edelstein, S., and Lippman, L. "Sugar chromatography studies in recurrent Candida vulvovaginitis" (*J. Reprod. Med.* 1984, 29:441).

2   Falagas, M., Betsi, G., and Athanasiou, S. "Probiotics for prevention of recurrent vulvovaginal candidiasis: a review" (*J. Antimicrobial Chemotherapy* 2006, 58:266-272).

3   Horowitz, B. Edelstein, S., and Lippman, L. "Sexual transmission of Candida." (*Obstet. Gynecol.* 1987, 69:883).

4   Falagas, M., Betsi, G., and Athanasiou, S. (2006).

5   Kontiokari, T., Nuutinen, M., and Uhari, M. "Dietary factors affecting susceptibility to urinary tract infection" (*Pediatr. Nephrol.* 2004, 19:378-383).

6   Shorter, B., Lesser, M., Moldwin, D., et al. "Effect of comestibles on symptoms of interstitial cystitis" (*J. Urology* 2007, 178:145-152).

7   Lee, J., and Hopkins, V. *What Your Doctor May Not Tell You about Menopause* (New York: Warner Books, 2004, p. 97).

8   Abraham, G., personal communication to M. Shannon (1999).

9   Lee, J., and Hopkins, V. (2004, p. 396).

10 Ito, T., Polan, M., Whipple, B., et al. "The enhancement of female sexual func-
    tion with ArginMax, a nutritional supplement, among women differing in meno-
    pausal status" (*J. Sex & Marital Therapy* 2006, 32:369-378).

11 Lark, S. "Lift Your Libido" (*Women's Wellness Today* 2008, 15(7):6-7).

12 Lark, S. (2008).

CHAPTER 14

1   Abraham, G., personal communication to M. Shannon (April 10, 1991).

2   Davis, A., *Let's Get Well* (New York: Harcourt Brace Jovanovich, Inc., 1972, pp.
    22-31).

3   Travis, J., "Probing the cause of after-baby blues" (*Science News* 1995, 148:15).

CHAPTER 15

1   Wong, W., Thomas, C., Merkus, J., et al. "Male factor subfertility: possible causes
    and the impact of nutritional factors" (*Fertil. Steril.* 2000, 73:435-442).

2   Sheweita, S., Tilmisany, A., and Al-Sawaf, H. "Mechanisms of male infertility:
    Role of antioxidants" (*Current Drug Metabolism* 2005, 6:495-501).

3   Comhaire, F., Cristophe, A., Zalata, A., et al. "The effects of combined conven-
    tional treatment, oral antioxidants and essential fatty acids on sperm biology
    in subfertile men" (*Prostaglandins, Leukotrienes, and Essential Fatty Acids* 2000,
    63:159-165).

4   Tremellen, K. "Oxidative stress and male fertility–a clinical perspective" (*Human
    Reproduction Update 2008*, pp. 1-16).

5   Tremellen, K. (2008).

6   Sallmen, M., Sandler, D., Hoppin, J., et al. "Reduced fertility among overweight
    and obese men" (*Epidemiology* 2006, 17:520-523).

7   Kaukua, J., Pekkarinen, T., Sane, T., et al. "Sex hormones and sexual function in
    obese men losing weight" (*Obesity Res.* 2003, 11:689-694).

8   Frisch, R. *Female Fertility and the Body Fat Connection* (Chicago: University of
    Chicago Press 2002, p. 35) In referring to extreme weight loss in men, at the
    point of loss of sperm production, Dr. Frisch writes, "They look like skeletons."

9   Tremellen, K. (2008).

10 Tremellen, K. (2008).

11 Sheweita, S., Tilmisany, A., and Al-Sawaf, H. (2005).

12 Chavarro, J., Toth, T., Sadio, S., et al. "Soy food and isoflavone intake in rela-
    tion to semen quality parameters among men from an infertility clinic" (*Human
    Reprod.* 2008, 11:2584-2590).

13 Chavarro, J., personal communication to M. Shannon (Jan. 3, 2009).

14 Tremellen, K. (2008).

15 Harris, W., Harden, T., and Dawson, E. "Apparent effect of ascorbic acid medication on semen metal levels" (*Fertil. Steril.* 1979, 32:456-457).

16 Dawson, E., Harris, W., Rankin W., et al. "Effect of ascorbic acid on male infertility" (*Ann. New York Acad. Sci.* 1987, 498:312).

17 Dawson, E., Harris, B., Teter, M., et al. "Effect of ascorbic acid supplementation on the sperm quality of smokers." (*Fertil. Steril.* 1992, 58:1034-1039).

18 Song, G., Norkus, E., and Lewis, V. "Relationship between seminal ascorbic acid and sperm DNA integrity in infertile men" (*Int. J. Andrology* 2006, 29:569-575).

19 Wong, W., Merkus, H., Thomas, C., et al. "Effect of folic acid and zinc sulfate on male factor subfertility: a double-blind, randomized, placebo-controlled trial" (*Fertil. Steril.* 2002, 77:491-497) .

20 Maret, W., and Sandstead, H. "Zinc requirements and the risks and benefits of zinc supplementation" (*J. Trace Elements in Medicine and Biology* 2006, 20:3-8).

21 Beckett G., and Arthur, J. "Selenium and endocrine systems" (*J. Endocrinol.* 2005, 184:455-465).

22 Keskes-Ammar, L., Feki-Chakroun, N., Rebai, T., et al. "Sperm oxidative stress and the effect of an oral vitamin E and selenium supplement on semen quality in infertile men" (*Archives of Andrology* 2003, 49:83-94).

23 Scott, R., MacPherson, A., Yates, R., et al. "The effect of oral selenium supplementation on human sperm motility" (*Br. J. Urology* 1998, 82:76-80).

24 Comhaire, F., Cristophe, A., Zalata, A., et al. (2000).

25 Suleiman, S., Ali, M., Zaki, Z., et al. "Lipid peroxidation and human sperm motility: protective role of vitamin E" (*J. Androl.* 1996, 17:530-537).

26 Calloway, D. "Nutrition and reproductive function of men" (*Nutrition Abstracts and Reviews/Reviews in Clinical Nutrition* 1983, 53:373).

27 Tremellen, K. (2008).

28 Comhaire, F., and Mahmoud, A. "The role of food supplements in the treatment of the infertile man" (*Reprod. BioMed. Online* 2003, 7:385-391).

29 Comhaire, F., and Mahmoud, A. (2003).

30 Comhaire, F., and Mahnoud, A. (2003); Conhaire, F., El Garem, Y., Mahmoud, A., et al. "Combined conventional/antioxidant 'Astaxanthin' treatment for male infertility: a double-blind, randomized trial" (*Asian J. Andrology* 2005, 7:257-262) [Astaxanthin is a red pigment that gives the pinkish color to many seafoods. It is a carotenoid; that is it is a fat-soluble nutrient related to the beta-carotene. (***www.astaxanthin.org***)]

31 Lenzi, A., Lombardo, F., Sgro, P., et al. "Use of carnitine therapy in selected cases of male factor infertility: A double-blind crossover trial" (*Fertil. Steril.* 2003, 79:292-300); reviewed in Agarwall, A., Nallella, K., Allamaneni, S., et al. (2004).

32 Sallmen, M., Sandler, D., Hoppin, J., et al. (2006).

33 Krassaa, G. "Male reproductive function in relation with thyroid alterations" (*Best Practice & Research in Clinical Endocrinology and Metabolism* 2004, 18:183-195).

34 Kumar, A., Chaturvedi, K., and Mohanty, B. "Hypoandrogenaemia is associated with subclinical hypothyroidism in men" (*Int. J. Andrology* 2007, 30:14-20).

35 Stogdill, B., personal communication to M. Shannon (July, 1989).

36 Balch, P. *Prescription for Nutritional Healing*, 4th ed. (New York: Avery Press, 2006, p. 655).

37 Balch, P. (2006).

38 Rohrman, S., Giovannucci, E., Willett, W., et al. "Fruit and vegetable consumption, intake of micronutrients, and benign prostatic hyperplasia in U.S. men" (*Am. J. Clin. Nutr.* 2007, 85:523-529).

39 Pytel, Y., Vinarov, A ., Lopatkin, N., et al. "Long-term clinical and biologic effects of the lipido-sterolic extract of Serenoa repens in patients with symptomatic benign prostatic hyperplasia" (*Advances in Therapy* 2002, 19:297-306).

40 Pytel, Y., Vinarov, A ., Lopatkin, N., et al. (2002).

41 Fleshner, N., Zlotta, A. "Prostate cancer prevention" (*Cancer* 2007, 110:1889-1899).

42 Cheung, E., Wadhera, P., Dorff, T., et al. "Diet and prostate cancer risk reduction" (*Expert Rev. Anticancer Ther.* 2008, 8:43-50).

43 Cheung, E., Wadhera, P., Dorff, T., et al. (2008).

44 Vaishampayan, U., Hussain, M., Banerjee, M., et al. "Lycopene and soy isoflavones in the treatment of prostate cancer" (*Nutrition and Cancer* 2007, 59:1-7).

45 Chavarro, J., Stampfer, M., Campos, H., et al. "A prospective study of trans-fatty acid levels in blood and risk of prostate cancer" (*Cancer Epidemiol. Biomarkers & Prevention* 2008, 17:95-101).

46 Clark, L., Combs, G., Turnbull, B., et al. "Effects of selenium supplementation for cancer prevention in patients with carcinoma of the skin: a randomized controlled trial" (*JAMA* 1996, 276: 1957-1963); Combs, G., and Gray, W. "Chemopreventive agents: selenium" (*Pharmacol Ther.* 1998 79:179-182).

47 Heinonen, O., Albanes, D., Virtamo, J., et al. "Prostate cancer and supplementation with alpha-tocopherol and beta-carotene: incidence and mortality in a controlled trial"(*J. Natl. Cancer Inst.* 1998, 90:440-446).

48 Mettlin, C., Natarajan, N., and Huben, R. "Vasectomy and prostate cancer risk" (*Am. J. Epidemiol.* 1990, 132:1056-1061); Rosenberg, L., Palmer, J., Zauber, M., et al. "Vasectomy and the risk of prostate cancer" (*Am. J. Epidemiol.* 1990, 132:1051-1055); Giovannucci, E., Ascherio, A., Rimm, E., et al. "A prospective cohort study of vasectomy and prostate cancer in U.S. men" (*JAMA* 1993, 269:873-876); Giovannucci, E., Tosteson, T., Speizer, F., et al. "A retrospective cohort study of vasectomy and prostate cancer in U.S. men" (*JAMA* 1993, 269:878-882).

CHAPTER 16

1 Carmichael, A. "Can Vitex agnus castus be used for the treatment of mastalgia? What is the current evidence? (*ECAM* 2008, 5:247-250).

2 *The Art of Natural Family Planning Premenopause Student Guide* (Cincinnati, OH: The Couple to Couple League, 2009) p. 26.

3 Cordain, L., Lindeberg, S., and Hurtado, M. "Acne vulgaris: a disease of Western civilization" (*Arch. Dermatol.* 2002, 138:1584-1590).

4 McIntosh, M.E. "Treatment of women with the galactorrhea-amenorrhea syndrome with pyridoxine (vitamin B6)" (*J. Clin. Endocrinol. Metab.* 1976, 42:1192).

5 Kapcala, L. "Galactorrhea and thyrotoxicosis" (*Arch. Intern. Med.* 1984, 144:2349).

6 Ryan-Harshman, M., and Aldoori, W. "Carpal tunnel syndrome and vitamin B6" (*Canadian Family Physician* 2007, 53:1161-1162).

7 Siega-Riz, A., Promislow, J., Savitz, D., et al. "Vitamin C intake and the risk of preterm delivery" (*Am. J. Obstet. Gynecol.* 2003, 189:519-523).

8 Prior, C., Vigna, Y., et al. "Spinal bone loss and ovulatory infertility" (*NEJM* 1991, 323:1221-1227).

9 Streeten, E., Ryan, K., McBride, D., et al. "The relationship between parity and bone mineral density in women characterized by a homogeneous lifestyle and high parity" (*J. Clin. Endocrinol. Metab.* 2005, 90:4536-4541).

10 Rothman, K., and Moore, L. "Teratogenicity of high vitamin A intake" (*NEJM* 1995, 333:1369-1373).

11 Bruchalsi, J. (personal communication to M. Shannon, October 6, 2008).

Index

and miscarriage 166
and sexual desire 184
causes of 107
consequences of 107
medical intervention for related infertility 109
during premenopause 181
Body Mass Index (BMI) 108, 166–167
and the NFP chart 108
normal, but underfat 108
Body weight
and bone health 188
and loss of cycles 108
and PMS 76
Bone Builder 188
Bone density test 239
Bone health
during premenopause 186
nutrition for 187
Borage oil 186
Brain cancer, childhood 169
Brain development 6
Brain fog
and adrenal function 186
and B vitamins 152
postpartum 158
Brain function 4, 10
Brandt, Frederic, M.D. 191
Breadmaker 30
Bread recipe 31
Breakfast 17, 19
Breakthrough bleeding 80
Breast cancer
and estrogen dominance 119
and night shift work 129
Breastfeeding x, 20
and amenorrhea 94
and anovulatory cycles 94
and aspartame (Nutrasweet) 51
and fertility 94
and folic acid 171
and FSH and LH 94
and low basal temperatures 157
and luteal phase deficiency 94, 96
and osteoporosis 238
and postpartum bleeding 82

and prolonged mucus 233
and protein needs 6
and sleep 58, 205
nutrition 155
Breastfeeding and Natural Child Spacing 20, 243
Breast pain 231
Breast self-examination 237
Breasts, sore 70, 231
and high estrogen 182
Brewer diet 145, 156
Brewer, Gail Sforza 249
Brewer, Tom, M.D. 145, 148–149, 249
Broda O. Barnes, M.D., Research Foundation, Inc., The 103, 256
Bromelain 90
Bromocriptine 236
Brown bleeding
post-menstrual 104
Bulimia 107, 109
Buying clubs 26
B vitamins
and estrogen levels 69
and male fertility 221
for PCOS 116

C

Caffeine 15–16, 50, 71, 131–132, 135, 188, 266
and adrenal function 186
and anxiety 15, 56
and bladder pain 196
and blood sugar levels 209
and breastfeeding 156
and chocolate 50
and fertility 131
and male fertility 219
and melatonin 130
and migraines 232
and miscarriage 16, 164
and PMS 16
and prolonged mucus 235
and seeking pregnancy 142
and sleep 15, 186
and sore breasts 231

Dreams
and vitamins, minerals, fish oil 56

Dr. John Lee's Hormone Balance Made Simple: The Essential How-to Guide to Symptoms, Dosage, Timing, and More 185, 245

Drugs
and melatonin 131

Dry mouth
and aspartame (Nutrasweet) 51

Dysmenorrhea. *See* Menstruation, painful

E

Eclampsia 145
and vitamin B6 151

Edema 153
during pregnancy 144, 151
other strategies 153

Effects of Light on the Menstrual Cycle, The 131, 248

Egg
and cholesterol 52
protein content 47

Eicosapentaenoic acid (EPA) 10, 36

Ellis, John, M.D. 151, 237, 250

Ely, Leanne 29, 34, 243

Emotional nurturing
during postpartum 155

Endometriosis 88–90
and luteal phase deficiency 89
and PMS nutritional strategy 89
and prolonged or heavy menstruation 80
and yeast overgrowth 123
enzymes for 90
herbal remedies for 90
other helps 90

Endometriosis: A Key to Healing through Nutrition 90, 245

Endometriosis Association, The 91, 256

Endometrium
defined 62

Energy 205

and adequate sleep 205
and blood sugar levels 207
and exercise 206
and stress 206
decreased during premenopause 185
during pregnancy 151

Enlarged ovaries
as symptom of PCOS 111

Enzymes
digestive
for morning sickness 144

EPA 10, 25, 37, 222. *See also* Eicosapentaenoic acid
in fish oil vs. flax oil 54

Epididymis 65
and vitamin A deficiency 221

Epinephrine 185, 206–208, 211

Equal 51. *See also* Artificial sweeteners

Erasmus, Udo, Ph.D. 154

Erectile dysfunction 219, 223–224
and age 228

Essential fatty acids 6, 10, 12, 35
and blood sugar levels 209
and flax oil 7
and insulin resistance 116
and male fertility 221
and prostate gland 225
and thyroid function 102
defined 36
sources of 36

Estrogen 7
and fibroid tumors 237
and melatonin 129
and overweight 199
and pear shape 119
in men 222
low
and pain during intercourse 202
as cause of hot flashes 183
replacement 273–274

Estrogen cream
natural, for vaginal dryness 184

Estrogen dominance 119, 182
and fibroid tumors 81
and progesterone 69

related to low thyroid function 100

vitamin B6 for 97

Gallbladder

and high estrogen 182

Gardening 28

Gardening Without Work 28, 244

Garden vegetables 3

Genetics & Disabilities Diagnostic Care Center 258

Genital pain 123, 194

Get the Sugar Out! 15, 18, 51, 118, 243

Ginger 143

Gittleman, Ann Louise 15, 18, 49, 51, 186, 243, 250

Gluten 31, 133–134

and celiac disease 167

-free foods 26

implementing 135

sensitivity 134

Glycation 191

Glycemic Index 114–115

GnRH

affected by low body fat 106

effect on FSH and LH 106

Goiter

hypothyroid 105

postpartum 156

Goldfarb, Herbert A., M.D 277

Gonadotropin releasing hormone analogues (GnRH-a)

for endometriosis 90

Grant, Ellen, M.D. 128

Grapefruit seed extract

for yeast overgrowth 127

Graves' disease 105

Growth retardation

and folic acid 170

Guaifenesin 267

H

Hair

body 112. *See also* Hirsutism

Hair loss 99, 240

Haploid cell

defined 63

Hargrove, Joel, M.D. 89

Harvard School of Public Health 71, 219

Hashimoto's thyroiditis 100, 102

Headache 14, 16, 18–19

and artificial sweeteners 209

during menstruation 86

Health and Healing 259

Health food shops 25–26, 42

Heart defects

congenital 169

Herbs

for prostate enlargement 226

Herpes virus

and arginine 199

High fructose corn syrup 14

Hilgert, Jackie 21, 243

Hip fracture 187, 189

risk of 238

Hirsutism 114, 119

as symptom of PCOS 111

defined 112

Homocysteine 150

and birth defects 170

and Down syndrome 174

and exercise 117

and male fertility 221

and miscarriage 172

and PCOS 116

and preeclampsia 150

Hopkins, Virginia 59, 245, 249–250

Hormonal birth control 193. *See also* Birth control pill

and low sexual desire 200–201

and yeast infections 193

discontinuing 234

Hormonal testing 75

Hormone replacement therapy 48

Hospital for Sick Children, The 171

Hot flashes 183

related to childbirth 183

related to weight loss 183

W

ABOUT THE AUTHOR

Marilyn M. Shannon, M.A.

Marilyn McCusker Shannon holds a master's degree in human physiology with a minor in biochemistry from Indiana University's Medical Sciences Program. She is a tenured, part-time instructor of biology at Indiana University Purdue University at Fort Wayne, Indiana, where she has taught human anatomy and physiology for the last 25 years.

Marilyn and her husband Ron have been a Teaching Couple for the Couple to Couple League for Natural Family Planning (NFP) since 1982. Her interest in the impact of nutrition on reproductive health is an outgrowth of her educational background and her experience as an NFP instructor. She has written many articles on nutrition and fertility for the Couple to Couple League's magazine, *Family Foundations*, and has spoken widely on this topic. She was awarded the Couple to Couple League's Edward M. Keefe, M.D. Award for the Scientific Advancement of Natural Family Planning following the first edition of *Fertility, Cycles & Nutrition*.

Ron and Marilyn are the parents of nine children, ages 30 to 3. Their seventh and ninth children were adopted as babies, and their eighth was born to them shortly before Marilyn's 48th birthday. The Shannons live on a small farm in Indiana , where the family interests include raising dairy goats, sheep, and chickens, gardening, and beekeeping. Their homestead is also the birthplace of several of their children.